AF606585

20 078 508 93

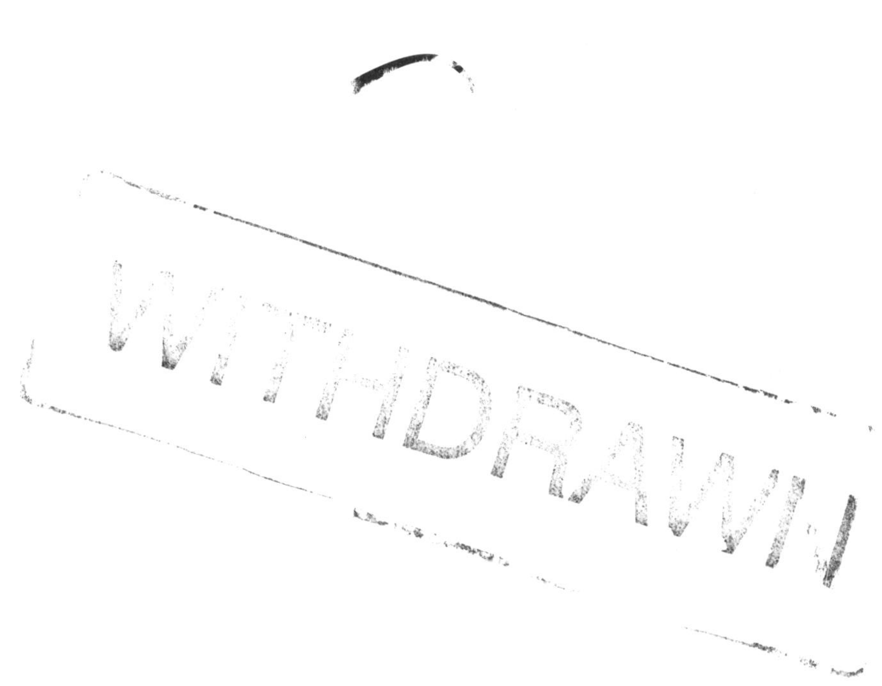
WITHDRAWN

PUBLIC HEALTH IN THE 21ST CENTURY

PALLIATIVE AND NURSING HOME CARE: POLICIES, CHALLENGES AND QUALITY OF LIFE

PUBLIC HEALTH IN THE 21ST CENTURY

Additional books in this series can be found on Nova's website under the Series tab.

Additional E-books in this series can be found on Nova's website under the E-books tab.

HEALTH CARE ISSUES, COSTS AND ACCESS

Additional books in this series can be found on Nova's website under the Series tab.

Additional E-books in this series can be found on Nova's website under the E-books tab.

PUBLIC HEALTH IN THE 21ST CENTURY

PALLIATIVE AND NURSING HOME CARE: POLICIES, CHALLENGES AND QUALITY OF LIFE

SAMUEL E. PLUNKETT
EDITOR

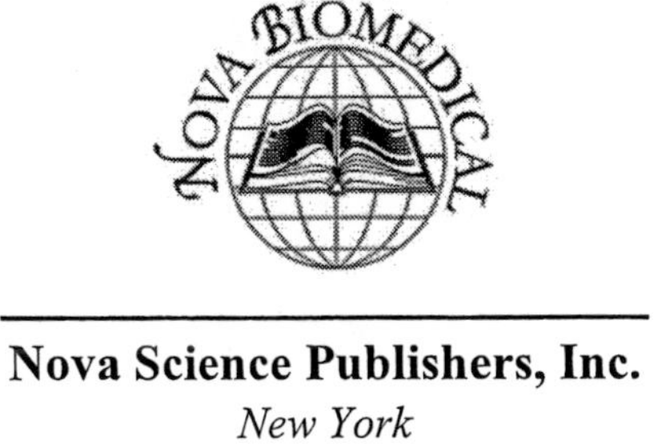

Nova Science Publishers, Inc.
New York

For permission to use material from this book please contact us:
Telephone 631-231-7269; Fax 631-231-8175
Web Site: http://www.novapublishers.com

Additional color graphics may be available in the e-book version of this book.

LIBRARY OF CONGRESS CATALOGING-IN-PUBLICATION DATA

Palliative and nursing home care : policies, challenges, and quality of life
/ editor, Samuel E. Plunkett.
p. ; cm.
Includes bibliographical references and index.
ISBN 978-1-61122-417-7 (hardcover)
1. Palliative treatment. 2. Nursing home care. I. Plunkett, Samuel E.
[DNLM: 1. Palliative Care. 2. Nursing Homes. WB 310]
R726.8.P3425 2010
362.17'5--dc22
2010041311

Published by Nova Science Publishers, Inc. † New York

Contents

Preface		**vii**
Chapter 1	Identifying the Palliative Care Needs of Home-Based People with End-Stage Dementia and Their Caregivers *Barbara Anderson and Debbie Kralik*	**1**
Chapter 2	Mental Distress in AIDS-Orphaned Children: The Efficacy of Natural Mentoring Palliative Care *Francis N. Onuoha*	**31**
Chapter 3	Quality of Sexual Life of Nursing Home Residents *André Dupras*	**63**
Chapter 4	Back to the Future: A Research Journey in Haematology and Palliative Care *Pam McGrath*	**87**
Chapter 5	The Changing Role of the Licensed Practical Nurse in Nursing Home Care *Aggie T. G. Paulus and Arno J. A. van Raak*	**101**
Chapter 6	Special Considerations for Providing Care for Obese Nursing Home Residents *Holly C. Felix, Christine Bradway, Irene Fleshner, Amy Heivly and Lawrence S. Powell*	**117**
Chapter 7	Palliative Care and Dementia: Is a Good Death Possible at Home? *Barbara Anderson*	**131**
Chapter 8	Where and How Non Oncological Respiratory Patients Die: A Palliative Answer *Michele Vitacca and Luca Barbano*	**145**
Chapter 9	Can Data Envelopment Analysis Be Used to Study Performance Efficiency in Nursing Homes? *Daniel G. Shimshak*	**161**

Chapter 10 Quality of Life for Older Persons Living in Nursing Homes: A Cross-Sectional Study **175**
Mimi Tse and Vanessa Wan

Chapter 11 Neonatal Palliative Care: New Practice, New Challenges **191**
Pierre Bétrémieux and Umberto Simeoni

Chapter 12 Depression and Mood Distress among Female Patients with Gynecological Cancer in a Programme of Palliative Cancer Care **201**
L. Slovacek

Index **209**

Preface

This book examines the policies, challenges, and quality of life issues in palliative care and nursing home care facilities. Some topics discussed in this compilation include: identifying the palliative care needs of home-based dementia patients and their caregivers; the functions of sexuality in older adults living in nursing homes and increasing awareness of staff and family members to this issue; haematology and non-oncological respiratory patients in palliative care; the changing role of the licensed practical nurse in nursing home care; obese nursing residents and their special considerations; gynecological cancer and palliative cancer care; and neonatal palliative care.

Chapter 1 - Introduction: Dementia is a challenge facing the health care systems of countries around the world. By 2050, the number of people affected has been estimated to be over 100 million world wide. In 2005, the Australian Commonwealth Government declared dementia as a national health priority in recognition of its increasing impact with respect to prevalence and health costs. Due to the historical association with cancer care and the lack of recognition of dementia as a terminal illness, the palliative care needs of people with end-stage dementia have taken time to be addressed. This chapter reports the findings of an Australian research project, funded the National Health and Medical Research Council, which sought to identify the palliative care needs of home-based people with end-stage dementia and their carers.

Findings: Interviews with carers, medical professionals and representatives of service organisations, revealed that the context in which care was provided was one of extended duration, during which the carers, at significant personal cost, tried to fulfil the desire of the person with dementia to remain at home. With respect to the palliative care needs of people with end-stage dementia and their carers, these needs included receiving a diagnosis of dementia and referral to specialists, supports for carers and in-home services such as carer respite, assistance with activities of daily living and equipment, including hoists and shower chairs. There was also recognition that services should be appropriately structured such that the changing needs of people with end-stage dementia and their carers can be addressed in a timely manner.

Conclusion: the incidence of dementia is increasing worldwide, with its associated impact on health costs. For those home-based people with end-stage dementia, who wish to die at home, it is vital that there are appropriately structured community resources to assist their carers as they seek to fulfil this desire.

Chapter 2 - Every 2.2 seconds a child tends to lose a parent somewhere around the world to the vagaries of life (CSCV, 2010), particularly war, illicit drug use, traffic accident, famine, hunger, and disease. However, in contemporary times, the probability of parent loss worldwide and in sub-Saharan Africa specifically has been compounded by the prevalence of HIV/AIDS. Of the world's estimated 17.5 million AIDS-orphaned children, about 75% of them are in sub-Saharan Africa (UNAIDS, 2009).

Chapter 3 - The goal of this review article is to discuss the meanings and the functions of sexuality of older adults living in nursing homes and to increase awareness of staff and family members to these issues. Although nursing homes are increasingly recognized as provider of sexual health services, there is evidence that a majority of residents do not receive the services.

The article tackles the subject of the sexual well-being of nursing home residents by proposing theoretic and practical tools in order to guide professional interventions. Sexology may contribute to enhance quality of sexual life by helping nursing homes to ensure the physical, psychological and social well-being of their residents with regards to sexuality. They can achieve this goal by integrating sexual rights in the cultural change movement of nursing homes.

The sexual modernization of nursing homes is described first by specifying the project's purpose with the presentation of the historical and social context, second by observing the present situation with a description of the attitudes and behaviors of residents and staff, third by choosing strategies for change such as *setting a general goal that must be clarified in a sexuality policy and a staff training program, preserving sexual identity of residents entering institution, and finally establishing a research structure. It is concluded that listening to sexual needs of residents is necessary for the enhancement of their quality of sexual life.*

Chapter 4 - For many years, increasing research evidence has indicated that the discipline of palliative care, recognised as best practice in end-of-life care, is not integrated adequately into adult haematology. Research indicates that most haematology patients are likely to die in acute care health care settings, exposed to an escalation of invasive technology, aware that they are dying but with no knowledge of or referral to palliative care, in hospital situations that are not designed to be responsive to the support or spiritual needs of terminally ill patients or their families. This chapter provides an overview of a program of psycho-social research that for over a decade has not only increased awareness of the problem by documenting the end-of-life experience of haematology patients and their families, but has also contributed to a solution through the development of a model for the integration of palliative care in haematology. The discussion will follow the program's journey of research starting with consumer work directly related to end-of-life concerns in haematology including work on post-traumatic stress, spiritual pain, bereavement, relocation for specialist treatment, informed consent, supportive care and carers' issues.

The journey concludes with the description of a research-*based* model for health professionals developed to inform the integration of palliative care and haematology that is now disseminated and informing practice both nationally and internationally. In short, the reader is taken on a journey back to the future to see what was, what is and what can be in relation to the provision of appropriate supportive and palliative care for haematology patients, their families and the health professionals who care for them.

Chapter 5 - Traditional care for older people is increasingly being substituted or supplemented by care arrangements such as integrated care. The ageing of the population, economic pressures and social developments are among the primary reasons. To match the emerging range of care arrangements, changes in the traditional role performed by the licensed practical nurse (LPN) are considered both likely and necessary.

To find out if LPNs perform a different role in traditional and emerging care types, the main goal of this chapter is to compare this role in three varieties of care for older people: traditional care, transitional care and integrated care. Between 1999 and 2003, data were assembled in three nursing homes in the Netherlands. Each home represented one type of nursing home care. At three measurement points (each lasting 14 consecutive days), LPNs (on average 177 per measurement) registered the type, frequency and duration of activities delivered to older people with somatic and psycho-social problems. Data-analysis showed that the more nursing home care became integrated, the more (frequently) the LPN became involved in indirect care activities and in activities for psycho-geriatric residents. Some parts of the role of the LPN, however, did not differ between the care types. On the basis of these results it can be concluded that the licensed practical nurse, to a limited extent, performed a different role in different types of care. In all care types, however, the LPN also remained a generalist. In view of these results, the future role of the LPN is not expected to become less important in emerging care types.

Chapter 6 - The demographics and care needs of nursing home residents in the United States (US) are changing. Nursing homes are now seeing increasing numbers of obese (body mass index [BMI] $\geq$ 30) persons seeking long-term care. Current estimates indicate approximately 25% of nursing home residents are obese, and this percentage is likely to increase as rates of obesity among the US pre-elderly (55-64 years of age) and elderly ($\geq$65 years of age) population increases. The experience of providing care for obese patients in hospital settings reveals that obese patients often have complex medical profiles with multiple co-morbidities, unique care needs, and greater health care resource utilization. Emerging research reveals that the differences in the process of care between obese and non-obese patients experienced in hospital settings persists into nursing home settings and presents unique care challenges for the long-term care system, such as the need for bariatric medical supplies and equipment, increased staffing levels, and greater personal care assistance. This chapter will review this emerging research on the long-term care needs of obese persons in the US, present several case studies to highlight specific care needs of obese residents around continence care and bathing, review best practices and OSHA worker safety recommendations for patient handling, and conclude with the description of a model program to provide quality care for obese nursing home residents (developed and implemented at Genesis Healthcare Corporation).

Chapter 7 - Introduction: The suggestion has been made that modern medicine has diverted attention from preparing for death and helping people to die a good death. The branch of medicine which has addressed the care of the dying, palliative medicine, has seemed to give the impression that dying can be dignified through the management of terminal pain. However, many patients dying from cancer and non-cancer diagnoses have a range of symptoms which are less easily managed in old age. The principles of a good death have been outlined and are used to answer the question “Can people with end-stage dementia have a good death at home?”

Conclusion: there are complex issues associated with the care of people with end-stage dementia at home, including the difficulties in prognostication. However, with committed informal carers, supported by appropriately funded home care organisations, and the use of advance care plans to minimise hospital admissions and unnecessarily invasive interventions, the desire of people with end-stage dementia to die a good death at home can be fulfilled.

Chapter 8 - Death due to respiratory diseases is high, being chronic obstructive pulmonary disease (COPD) an important risk factor for death. The COPD dying trajectory is often unknown. Commonest cause of death after Intensive Care Unit (ICU) discharge is respiratory failure, while respiratory causes for death are often under-diagnosed. Among COPD patients, a lot of subjects may be defined under palliative and at risk of end of life conditions.

Three different situations emerge depending on the fact that patient is in hospital, at home or using mechanical ventilation. The hospital scenario often offers a high percentage of respiratory patients receiving end of life decisions by different professional figures involved in end of life (EOL) strategies. Major difficulties are represented by death prediction, particularly in those patients admitted in ICU, or by interaction with patient expressing different preferences for a life support or having a poor level of discussion among doctors and between doctors and patients. A second scenario is represented by chronic respiratory patients at home. More than 68% of all COPD admissions and 74% of all days in-hospital occurred in the 3.5 years before death, indicating longer stays closer to death. The last 6 months of life accounted for 22% and 28% of all COPD admissions and days, respectively. Poor symptom control remains an important cause of distress. The most frequent cause of death after discharge is heart disease. Lack of surveillance and inadequate services with absence of palliative care is a routinely experience. The more frequent request from COPD patients is education on diagnosis and disease process, treatments, prognosis for survival, quality of life and advance care planning. They do not receive holistic care as patients with lung cancer. The last scenario is relative to patients with home mechanical ventilation. Despite these patients are usually pleased about their chose, they are well confident about the high burden imposed to their caregivers. Moreover, for these patients dyspnoea and secretion encumbrance remain the main unresolved symptoms. In comparison with mechanical invasively ventilated patients, non invasively ventilated patients are more aware of prognosis, use more respiratory drugs, change ventilation time more frequently and die less frequently when under mechanical ventilation.

Palliative home care programs and Hospice admissions for EOL care in respiratory patients are insufficient or absent. Individual approach to patients with non homogenous disease is often necessary. Hospital and home palliation protocols (milestones, skills and interventions) for non-oncological respiratory patients are urgently needed.

Chapter 9 - One area that has been the focus of growing attention has been the nursing home sector, which constitutes a large and increasingly costly segment of the health care industry. Nursing home administrators have come under great pressure to control costs while maintaining or increasing the quality and level of care. However, administrators in the industry have had difficulty in developing a useful measure of nursing home performance and strategies for improving nursing home care. Currently, large amounts of data are collected on numerous aspects of performance, including cost, utilization, case-mix severity, and quality. These data are typically compiled into summary reports that are prepared on a regular basis for individual nursing homes. Often values on these profile reports are benchmarked against normative values representing averages for other nursing homes in the state, region, or nation. It is anticipated that nursing homes will use the results of these benchmark reports to identify aspects of their performance that may need improvement.

There are some inherent problems with this technique for evaluating nursing home performance. First, it is cumbersome to inspect a long list of performance measures and their rankings compared to other homes. Second, without an objective means of prioritizing or combining the various measures, it is difficult to determine which nursing homes are performing well overall. Finally, this technique provides very little guidance on how nursing homes can change their operations to improve their performance.

Given the limitations on existing techniques, it is apparent that the nursing home industry needs better tools for converting the vast amounts of available data into information that is useful for managers. Here the authors will discuss the possibility of using Data Envelopment Analysis (DEA) for studying performance in nursing homes. DEA is a mathematical technique that converts multiple input and output measures into a single comprehensive measure of performance. Thus, DEA can calculate a single "performance rating" for each nursing home. Not only can DEA evaluate the utilization efficiency of a nursing home's resources, but it can construct performance targets for each home based on a comparison with a selected group of the best-performing nursing homes. In this way, DEA can help administrators of nursing homes to conduct a comprehensive evaluation of their performance and to devise strategies for improvement.

Chapter 10 - Background: Given the increasingly ageing population ad the impact of diseases and disabilities during the ageing process, the need of older persons for some form of alternative accommodation and residential care facilities is expected to rise. The Hong Kong Association of Gerontology (2004) estimates that 5.5% of people aged 65 or older need institutionalized care for their later life.

Aim: To explore quality of life among older persons living in nursing homes

Method: This was an exploratory cross-sectional study. Six nursing homes were approached and 365 older persons invited to join the study. A questionnaire was administered to them to collect information on their demographic data, bowel habits and pain situation. The authors also investigated their physical function (assessed using Barthel ADL Scores and Elderly Mobility Scores) and psychological condition, including life satisfaction, depression, happiness and loneliness (using the Life Satisfaction, Geriatric Depression, Happiness and UCLA Loneliness Scales).

Results: There were 365 older nursing home residents (248 female and 117 male, mean age 84.7 ± 6.73) in the study, of whom 249 (70%) suffered from pain, mean pain scores of 4.55 indicating medium pain intensity. The location of pain was mainly in the knee, back and shoulder, possibly affecting the older persons' physical function and psychological health. Those with mildly limited physical function had Barthel ADL Scores of 16.55 ± 4.75 (mostly those with difficulty bathing and climbing stairs) and Elderly Mobility Scores of 14.55 ± 5.69 (difficulty walking 6 meters and functional reaching). As for their psychological health, they scored low life satisfaction 8.81 ± 4.05, mild depression 6.92 ± 3.93, fair happiness 17.70 ± 6.09, and moderate loneliness 42.83 ± 12.34. In addition, the correlation between the demographic data and the psychological parameters was tested: there was a weak positive correlation between age and depression, and weak negative correlations between gender and happiness (male older residents felt happier) and pain and depression (elderly people with pain felt more depressed than the group with no pain).

Conclusions and relevance to clinical practice: Overall, older persons suffer from moderate to severe physical and psychological impairment in nursing homes. Nurses and other healthcare professionals should encourage them to engage in various interventions to minimize these problems and enhance their quality of life at the end of their life journey.

Chapter 11 - The delineation of Palliative Care (PC) in newborns recently opened a new practice. In the past and for years, neonatologists did not consider Palliative Care at the beginning of life. Nevertheless End of life procedures did exist but referred to either withholding or withdrawing active treatments, or even to active ending of life in desperate circumstances (what we now would call neonatal euthanasia). Four main domains can be recognized in the field of neonatology: 1) Babies born between 22 and 25 weeks: palliative care is the good alternative to life support therapy in some cases where the medical context and the parents' wishes are not in favour of such choice; 2) Babies born to a mother who knows that an intractable malformation affects the baby and wants to continue her pregnancy and meet her living baby, so that she does not ask for Termination of Pregnancy (TOP). This approach is quite new in France, for example, and concerns 3 to 5 % of mothers who could legally ask for TOP. Midwives, obstetrician and neonatologists give comfort care to the baby and sometimes help the family to bring the baby back home (most of prolonged PC occurs in severe hypoplastic left heart syndrome); 3) PC may also find its place in the neonatal intensive care unit when a baby who has been resuscitated at birth finally shows a dramatic neurologic outcome at a time when he/she is still dependent on intensive techniques such as mechanical ventilation or hemodynamic support. Withdrawing mechanical ventilation may sometimes lead to death but sometimes not and PC is the response to these situations.4) Finally PC may also be considered in an emergency context in any of the three previous situations occurring suddenly. Paediatricians must then decide in a while what would be the best choice for the baby. Each context modifies the way PC is provided, although in all cases basic compassionate and comfort care is delivered. Special attention is needed to ensure that parents and sometimes extended family may really meet their newborn baby, have their religious wills completed and are accompanied by a multiprofessional team attentive to their physical and psychological needs. This is conducted in the place the baby lives in, either delivery room, neonatal ward or even home if possible.

Chapter 12 - Cancer can be characterized as uncontrolled growth of cells, which is of authonomous means. This cell proliferation is connected with defect of control mechanisms and alteration of cell diferentiation. Uncontroled growth of cell leads to expanding of affected tissue which can press the surrounding organs, or to gradual invasion to surrounding structures and to metastasis.

Thanks to the growing average lifetime occurence of carcinoma is raising. The number of people who survive the carcinoma is raising, too. Yet it is perceived as death judgement for many people which consider it as chronic or even incurable disease. In every case, it is a shock for a patient to hear such a diagnosis. Patient must tie with a sense of uncertainty of their future life, with undesirable side effects of anti-tumorous therapy, with a sense of isolation, stigmatization and guilt. Block cites that diagnosis af cancer evokes subexistence crisis in every affected individual. So it is needed to handel disease succesfully to use a supportive methods too, which could lead to regaining of certain control of patient over the situation.

In: Palliative and Nursing Home Care
Editor: Samuel E. Plunkett
ISBN 978-1-61122-417-7

Chapter 1

Identifying the Palliative Care Needs of Home-Based People with End-Stage Dementia and Their Caregivers

***Barbara Anderson*[1] *and Debbie Kralik*[2]**
[1]Senior Researcher, Research, Strategy and Growth,
Royal District Nursing Service of SA Inc, South Australia
[2]General Manager, Research, Strategy and Growth,
Royal District Nursing Service of SA Inc, South Australia

Abstract

Introduction: Dementia is a challenge facing the health care systems of countries around the world. By 2050, the number of people affected has been estimated to be over 100 million world- wide. In 2005, the Australian Commonwealth Government declared dementia as a national health priority in recognition of its increasing impact with respect to prevalence and health costs. Due to the historical association with cancer care and the lack of recognition of dementia as a terminal illness, the palliative care needs of people with end-stage dementia have taken time to be addressed. This chapter reports the findings of an Australian research project, funded the National Health and Medical Research Council, which sought to identify the palliative care needs of home-based people with end-stage dementia and their caregivers.

Findings: Interviews with caregivers, medical professionals and representatives of service organizations, revealed that the context in which care was provided was one of extended duration, during which the caregivers, at significant personal cost, tried to fulfil the desire of the person with dementia to remain at home. With respect to the palliative care needs of people with end-stage dementia and their caregivers, these needs included receiving a diagnosis of dementia and referral to specialists, supports for caregivers and in-home services such as caregiver respite, assistance with activities of daily living and equipment, including hoists and shower chairs. There was also recognition that services should be appropriately structured such that the changing needs of people with end-stage dementia and their caregivers can be addressed in a timely manner.

Conclusion: the incidence of dementia is increasing worldwide, with its associated impact on health costs. For those home-based people with end-stage dementia, who wish to die at home, it is vital that there are appropriately structured community resources to assist their caregivers as they seek to fulfil this desire.

Introduction

Dementia is a challenge facing the health care systems of countries around the world. Alzheimer's Disease International estimates that there are currently 30 million people with dementia, with 4.6 million new cases diagnosed every year. By 2050, the number of people affected has been estimated to be over 100 million worldwide (Prince, 2008).

In 2005, the Australian Commonwealth Government declared dementia as a national health priority in recognition of its increasing impact with respect to prevalence and health costs (Australian Government Department of Health and Ageing, 2008). In the United Kingdom (UK), a report into the prevalence and cost of dementia has recommended that dementia be made a national health and social care priority, reflected in plans for service development and public spending (Personal Social Services Research Unit, 2007).

In the United States of America (USA), it has been estimated that there are 3.8 million individuals with dementia, 2.5 million of whom have Alzheimer's disease (AD) (Plassman, Langa, Fisher, Heeringa, Weir, Ofstendal, Burke, Hurd, Potter, Rodgers, Steffens, Willis and Wallace, 2007). However, the Alzheimer's Association suggest that as many as 5.3 million Americans are living with this disease (Alzheimer's Association, year: not provided). In the UK, there are estimated to be approximately 700,000 people with dementia. AD is the dominant sub-type, particularly among older people and in women (Personal Social Services Research Unit, 2007).

Australian data indicate that almost 175,000 people had dementia in 2003, increasing to 190,000 in 2006. Of these 190,000 people, dementia was classified as 'mild' in approximately 96,000 (55%) people; as 'moderate' in 52,000 people (30%), and as 'severe' in 26,000 (15%) people. Of all Australians with dementia and living in households, 53.1% have 'mild' dementia; 2.6% have 'moderate' dementia, and 3% have end-stage dementia (Australian Institute of Health and Welfare (AIHW), 2006). These demographics reveal the challenge for community health and care services to develop services specifically for people with co-morbid chronic conditions and dementia.

The prevalence of dementia increases with age, doubling every five year increase across the age range (Personal Social Services Research Unit, 2007). The total number of people with dementia in the UK is forecasted to increase by 940,110 by 2021 and 1,735,087 by 2051, an increase of 38% over the next 15 years and 154% over the next 45 years (Personal Social Services Research Unit, 2007). In Australia, the prevalence of dementia has been projected to increase more than four-fold from 245,000 people in 2009, to approximately 1.13 million people by the year 2050. The incidence of dementia has been estimated to increase from 69,600 new cases in 2009 to 385,200 new cases in 2050 (Access Economics Pty Ltd, 2009).

The populations of China, India and Latin America are also aging rapidly. The number of older people in developing countries will have increased by 200%, as compared to 68% in the developed countries in the 30 years up to 2030. In the developing world, there is much more uncertainty about the frequency of dementia (Prince, 2008).

As the duration of dementia reported in a number of small Australian studies ranged from 6 months to 8 years (Australian Institute of Health and Welfare (AIHW), 2006) by implication, the 'severe' or end-stage dementia could last for more than 12 months. International studies have indicated that the prognosis for a person with dementia may last from between two to more than 15 years, with the end-stage lasting as long as two or three years (Birch and Draper, 2008).

Dementia

What Is Dementia?

Dementia is a term used to describe a group of diseases that affect the brain and cause a progressive decline in the ability to think, remember and learn (NSW Department of Health on behalf of Australian Health Ministers' Conference (AHMC), 2006).

The cognitive, psychiatric and behavioral manifestations of dementia may include:

- memory problems,
- communication difficulties through problems with speech and understanding language,
- confusion, wandering, getting lost,
- personality changes and behavior changes, such as agitation and repetition,
- depression, delusions, apathy and withdrawal (Australian Institute of Health and Welfarc (AIHW), 2006, p5).

While there are over 100 illnesses and conditions where the outcome is dementia, the most common types of dementia in Australia are:

- Dementia in Alzheimer's disease – approx. 50-70% of people with dementia, involving abnormal plaques and tangles in the brain.
- Vascular dementia, resulting from significant brain damage caused by cerebrovascular disease.
- Dementia with Lewy bodies, in which abnormal brain cells (Lewy bodies) form in all parts of the brain.
- Fronto-temporal dementia (e.g. Pick's disease), in which damage starts in the front part of the brain.
- Mixed dementia, in which features of more than one type of dementia are present (Australian Institute of Health and Welfare (AIHW), 2006, pp5-6).

In the US, Alzheimer's disease accounts for 50-80 per cent of dementia cases. The other types of dementia include Vascular dementia, mixed dementia, dementia with Lewy bodies and fronto-temporal dementia (Alzheimer's Association, year: not provided). In the UK, AD is considered to be the dominant subtype, particularly among older people and women (Personal Social Services Research Unit, 2007).

How Is Dementia Diagnosed?

There is no one diagnostic test for AD or most other causes of dementia. A range of tests and assessments are used to determine whether symptoms are consistent with certain criteria and exclude other possible causes. Assessment for dementia usually includes:

- Personal history.
- Physical examination and laboratory testing of blood and urine samples.
- Mental status evaluation, including cognitive testing.
- Radiological tests, including brain imaging techniques (Alzheimer's Association, 2008).

Currently, autopsy is the most accurate means of confirming a diagnosis of dementia (Black, LoGuidice, Ames, Barber and Smith, 2001), which is less than useful for people wanting confirmation of a diagnosis and assistance to live with the condition.

Providing the Diagnosis of Dementia

Medical professionals have acknowledged that providing the diagnosis of dementia can be difficult for reasons such as:

- difficulty of making an accurate diagnosis,
- challenge of imparting 'bad news',
- uncertainty about whether or not the person will understand what is being said,
- uncertainty about whether or not the person will retain information, and
- lack of options and referral points for follow-up support (National Collaborating Centre for Mental Health, 2007, p87).

However, there is growing acknowledgement of the need to diagnose dementias, such as AD, in the early stages. People who are diagnosed at this time have the potential to make choices and plan for their future care. Caregivers have the opportunity to learn about the disease and its ramifications, commence their adjustment to the diagnosis and plan ahead. Furthermore, there may well be ethical issues associated with the withholding of the diagnosis from patients (Leifer, 2003). Advantages of early diagnosis were identified by general practitioners (GPs) as including reduction of uncertainty about the diagnosis and then coming to terms with it, and time to organize support and plan for the future (Iliffe, Manthorpe and Eden, 2003).

In the UK, the National Service Framework for Older People has identified the importance of early diagnosis in enabling people and their family to respond effectively to the prognosis of dementia. However a study of Scottish GPs has revealed that almost all the GPs told the caregiver the diagnosis, but only approximately half of them told the person with dementia.

Furthermore, when the diagnosis of dementia was given to people with dementia, more than a third of the GPs used euphemistic terms, such as memory problems or confusion when describing the illness (Downs, Clibbens, Rae, Cook and Woods, 2002).

In Australia, three linked qualitative research projects have found that GPs did not consider that an early diagnosis of dementia was especially important and acknowledged the harm that such a diagnosis may cause to some people (Hansen, Hughes, Routley and Robinson, 2008).

What Are the Characteristics of End-Stage Dementia?

Dementias are known to vary greatly in their course and rate of progression among individual patients. However, there are consistent signs and symptoms, indicating the final stages of dementia (Shuster Jr, 2000).

Hancock, Chang, Johnson, Harrison, Daly, Easterbrook, Noel, Luhir-Taylor and Davidson (2006) summarize the work of a number of authors, which suggests that end-stage dementia is characterized by:

- dependence in activities of daily living, requiring the assistance of caregivers to survive,
- severe impairment of expressive and receptive communication, often limited to single words or nonsense phrases,
- loss of the ability to walk, followed by inability to stand, problems maintaining sitting posture and a subsequent loss of head and neck control,
- development of contractures because of muscle rigidity and de-conditioning,
- loss of ability to recognise food, self-feed and swallow effectively,
- bowel and bladder incontinence, and
- inability to recognize self and others.

Palliative Care in End-stage Dementia

Who Receives Palliative Care Services?

Australian data relating to patients admitted for palliative care in 1999-00 reveal that 69 percent of palliative care separations had a principle diagnosis of cancer (Australian Institute of Health and Welfare (AIHW), 2003).

Chatterjee (2008) acknowledges that as the philosophy and practice of palliative care has been based in the care of cancer patients, those dying of non-malignant diseases receive less of this type of care (Chatterjee, 2008, p29).

This observation is confirmed by a number of studies indicating palliative care being regularly provided to people with cancers, but not to people with end-stage dementia. For example, a survey of 796 hospice organizations in the USA, revealed that 46.3 per cent of deaths were from cancers, 42.4 per cent were from other chronic conditions, and 11.3 per cent were from dementia.

However, they note that dementia is a leading cause of death in the USA (Mitchell, Kiely, Miller, Connor, Spence and Teno, 2007). Similarly in the UK, there is growing evidence that people with diseases other than cancer, have difficulty accessing specialist palliative care services (Birch and Draper, 2008).

Although the principles of palliative care should be applicable to the care of people dying from dementia, many do not receive the same attention to symptom control and discussions about end-of-life care (Armitage and Evans, 2005). Unlike most people dying from cancers, those with end-stage dementia cannot verbally relate their symptoms, which can impact the assessment and management of their physical and psychological symptoms (Shega and Tozer, 2009).

What Are the Barriers to Quality End-of-Life Care?

Drawing on the work of numerous authors, Sachs, Shega and Cox-Hayley (2004) outline the key challenges to providing quality end-of-life care. Their work and that of others have been summarized, as follows:

Dementia Not Seen as a Terminal Illness

Identifying that a person is dying or terminally ill allows health professionals, patients and families to consider end-of-life choices and issues. However, professionals and families often do not see dementia as a terminal illness. They report the findings of a study, which found that although 70 per cent of families interviewed knew that the patient was dying, prior to their death, more than two thirds of these family members thought that the patient was dying of another cause, rather than dementia. The protracted course of dementia, with the gradual loss of cognition and function, are said to obscure the fact that the person is dying (Sachs *et al.*, 2004).

Nature of Advanced Dementia and Treatment Decisions

Many terminal diseases reach an advanced stage and then follow a recognizable downhill course over a number of days, weeks or months. However, with dementia, there are no reliable prognostic markers to predict life expectancy of less than 6 months. Hence, there is a reluctance to refer patients with dementia for hospice care. The trajectory of the dementia patient is a gradual decline in health status, interspersed by declines caused by acute illness (Sachs *et al.*, 2004).

This trajectory is graphically represented by the frailty (lingering expected deaths) group in Figure 1.

Lunney *et al* (2003) also identified that those who died in the frailty group were relatively more disabled throughout the last year of life.

After controlling for a range of factors, those assigned to the frailty group were more than eight times more likely to be dependent in activities of daily living, including bathing, grooming, eating and using the toilet, than those who died suddenly (Lunney *et al.*, 2003, p2390).

As the trajectory of dementia is unpredictable, the end-of-life phase may last for months or years, often without recognition or planning (Godwin and Waters, 2009).

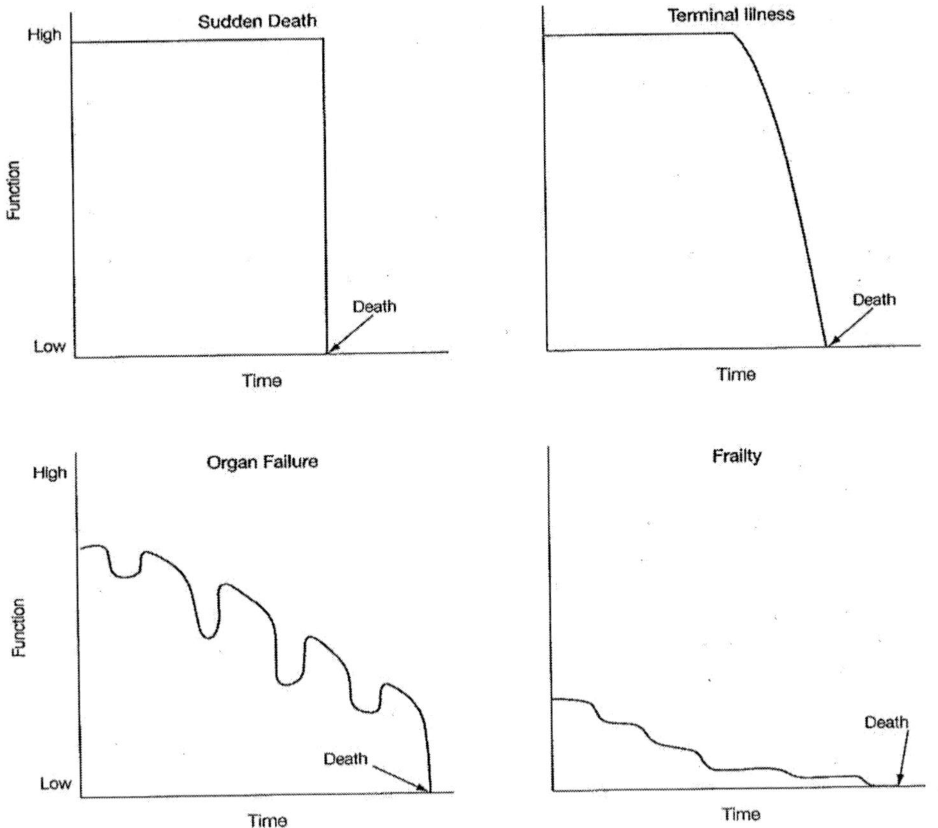

Figure 1. Theoretical trajectories of dying (Lunney, Lynn, Foley, Lipson and Guralnik, 2003, p2388).

Assessment and Management of Symptoms

As the patient's cognitive and communication abilities decline, assessment of symptoms becomes more difficult, which is particularly significant in the diagnosis and management of pain. Patients with dementia also demonstrate behaviors of concern. Symptoms to be managed may include anxiety, depression, paranoia and aggression (Sachs *et al.*, 2004).

Challenging Caregiver Stress and Bereavement Issues

Caring for someone with dementia is widely recognized as being particularly onerous. Sachs *et al* (2004) report that when compared to non-dementia caregivers, people caring for a person with dementia have reported more hours spent on providing care, greater detrimental effects on employment, more emotional and physical strain and increased probability of experiencing mental or physical health problems as a result of caregiving (Sachs *et al.*, 2004).

Health System Challenges

Sachs *et al* (2004) discuss the challenges for the US health system with respect to the provision of palliative care for people with dementia. They indicate that Medicare's policies create discontinuities in care for people with dementia, who experience recurring acute illnesses in conjunction with chronic decline. In Australia, the complexity of the health system also creates similar fragmentation and discontinuities in care for people with dementia and their caregivers.

A recently published study which investigated end-of-life care for people with dementia in a UK borough, Sampson, Harrison-Dening, Greenish, Mandal, Holman and Jones (2009) identified a number of key themes which included:

- pathway of care: holistic dementia care pathway needed to support staff in giving appropriate interventions at time of crisis, increase preventative services and reduce inappropriate admissions to the hospital. Greater coordination of care required and raised awareness and understanding was needed among professionals of the range of services available.
- advance care planning: rare in the borough.
- impact on caregivers: stressed and burdened by role. Array of services available difficult to access when needed, reporting that at times 'confusing' to know who to contact (Sampson *et al.*, 2009, p3).

Guidelines for Palliative Care in End-Stage Dementia

In the UK, the Social Care Institute for Excellence and the National Institute for Health and Clinical Excellence have combined to produce the NICE-SCIE Guideline on supporting people with dementia and their caregivers in health and social care. In the section, Palliative Care, Pain Relief and Care at the end-of-life for People with Dementia, the need for further research as to what constitutes good quality palliative care in dementia is acknowledged (National Collaborating Centre for Mental Health, 2007). However, a number of aspects are discussed, including:

- Artificial nutrition and hydration: Swallowing difficulties develop as dementia worsens; aspiration pneumonia is a possibility. Dysphagia can be managed conservatively by a combination of appropriately textured food and feeding techniques and appropriate posture.
- Fever and infection: Pneumonia is a common cause of death.
- Pain: In the final days of life, a palliative care pathway might encourage appropriate management of symptoms including pain.
- Services to support palliative care in dementia: Few in number, due in part to the problem of a lack of familiarity with dementia (National Collaborating Centre for Mental Health, 2007).

What Resources Are Required to Support End-of-Life Care in the Home?

Treloar, Crugel and Adamis (2009) observe that people with advanced dementia are seldom able to live and die at home in the UK. They also note that dementia services have been slow to adopt the concepts of palliative and end-of-life care, due partly to a lack of understanding of palliative care needs of these people. From their interviews with caregivers who had been supported to look after people who died at home, the key themes included:

- Care worker support: Caregivers experienced difficulty with the support received from care workers, who could be unpredictable in attendance, and there was little continuity of staff.
- Professional expertise:
  - Caregivers accessed a wide range of professional expertise, including old age psychiatry, which was considered as 'indispensable'.
  - Caregivers experienced difficulty in accessing GP services.
- Equipment needed:
  - Continence pads and sheets, commode and wheelchair rated as 'indispensable'.
  - Hospital beds, chair and pressure relieving cushions and electric hoists were rated 'very useful'.
- Feeding: In order to try and prevent weight loss, many techniques for maintaining the food intake were described, such as 'good, nutritious food well laid out', 'Irish stews', 'thickened soups'.
- Support and services: There was a need for a person who would visit regularly, advise and bring in other people, as necessary. Caregivers wanted a support team who understood the challenges of looking after a person with dementia.
- Inappropriate hospital admission: There was a desire to keep the people for whom they cared out of hospital. Negative experiences were reported when people had been hospitalized (Treloar, Crugel and Adamis, 2009).

What Are the Palliative Care Needs of Home-Based People with Dementia at End-Stage and Their Carers?

In this section, the findings of a research project, carried out in Australia, funded by the National Health and Medical Research Council, which sought to identify these needs, are reported (Anderson, Kralik, March and Briffa, 2010). Semi-structured interviews were carried out with a range of participants:

- Caregivers (n=18) who were either
  - currently caring for a relative at home with end-stage dementia,
  - had placed their relative in an aged care facility, or
  - had cared for a relative who had died either at home or in an aged care facility.
- Medical professionals: general practitioners (GP) (n=6) and a geriatrician (GT).
- Representatives (n=4) of organizations (SPs) providing services in the community to people with dementia and their caregivers.

Ethical approval was gained from the Human Research Ethics Committee of the University of South Australia to conduct this project.

A total of twenty nine interviews, lasting between 30 and 45 minutes, were transcribed and analysed thematically.

The findings presented here focus on the caregivers' responses, which have been augmented by the responses of the medical professionals and service providers, where appropriate.

In order to identify these needs, it is valuable to understand aspects of the environment in which participants have been providing care to people with dementia.

What Is the Context in Which Caregivers Are Looking after People at Home with End-Stage Dementia?

A number of sub-themes were identified in the caregivers' responses which included:

- desire and ability to stay at home,
- duration of care,
- behaviors of concern, and
- carer burden.

Desire and Ability to Remain at Home

A number of caregivers provided their thoughts about the desire of their relatives to remain at home. Admission to an aged care facility was generally viewed in a negative light, by both caregivers and people with dementia, when they had been able to communicate their thoughts about their place of care.

> I know she said a number of times over the years that she never wanted to go into a nursing home (she saw them as a place where some of her freedom would be taken from her, and she is a very independent woman). I don't want her to go to one because regardless of my lack of medical background or the quality of the facility, I can still give her better care at home. ... I want her to be here until she dies... you know, quietly in her sleep at the age of 95. (Caregiver 1)
>
> I knew he didn't want to go to a nursing home, because some of his friends had been in, and he always sort of dreaded it, and as long as we could manage, I didn't mind having him home...I felt it was my job to do it... it wasn't a question about it. (Caregiver 11)

One caregiver tried valiantly, albeit ultimately unsuccessfully, to look after her husband at home, desperately trying to fulfill the promise that they had made to each other that one would not place the other in an aged care facility. Another caregiver reported struggling with coming to terms with her decision to place her mother in such a facility:

> And I think the worst bit for me to cope with was putting her in the home. That was, I had to come to terms with that. And now that I know that she is being looked after, it's made it easier. Even so, I still think, this is her home, she should be home. (Caregiver 13)

Several of the GPs acknowledged the value of people with dementia remaining at home as long as possible:

> I try and keep them at home as long as it's comfortable for them and their caregivers. We've just in the last couple of weeks had a few who had to transfer to a nursing home because they could no longer manage... in a nursing home,... to me, they seem to deteriorate a little bit more quickly than when they were at home ... (GP2)
>
> It would be good if they could be kept at home, but it's not always a quick process and you can think they might be end-stage dementia, but ... 'til time of death, it can still

be quite a long, drawn out process and quite, quite stressful and quite debilitating ...(GP1)

One GP suggested that there should be flexibility in the approach of people to the most appropriate place of care:

> ... I think that sometimes people have expectations, ... I'll never let you go into a nursing home or might have made some kind of statement – enacting a promise to ... and yet, sometimes the level of care that can be provided in a home situation is not as good as what can be provided in a nursing home, just through exhaustion and through a lack of facilities. If people can stay at home until the end and that's their wish and they're able to follow it through, that's great, but I know that it's a very difficult ask, ... [s]ometimes you have to go with ... the way things pan out ... just have to be flexible, and change your plans according to what actually happens to you... I think, for most people, there comes a point where they will need extra care. (GP4)

Duration of Care

The slow decline of dementia is reflected in the caregivers' comments about the length of time that they had been looking after the person with dementia.

> ...the first indication really was in early 1998, [wife] began to have difficulty in naming objects, just every day objects.....[b]ut it did develop over the next months into confusion ... only minor things, but there was definitely a, a thing that was happening ...(Caregiver 10)
>
> January 2000 officially, but the previous 3 or 4 years, he was obviously unwell. He had a personality changes, and he was getting forgetful, and very suspicious and nasty... (Caregiver 11)
>
> We've been together since '94 and in '97, [partner] was showing signs of not being himself... forgetfulness...by 2000, he didn't know how many children he had or their names... so I suppose I've been looking after him 14 years. (Caregiver 17)

Behaviors of Concern

A number of caregivers recounted a range of behaviors of concern, which included violent behavior and incessant talking.

Case Study 1: "A caregiver's story of denial and commitment"
This study highlights a number of themes:

- Caregiver denial as to the true condition of the person with dementia.
- Danger of promising partners that they would not be put in an aged care facility and the sense of betrayal experienced when such promises cannot be kept.
- Exhausting nature of caring for a person exhibiting a range of behaviors of concern, including violence.
- Value of creative care co-ordinators and caregiver support groups.
- Sub-optimal care provided on admission to hospital.
- Social isolation experienced by caregiver.
- Eventual recognition that admission to an aged care facility is necessary.

Case Study 1. "A Caregiver's Story of Denial and Commitment": as related by Caregiver 15

We moved to a different town to be near my daughter, who has been absolutely wonderful through all this. I took my husband to a new doctor for a check-up. He said to me, 'I believe your husband has the beginnings of dementia'. I almost didn't want to believe it. I knew things had been going wrong for at least 2 years prior to this. However, you lie to yourself, that you can manage this. I was a nurse. I could do anything. I knew what to do in these cases. This attitude was so silly. The doctor also said to me, 'if you don't get your husband into a nursing home, you'll be dead first'. I didn't take any notice of him. I thought, 'I love him'. I had made a promise that we'd never go into a nursing home, and so, I was not going to do that.

Eventually, I got in touch with an organization supporting people in their homes. The coordinator was absolutely wonderful. She knew how touchy my husband was, so we arranged the first meeting with him in a coffee shop down in the town, under the guise of meeting a new friend of mine. This was the cleverest thing she could have done, because there was no way she could have come home at that time, he was so violent, he would have attacked her. It wasn't very pleasant living in a house where you couldn't have any knives, apart from the ones which could have only damaged your skin surface if he tried to stab you with them. Any sharp knives used for cooking were kept in the shed, which I used to keep locked. You never knew if he was going to turn funny.

I can remember one really awkward day. My husband refused everything. He wouldn't have a shower; wouldn't have a shave; wouldn't have anything. When it got to night time, he suddenly decided that all the beds in the house had to go into the shed. I have no idea why they had to be moved, but anyway, just to placate him, I took some bed linen out there, but no, that wasn't enough, the beds had to be moved too. We got halfway across the lawn with the beds, and then he decided that it was going to rain. He just dropped them there. I spent the rest of the night getting the beds back indoors and got myself a hernia. The following day, I went down to get some milk, so I said, 'I won't be long now, you wait here, I'll go down and get some milk'. When I got back, I found that he'd had all the photographs that we possessed in the dust bin and had poured petrol on them. Every photograph we possessed! Wedding photographs, insurance policies, everything out of the safety box put into the bin and set alight. I said to him, 'What did you do that for?' 'Oh, that's not me' he replied.

The hernia was really bad and I was rushed into the hospital in an emergency. My daughter came over to stay with her father and he spent the night trying to get in bed with her, which was really distressing. Her husband came and put locks on all the doors, on the inside. This experience has spoiled her last pictures of her dad, which I feel is the worst thing I did to her. It just went from bad to worse from then on.

That's when I realized I had to get some help. The coordinator had been telling me for some time that I really ought to get some more help, but I wouldn't listen. However, she's now become a friend that I would listen to, first time, but then, I thought I knew it all.

Living with someone like that is quite horrendous. I went along to caregivers' meetings. I felt ashamed sometimes, telling them about my husband's behavior. I don't know why we bear the shame, when it isn't us doing it. However, I received the most wonderful support from the coordinator and the care group. The coordinator just seemed to understand how my husband was. She never pushed him. He never got to hate her, like he did most other people.

He went down the street and wee'd over people's cars, in the middle of the mad shopping hour. He tried to shut my head in the car door, but I still didn't want to see him go into a nursing home. Unfortunately, the worst thing that happened was when he tried to shut my head in the car door, I screamed and the next door neighbor sent for the police, who took him away. He went into hospital, which was horrendous, it really was. He was there for 8 weeks. I went down there early one morning, thinking that I could catch him when he wasn't quite so hett up. He was sitting eating a bowl of cold tinned spaghetti. He was unshaven and was sitting there in a revolting hospital gown with spaghetti all over it, plus all over him. It sounds ridiculous to say, but that distressed me more than his attacking of me did. That such an immaculate dresser, such a precise and positive man, could be like that was the cruellest cut of all, I think.

I found I lost my friends. The most wonderful one was somebody that had been a next door neighbor. We were moving a shed in the garden one day and suddenly my husband decided to attack him. My husband was 6' 3" and no light weight, but the neighbor was a very strong man. He just literally held my husband's arms by the side, put his face right in his and kept on saying, 'I'm your friend, I'm your friend, I'm [name]. In the end, he got him calmed down. However, the poor man, he could not see my husband in the street, he could not come to visit us at all. Every time he did, my husband went for him. When he attacked our neighbor, who had proved to be a really great friend to us, I realized that if he was going to hurt others, I had to let him go, for his sake, not mine.

It took about 3 months of hell before he was placed in a nursing home, where he died 9 months later. I was bigoted to think that I could manage him. I still get a sense of betrayal to a certain extent, but I couldn't have done anything else but put him in a home. The way I came to accept it in the end was that I didn't mind if he hurt me, but, by golly, he wasn't going to hurt anybody else. It was the acceptance of it that was so hard and you feel so alone. It was 52 years of marriage when my husband died, 50 years of it was all washed away. You were living with the photograph of the person you'd known all your life. It wasn't him any more. My daughter said, 'my father died 5 years ago'.

I was a fool. I should have given up before that and had him in a nursing home. It's something we need to get through to more people to be able to let them go, if you love them.

Another behavior of concern described by a caregiver was her mother's incessant talking:

> Oh, she could talk 24 hours… I mean, um, generally, she'll have breakfast, she'll go to sleep, she would normally be asleep now, and she'll have a snooze maybe 'til lunchtime, and then she'll wake up and she'll stay awake maybe 'til half past nine… she's not always consistent. And she can wake up at half past seven, start talking, and go until half past seven the next morning. So she can do it all night … some of it will be pleasant, you know, so sometimes she'll sing, and other times, she'll be very aggravated, very angry… screaming at the top of her lungs so much that she can barely talk the next day …well, I don't get to sleep, … you're awake all night with a headache… there's nothing you can do. (Caregiver 1)

Caregiver Burden

Caregiver burden manifests in a number of ways, such as reduced participation in the workforce, physical injury, impact on family life and emotional distress.

Caring responsibilities impacted on the ability of several caregivers to participate in the workforce. One caregiver took a lower paid position to allow her to continue her caring responsibilities, while another caregiver spent 18 months away from work caring for her mother.

> ... and I left that position [managerial position] in November because I just couldn't keep it all going… [s]o I came back to a Level 2 position in the city. (Caregiver 4)
>
> … the last 18 months, I took off work without pay to look after her. … (Caregiver 13)

A back injury experienced by a caregiver's son, in the course of his caring duties, meant that external assistance had to be obtained to help with showering:

> We had [organization] come and shower him in the end because we used to lead him… to the bathroom, sit him on a chair there… that would take the two of us to lead him there or put him in the wheelchair and bring him back… but in the end, we needed more help because [son's] back went… he couldn't help any more with that sort of

lifting... he was heavy. Although he wasn't a heavy person, but it was a dead weight... he couldn't help himself... it only lasted six months or maybe a year. (Caregiver 11)

The ability of one caregiver to participate in activities of her wider family was largely dependent on her mother's state of health:

I have 5 grandchildren, I would love to be part of their lives, but sometimes, I've also had to put them... on the side, because at the time, that I think, 'ok, I've made arrangements, I'll do this'. Mum's not well, and you can't leave her...[s]o then you just don't go. (Caregiver 3)

The emotional toll taken on caregivers was reflected in comments such as the following:

I, at the end, got cranky and crying because I was exhausted ...(Caregiver 5)

I found it very stressing, very, very stressing. I think I was even going through a bit of a depression,... because seeing my mother like that, not quite understanding it all, not having any freedom. I didn't really want freedom because I wanted to make sure that she was looked after, and I was a bit possessive and my brother, he was good. He'd come up and give me a hand, but ... at night time, she'd got her night and day mixed up. So she was awake during the night and that meant I was awake, and she'd come into my room, about 100 times a night and wake me up... it was really a difficult time...(Caregiver 13)

The geriatrician highlighted the toll on the health of caregivers:

... the carers get run down... [a]nd so ... carer health, mainly through night-time ... behavioral issues... or behavioral issues during the day... I think that seems to be the... the number one factor, I think, that will push people to make that final sort of 'out'. (GT)

What Are the Palliative Care Needs of People with Dementia and Their Caregivers?

Palliative care needs of people with end-stage dementia and their caregivers included:

- diagnosis and specialist referral,
- planning for the future,
- caregiver supports,
- resources received, and
- services required.

Diagnosis and Specialist Referral

Several caregivers recounted difficulties in obtaining a diagnosis from their GP, with a number of caregivers relating the need to change GPs in order to obtain a diagnosis. Caregivers valued knowing the cause of the changes in behavior in the person with dementia, even if there was no cure available. For other caregivers, diagnosis of dementia was a relatively straightforward matter. Due to certain family situations, one person with dementia was not told of the diagnosis, while for other people with dementia, the diagnosis did not actually mean anything to them. Referrals to specialists were often difficult to obtain.

Case study 2 "A caregiver's story: the quest to find out what was wrong".

The experience of this caregiver highlights a number of issues:

- difficulty in obtaining diagnosis from GP,
- inappropriate specialist referral,
- need to seek assistance from another GP, and
- referral to appropriate specialist to provide diagnosis.

Case Study 2. "A caregiver's story: the quest to find out what was wrong" – as related by Caregiver 18

It was very hard to get diagnosis from the GP. It was our second marriage and my wife's eldest son came to me one day, saying that her 3 children had been talking together and that they were worried about their mum. Now my wife had spent her life looking forward to having grandchildren. She loved kids, but her son said, "Look, we're worried about Mum. She doesn't seem to have the enthusiasm for the grandchildren that we expected." I said, "Oh, it's possibly the change of life", but never having been through it with a woman, I didn't know what to expect, so I said, "I'll take her to the doctor and get her checked out."

And so we went to her GP who had known her for 28 years and delivered her children and he said, "Oh, change of life." The GP did all sorts of tests and as nothing came back, he sent her off to another doctor, who might have had a different opinion. "Doctor" in inverted brackets! We told him the story, and he thought it was a big joke. He asked her a lot of questions, and eventually he sent us off to a psychiatrist for a psychiatric assessment. When we went back, he said, "Oh, well, she's not mad." To which I replied, "I know she's not mad. You're the bloody idiot that's mad", thinking that she had something wrong with her. We went back to the GP and asked him what sort of shrink he'd sent us to and he didn't answer. "Well, you're as bad as he is." I said, "As far as I'm concerned, you're finished." I walked out of the consulting room and went to the receptionist and said, "I want to see another doctor in the complex."

I managed to see another GP the following day who was able to access all my wife's files, so he knew the history. The first thing this GP said was, "Have you seen a neurologist?" "No", I said "you guys are the experts. The other doctor sent us to a witch doctor" He said, "We'll get you to see a neurologist". I rang this neurologist. Now this was in May or June, but I couldn't get in until October and so I rang the surgery back, and said, "Pass a message on to the doctor that I can't get in to see the neurologist until October." Well, about 20 minutes later, the phone rang. It was the GP that I'd seen saying, "You've got an appointment next Tuesday, can you make it?" I replied, "Yeah, no worries." He said, "Well, I've made an appointment with me for Thursday. Go and see the neurologist Tuesday, come and see me Thursday." We went to the neurologist, who I've since found out, has a lot to do with the Alzheimer's Association and Parkinson's Disease. Anyway, within 20 minutes, she told me that my wife was in early stages of dementia and early stages of Parkinson's. Within 20 minutes!

The experiences of caregivers who readily obtained a diagnosis indicate that GPs often referred the client to a specialist for confirmation.

> ... the doctor ran the standard memory test, which mum failed miserably, and announced straight away that mum had Alzheimer's. No [referral to geriatrician]. (Caregiver1)
>
> And in 1999, I did ask her [wife] to see her doctor, and fortunately, her doctor's mother had dementia, so that put us off on the right foot, really, she, she twigged almost immediately that there was a distinct possibility that there was going to be dementia developing, ... Her diagnosis was that it was a dementia and she arranged for an appointment for her with a neurologist and he did the usual tests, the mini mental and all the rest of it and his conclusion was that it was dementia, but of the fronto-temporal region of dementia and he recommended a doctor [name], who is researching memory

> loss, mainly at [hospital], and we had quite a few consultations with doctor [name]...(Caregiver 10)

GPs also discussed issues involved in the provision of a diagnosis to their patients and families. This GP had mixed opinions about the provision of a diagnosis, as he realized that such a diagnosis had different implications for people in different living situations and cultural groups:

> I could say 'yes' and 'no'. For some patients, and particularly their families, it's very important that they do get that diagnosis and it has very practical implications in just terms of medication and services. So if somebody doesn't have a formal diagnosis, then they don't have access to some of the services, so that would be a 'yes'. From a possibly a taboo subject, to label somebody as having Alzheimer's or whatever, particularly if they're living on their own or if they're ... an elderly couple, just the two of them with very little supports, a lot of the times, they don't actually like that diagnosis, because the fear is, as soon as it's diagnosed, they have to go into a home. Plus, sometimes family don't like to have grandma or their parent having that diagnosis because it's just taboo within that particular group, ..[p]articularly, we've got quite a big [cultural group] [in this practice] and depression and psychological things, they're ok, if they're attached to trauma, but to degeneration and old age, it isn't appropriate, because the older person is meant to be very wise ... and so having a diagnosis of dementia isn't appreciated. (GP3)

The geriatrician highlighted the limitations of the diagnostic tools currently available

> I suppose the biggest problem is that our diagnostic tools are still relatively crude...(GT)

Planning for the Future

Several caregivers recounted that they knew the wishes of the people, for whom they cared, with respect to the care to be provided at end-of-life, for example:

> ... they [parents] were very, very clear about what they wanted their end-of-life to look like, and so all the Wills were done, all the Enduring Power of Attorney, Guardianship, everything that you could do 10 years ago... we actually had all the paperwork all set up ready to go...which is really quite important when you're looking at end-stage dementia, because I was able to be very clear, and my brothers were able to be very clear about what the end stage would look like, ...(Carer 4)

However, for most of the caregivers, it was not a subject that had been able to be discussed mainly due to the lack of acceptance of the person with dementia of their condition.

> ... [i]n terms of her recognizing her own illness - in the early days she refused to accept it was happening, and would become angry if it was mentioned. So no specifics were ever gone into once the problem arose. (Caregiver 1)
>
> [advance care planning discussions] there was nothing wrong with him! No, No, No, he said 'just a bit of a memory lapse now and then...' he said 'there's nothing wrong with me'. (Caregiver 11)

For several caregivers, day-to-day care was all-consuming, with no thought given to the future:

[too late for discussions about advance care planning] yes, because we really didn't know… we'd just been coasting along and 'as it comes up, we'll handle it'. I think, in some ways, it's better, because if you knew what was ahead of you… I would have run a mile, I think. (Caregiver 17)

I don't think I was even contemplating that [advance care planning] at that stage… it was more of 'what can I do now?' not 'what will we have to do in the future?' (Caregiver 18)

Caregiver Supports

Caregivers related a variety of ways in which they received support, included avenues of support and counselling.

Avenues of Support - Formal and Informal

Caregivers highly valued the support received through formal support groups from organizations such as Alzheimer's Australia SA. The informal support received from relatives and friends was also widely acknowledged as invaluable in helping caregivers sustain their caring duties.

Other caregivers acknowledged the value of attending formal support groups:

We have these support groups and they're very helpful. We support each other, it really is very good … (Caregiver 7).

… [j]ust to hear how others were coping with things, … a huge feeling of guilt that a caregiver had by sometimes not being patient and being impatient and but to talk it over and hear what the others had to put up with and how they coped … I couldn't stress that enough, that meeting was very, very beneficial. (Caregiver 15)

Family Support

Emotional and physical support from family was fundamentally important for caregivers, to assist with care and reduce the burden and stress associated with being a full time caregiver.

I have two brothers… They're very supportive. … if I need them, they'll come. … like I've just been to Canberra… they've taken a turn each at night, and have moved in. Dad's also a Diabetic and on insulin, so, in actual fact, [name], my sister-in-law is a Registered Nurse, so she comes in and gives the insulin at night. (Caregiver 4)

I was lucky because my family, they are very supportive, my daughter, my son, my brother, all fantastic, they're all here to help. (Caregiver 13)

However, supportive relationships were also challenged:

I have a very supportive husband, but I find too, at times, it does affect our relationship. I mean he's very patient, he's understanding, but you know, I kind of put him on the back burner at times, …(Caregiver 3)

Not all friendships survived the challenges inherent in dementia. Several caregivers related that they lost some of their friends during this time.

I found I lost my friends... (Caregiver 16)

One caregiver related how she had used the Internet initially to cope with the effort of caring. A caring network had gradually developed, which provided the support she needed before she received any respite services.

Case study 3. "A caregiver's story: finding support on-line" – as related by Caregiver 1

My mother has dementia and for more than 3 years, I had been looking after her entirely on my own, without any respite or support whatsoever.

However, in a rather convoluted way, I built up a support network on-line. Late one night, I was on what I think was a movie website. I joined in some sort of forum and provided the name of a movie, which another participant loved, but couldn't remember the name of. We then started talking about the movie, the director and his other movies, and books that it was based on and blah, blah, blah, blah, blah... We just got to know each other. Then, on occasion, this person said, "I care for my mother." To which I replied, "Oh, yeah, so do I, mine's got dementia." And back came the reply, "Yeah, so has mine."

Gradually, other people joined our discussions. They were people that have gone through similar experiences or have something themselves, like MS or Motor Neurone or something like that, so that they were the person being cared for, rather than the caregiver. One of the participants then created an invitation-only website for about 30 of us. We're from all over Australia. Most of the people are in Queensland and New South Wales, but there are a couple over in WA, and one other in South Australia, a couple in Tassie.

We go online, and say "good morning", and not talk about our caring responsibilities or health issues, just say, "Oh, what are you doing today?" - the ordinary chit-chat. And then, somebody will say, "Had a drama last night".

When Mum broke her hip, it was my first contact. I love going on-line. I wrote "Mum's had a fall and I can't assess what's wrong with her. What do I do?" And I had all these calming voices coming back at all hours of the night, because there's always someone staying up late.

We share information by referring each other to different websites. Someone will say "Hey, have a look at this," and then you go and look at it.

We've become a really close group. I think the youngest is in her twenties, and the eldest is late 60s. We send each other birthday and Christmas presents, and cards. Some members of the group on the east coast have visited each other. Someone in Sydney has gone up to Queensland and stayed with somebody up there and had a ball.

And so, that was my entire support, on-line, because I had no respite. However, after mum broke her hip in September last year, I received an 'Extended Aged Care at Home' package and now, I have some respite.

Counselling as a Coping Strategy

A number of caregivers related that they had received counseling services to assist them to cope with their caring responsibilities and acknowledged the value of such services:

I have been having some counseling. I spoke to the Alzheimer's, the counselor there... [counseling] excellent, excellent, yes, very good and I also, through my doctor, I've been seeing a psychologist to help me deal with issues, set up strategies how to deal with, with my emotions and ... conflicts within the family, ... like sometimes you feel like stamping your feet and saying 'I don't want to be here'. (Caregiver 3)

I did have a one-to-one interview with somebody at the Alzheimer's Association.... She was very good and we talked through a lot of things. (Caregiver 6)

One caregiver related a negative experience with a counselor, whom she saw for advice about how to cope with her husband's behavior. The advice to leave the relationship however was not appreciated.

Services Received

Caregivers accessed a range of services that allowed them to continue to look after their relatives at home. These services were received in a variety of forms, ranging from government-funded co-ordinated packages of care, accessing a range of services and privately funded care arrangements. Respite and assistance with showering were the most commonly utilized services, followed by assistance with feeding and continence. The services received by people with dementia and their caregivers are summarized in Table 1.

Table 1. Services received by people with dementia and caregivers

Carer No	Respite	Shower-ing	Feeding	Contin-ence	Dom duties	Equip-ment	HP support	Priv Nursing
1	✓	✓	✓	✓		✓	✓	
2	✓	?	✓	?	✓			
3	✓	✓	✓	✓	✓		✓	
4	✓	✓				✓	✓	
5	✓	✓	✓	?		✓	✓	✓
6	✓							
7	✓	✓						
8								✓
9	✓	✓	✓	✓	✓			
10	✓							
11		✓	✓	✓		✓	✓	
12	✓	✓						
13	✓	✓	✓	✓				
14	✓	✓	✓	✓				
15	✓	✓						
16	✓	✓						
17	✓	✓	✓	✓	✓	✓		
18	✓	✓	✓	✓	✓	✓	✓	

?: not explicitly discussed, however reasonable to assume that help was also received with these aspects of care.

Comments of caregivers about each of these services are provided in the following sections:

a. Respite

Caregivers provided details of the respite they received and how they used this time. This respite was provided in a number of forms: in-home care, external day care, and overnight and longer duration respite. A number of the caregivers acknowledged the limited number of hours of in-home care worker support available to them and the need to use this time as efficiently as possible. Indeed, it is often a busy time for the caregiver during those "respite" interludes.

> I get 4 hours respite on Monday, and 3 hours on Friday, but I cut it an hour short so I come back, an hour earlier so I've got the helper here to help me toilet Mum... I get 2 hours and 3 hours instead of...no, I can't get on the train and go somewhere... mainly I sort of use that time to just get as much shopping done as I possibly can and you know, get the prescriptions, and ... if I have to see a doctor or whatever ... as soon as I leave my front door, I'm like 'Okay, where do I got to first?" I try to make it... so I'm not doubling back... and I go with lists, so you know, I'm not wandering around wondering 'what do I need?' (Caregiver1)

A number of caregivers valued respite, in the words of one caregiver:

> And then, I did a marvelous thing, I got him booked into the [organization] day care and they were able to take him 3 times a week, well to begin with it was only once, and then eventually three, and I'd drop him there at 10 and pick him up at 3, and that was absolutely wonderful, for me and I knew that he was looked after and fed, and they were so sweet there...(Caregiver 5)

The value of overnight respite was acknowledged by one caregiver:

> ... we've got just across the road... a respite cottage, where you can actually have an overnight... it's not a bad place to be and [husband], he went there for day care originally, with a buddy, ... and then eventually they asked me would I like him to have an overnight, which was a bit hard. I'm not very good at letting go, ... [husband] goes there usually once a week, sometimes he stays 2 nights. I find the 2 nights are brilliant, because ... he doesn't go usually until lunch time, he's so slow in the morning. I don't push him. If I have Wednesday afternoon, and then Wednesday night, ... is normal, I don't sleep very well, but then I have all day Thursday, and Thursday night, I usually die. My psyche tells me 'it's ok, you can go to sleep'. But by Friday morning, I really want to go and bring him home, it's long enough... for me. He's always happy to come home. They say he's happy there, but the minute I walk through the door he'll say, 'We're going home. Let's go'. (Caregiver 9)

While respite services were generally found to be valuable, there were a number of reports of unsuccessful placements due to the behavior of the person, or less that adequate care provided for the person, which added to their caregiver's burden, rather than lightening it.

> ... we had first respite three years ago, and it's been all downhill since, I'd have to say. He went into respite for 2 weeks, as everybody says you're supposed to have a break, he went to an aged care facility, I didn't go anywhere. I stayed home. The second week, ... they rang me and said he'd had a fall. They found him at the side of the bed and when I went over there, he was kind of semi-conscious, and then he wasn't conscious,

and I couldn't wake him up. They'd already had him seen by a doctor, but the doctor had just said he'd had a fall, but he was coming back to see him and he came while I was there and called an ambulance straight away. Came up here to [hospital a] for a scan, which didn't show anything. They thought he might have had a stroke, and then I had him transferred to [hospital b] because they wanted to admit him and we live on the same street as [hospital b], so that was the place to be. When they admitted him there, they found a pressure sore on his heel, it measured 6 x 5 cm, so he'd obviously had a lot of time in bed. And it became very infected and he just went down hill from that. They had to teach him to walk again and he's just never been the same person since.... [h]e'd gone in there totally ambulant ... he was probably walking 10kms at least a day. Since then, he's been in need of a lot of care. (Caregiver 9)

b. Showering

The majority of caregivers had to assist the person with dementia with showering. Indeed, assistance with showering was an important part of most of the care provided through care packages.

I had one [caregiver] this morning to help me with her wash and it's good having that ... I find, say after a long weekend like Easter, when I may not get help, and I'm just doing it... even with the lifter by myself, I find by the end of a four day weekend, my back is killing me, you know, because I am still bending over and all that sort of thing, so it takes twice as long. When I've got a person, it takes half as long and there's someone else doing half the bending down, and it just gives me relief... physical relief, when someone else is helping. (Caregiver 1)

And then they sent somebody to help me...they'd said 'we'll send someone to help you shower him.' And I said, 'no, its okay, I can manage'. He wasn't too bad, but then he got very boisterous and dangerous in the shower, so the girl came twice a week to help me shower him... (Caregiver 14)

c. Cooking and Feeding

Assisting people with dementia to eat was another vital task performed by some of the caregivers. Difficulties with swallowing, soft foods, such as purees, soups, ice creams and jellies were often provided.

He loves jellies and ice-cream and purees, so we have pureed soup made out of vegetables and meat. Tonight we're having chicken meatloaf and mashed potato... (Caregiver 4)

...and then I thought why isn't he swallowing his pills? Why is he crunching them? And then I realized that he didn't know how to swallow, ...(Caregiver 5)

He's still young, he's not 63 yet. ... I have to feed him, ... we're not sure [whether he's forgotten how to swallow], (Caregiver 9)

I'd feed him because he'd either spill the food everywhere, and just wouldn't eat it... towards the end, it was vitaminized because he used to gag on things and start coughing ... (Caregiver 11)

d. Continence

The majority of people with dementia had difficulties with maintaining continence, with associated impact on their caregivers' workloads and in some cases, finances. However, a number of caregivers received continence aids through the Continence Aids Assistance Scheme, funded by the Australian Government.

...[coordinator] brings all mum's continence products... would cost a fortune otherwise... (Caregiver 1)

He [husband] became incontinent, and through that government incentive, I was able to get the packs of pull-on pants and so forth. So that became a large part of the day, coping with all that. ... there was always a load of washing to do every day, because although he wore those things, they weren't always adequate. (Caregiver 6)

f. Equipment

Caregivers received a range of equipment through their packages of care that allowed the person with dementia to remain at home with reasonable degree of safety:

an occupational health person came around and she was useful... very useful and very good...she got whatever I asked her for and that was no hassle for her. It started off with the cot sides and then she got me the daybed, and the lifter and... the shower chair and the swivel chair... whatever I needed... it would arrive within a couple of days...so we were very fortunate that way... and I didn't have to pay for it ... that was a big help. (Caregiver 11)

[partner's] got an EACH-D package ...[i]f I need equipment or anything, all I have to do is say to the coordinator ... and it would be here the next day... that's like the bed and the air mattress, and the shower chair... and the wheelchair he's sitting in... (Caregiver 17)

h. Private Nursing Care

A number of caregivers reported purchasing private nursing care.

And [palliative care specialist] came and assessed him, ... [he] would come every day, and [name] and her caregivers [from private nursing organization] would look after him. They were absolutely amazing, ... He was clean and they washed him and if he wanted a drink, they'd give him one or if he wanted a whisky, they'd give him one, ...they were here ... mostly at night,... for about 6 days. (Caregiver 5)

And so mum lived in the unit for a couple of years before she couldn't cope there anymore and ... then we employed [private nursing organization] ... massive cost, like it cost $300,000.00, the care we used ... (Caregiver 8)

Services Required

The nature of dementia itself means that it was not always possible to determine the nature of services required, as recounted by this caregiver in Case Study 4.

Case Study 4: "A caregiver's dilemma: what services do I need?"
This case study highlights a range of issues:

- importance of tailoring care to the specific needs of each person with dementia and caregiver,
- need to ensure all care workers are appropriately trained,
- variability of care needs, and
- value of help received.

Case Study 4. "A Caregiver's Dilemma: what services do I need?" - as asked by Caregiver 9

It has only been in the last 2 weeks, for 3 or 4 mornings, depending on the week, that a care worker comes in about 9 in the morning. Steve doesn't always get up until later, but I try to make him get up while they're here. I shower him and they'll make the bed, because the bed always needs to be changed. We get the continence aids through the Government scheme, but they don't last very long. In our case, that's about 3 months' supply. I am a bit fussy about keeping him especially clean. I don't like anything wet or smelly. I know when he goes for respite once a week, he always comes home wet.

I'm desperate to get more help at home. We have been assessed for an 'Extended Aged Care at Home' package, which I believe is up to 30 hours a week of help, and lots of other bits and pieces as well. The organzsation has got funding for it, but they haven't got it set up properly yet.

I get 3 hours' respite on a Tuesday afternoon, which is great but in 3 hours, you can only go somewhere locally, have a cup of coffee with somebody, but most of my friends don't live locally, some of them are there, others are in town. And so in 3 hours, I can't get to do anything social. Although I don't want to say I don't want the 3 hours, it's not really what I want.

The package coordinator and I have talked about the 'Extended Aged Care at Home' package and she thinks when it comes into place, I should ask for a bit of help every morning. That help is great, because, while I'm showering Steve, they strip the bed and remake it, and the majority of them put it in the washing machine. There's one person who needs to be stood over, but I think that's care workers, some are much better than others. On that particular day, it's like 'why did we bother?' One of the care workers is really good. The washing goes in the machine. By the time we're out of the shower, the bed's made, she's folded up the washing from the clothes airer, and she's probably in the kitchen. She knows what Steve has for breakfast and so, she's got the Weetbix out, the bowl, and it's like, wow! That's great help, because normally I'd bring him out of the shower and then I've got to do all of that, so you've got another three quarters of an hour of those things, plus trying to feed him. Before that help came, I could still be doing that stuff at midday. As well as that, we've finished breakfast, now it's a trip to the toilet – it's just like that constant thing.

I really want that help; it is so useful. I can't believe how useful, because at first, I thought 'I don't want somebody in my house every day, what are they going to do?' It's this intrusion all the time and as I say, some of them are great and some of them, not so. When I first met the care worker who's probably the best, she smelt of cigarette smoke, which put me off immediately. I thought that she was a bit of a rough diamond, but she's fantastic; she just gets on with it. She's great with Steve, most of them are great with Steve, actually. They all seem to be good at being nice to people.

The coordinator and I have talked about instead of having respite on Monday and Tuesday afternoons, have the whole day on Monday; get somebody to come in and be here after his shower, and stay here until 4 o'clock or something, so I can take off, meet somebody, do something. The other thing that I'm not sure about at the moment is whether it's possible to have somebody come in during the evening. I love theatre, and I don't go very often. It would be nice to sometimes say, 'This is on, I'd love to go and see it' and get somebody to come in the evening and be here, but that's Steve's most difficult time. He gets really restless. They call it 'sundowning', don't they? From about 2.30 in the afternoon, he's up and down, will go to the loo 53 times and just wander around. I usually take him for a drive, which calms him. And so, that could be quite hard for someone. I think that the person who comes on Tuesday afternoon, from 2 'til 5, is finding it a bit hard. She doesn't quite know how to deal with it. She is allowed to take him for a drive, but she said to me, 'he doesn't sit still'. I know and I thought 'you've only got 3 hours!'

When you need help, it's never there. I've had situations where the caregiver's just left and I've gone to hang washing out. I've come back in; Steve's gone to the loo, he's come out into the bedroom and sat on the bed, so it's everywhere and the caregiver's gone! You can't ring a bell and say 'can you just do that, while I do this' and of course, he's distressed because of what's happened. And so I'm trying to get him back into the bathroom and maybe even into the shower, again and the bed needs to be done. And so, to me, that's the hardest part, when it's all happening and the caregiver's just left. Why didn't you do that 10 minutes ago? What do I want? Well, what I want varies from day to day, really. I've even thought about accessing my superannuation; it would be really nice to have somebody here a few days a week, just to be here. But then, it wouldn't work, because if I come in early from respite, as I did yesterday, the minute I come in, I'm 'it'. And so, even if you've got somebody in your home 24 hours a day, that wouldn't really work either. Sometimes, I think what do I want? I don't know myself what I want, but I do know that what we're getting at the moment is not perfect, but it's much better than getting nothing at all. I want the best, but what is the best?

One GP suggested that increasing resources, such as respite and domestic assistance, would be valuable:

> … increasing the amount of respite available to carers would be good. Sometimes the amount of respite they get isn't really significant – it might be for an hour or 2 to go shopping. Perhaps give people to opportunity to go out for an evening, to spend some time with friends or family, go for an outing. … perhaps have access to day care for the patient… I've had patients who've been going to day care and it's been a relief for the carers, during that time, they get to do the things they need to do. Extra housecleaning services perhaps for carers because they still have to look after the house themselves, and everything else, … as well as their loved ones. (GP1)

Provision of information and expertise in palliative care and dementia management were seen as being valuable:

> If there was a specific agency for dementia, I think, it would be really excellent, because 'call up the dementia people'. Obviously, they would be people experienced in that area, because palliative care for dementia is different to palliative care for or for people with cancer, they're not necessarily in pain…so with some mental health training, would be beneficial, … [mental health and palliative care?]… yes, I mean it needs mental health and once people have been dealing with patients with dementia, for some time, the experience would be invaluable, for the patients, because they would see how the caregivers react. And unless you have dealt with someone with dementia and families that haven't dealt with it, I don't think that the people outside the immediate family really realize how difficult it is.… They're adults and they can be heavy, …very difficult to control, and they don't realize what they're doing, they don't realize what's right or wrong or harmful or not harmful. They need a lot of looking after and it's 24 hours. And caregivers often don't get much sleep because they worry about what's going to happen during the night. (GP2)

The representatives of service organizations also highlighted the need to have the flexibility to be able to respond quickly to the changing care needs of their clients, referred to as consumer directed care:

> It [money] should be [attached to the people] … to then buy in whatever they need from one organization, if that's what they want … you get frustrated that you can't do continuity of care for people... our experience is people won't change and get the level of care that they need. They'll put up with inadequate levels of care, rather than go to another organization.… [m]ore than 50% of the time, that's what people will chose to do, which is crazy, but you can understand why they do it. You're 80, you're in pain, you've got lots of chronic conditions – the last thing you need is another massive change in your life, and invite another group of people into your life with a different philosophy to the ones they had before or they've got different rules about this or different rules about that… you've got a tenuous hold on staying at home, the last thing you need is another big change, isn't it? (SP3)
>
> … my belief is that … if you need extra intensity of services for a period of time, you should be able to access it, … even for people with dementia, there'll be times where their behaviors are heightened and its more difficult, but then, they'll often change, a different group of behaviors will come in, which may not be so difficult for the carer to manage, so … they need a different type of service, but you're … locked in to what your funding … looks like, in other words, I'd like consumer directed care …, so that you can get what you want when you need it… (SP4)

The need to be able to provide additional resources to support families when death was imminent was also recognized by one service provider:

> And I think dying at home isn't a real alternative, for people, because of that lack of resources. So I think, lots of people won't do it, lots of people fully intend to want to do it for their family member, or the family are committed to doing it for their family member, but struggle right at that end because of that, the level of commitment that's required and the lack of support that they have. ... And I just don't think that there's any one program out there that can do it. As I said, it takes enormous resources from the family, some families don't have that level of resource. .... That's why I think a top-up palliative care package, is really what is required to help that person stay at home, with the opportunity to increase the services over a period of time, as needed. (SP3)

What is the Relevance of These Findings?

The findings of this research have confirmed a number of issues mentioned in the literature. With respect to the desire to die at home, while this preference had been expressed by a number of people with dementia when able to do so, in line with sentiments reported in Care of Patients with Dementia in General Practice (NSW Department of Health, 2003), there was recognition amongst caregivers, medical professionals and SPs that a diagnosis of dementia may result in admission to an aged care facility. The determination and commitment of a number of caregivers to keep their relative at home, for as long as possible, even into the late-stage, confirms the observations of Hughes, Jolley, Jordan and Sampson (2007) that such determination in addition to support received from local services is critical in allowing this to happen. However, ultimately, issues including safety associated with behaviours of concern and caregiver exhaustion eventually lead to admission to aged care facilities in a number of cases (Hughes *et al.*, 2007).

The duration of caring, lasting at least in several cases more than 10 years, highlights the unpredictability and extended nature of the disease and the protracted nature of the end-of-life phase (Lunney *et al.*, 2003; Birch and Draper, 2008).

The frustrations experienced by most patients and caregivers in this study in trying to obtain a diagnosis of dementia confirm the experience of other caregivers (Iliffe *et al.*, 2003; Iliffe and Wilcock, 2005). Also, a number of caregivers experienced a similar dismissive attitude towards them by their GPs as they discussed their concerns about the health of their relatives, as reported by Downs *et al.*, (2002). However, the time needed to make a diagnosis and the limitations of the diagnostic tools available, mentioned by the geriatrician, may also contribute to the difficulty in making an accurate diagnosis (National Collaborating Centre for Mental Health, 2007). Nevertheless, the provision of a diagnosis was important to allow services to be organized (Robinson, Emden, Lea, Elder, Turner and Vickers, 2009) and to have discussions about nature of care to be provided at end-of-life.

In contrast to the findings of Treloar *et al.*, (2009), a relatively small number of people with dementia in this study received referrals to geriatricians. However, in common with those of Treloar *et al.*, (2009), very few people with dementia and caregivers had completed advance care plans, for reasons such as discomfort of physicians and families to discuss death and dying (Godwin and Waters, 2009; Hancock *et al.*, 2006).

While all people with dementia had informal caregivers, either spouses/partners, or daughters, these caregivers reached the point along the dementia journey where additional support was needed. All of the caregivers in this study had accessed one or more services, while looking after their relative at home. These services included respite care, with care workers coming into the home, attendance at day care centres and extended respite in aged care facilities, which were generally acknowledged as being valuable.

One strategy commonly used by caregivers in enabling them to continue in their caring role was accessing information and support from others, through both formal and informal support services. Caregivers found support through formal support groups and informally from relatives and friends in their broader social networks. Indeed, family support was a key element in allowing caregivers to continue their demanding role at home. However, as also reported by Iliffe *et al.*, (2003), a number of caregivers reported experiencing shame and social isolation due to the reactions of friends largely to their husband or partner's behavior. In common with the findings of Sachs *et al.*, (2004), a number of caregivers had made substantial financial sacrifices to look after their relatives at home. Two caregivers had left the workforce, one for a period of 18 months and the other has been full-time caregiver for more than 3 years. Another caregiver sought a demotion, in order for her to be able to continue caring for her parents at home.

Caregivers accessed a range of services to support them in their caring role, ranging from government-funded programs, to government care packages, supplemented with private nursing services, to completely privately funded care. People with dementia were reported as needing help with activities of daily living, such as bathing, grooming, eating and using the toilet, having impaired communication skills and having lost the ability to recognize themselves and others, confirming the summary of the characteristics of end-stage dementia provided by Hancock *et al.*, (2006).

The types of resources required by caregivers identified by Treloar *et al.*, (2009) including continence aids and equipment were confirmed by caregivers in this research.

Caregivers, medical professionals and SPs provided a number of suggestions as to services which were needed which highlighted the need for packages of care to be tailored to suit the specific needs of people dementia and their caregivers and with the flexibility to be able to respond to the ever-changing needs of people with dementia and their caregivers. In common with the findings of Treloar *et al.*, (2009), some SPs suggested that dying at home was not an option in South Australia due to the intensity of resources needed to support caregivers during this time. Hence, a 'top-up' palliative care package to allow the provision of additional resources when death was judged to be imminent was advocated.

There was recognition among medical professionals that any extra support should be directed towards supporting caregivers in their caring role, in areas such as respite and domestic assistance. Information and expertise in palliative care and dementia management were also acknowledged as being needed.

Conclusion

The incidence of dementia is increasing worldwide. Due to its historical association with cancer care and the lack of recognition of dementia as a terminal illness, the palliative care needs of people with end-stage dementia have taken time to be recognized and addressed. Caring for people with end-stage dementia in the home is an onerous task, which exacts a high toll in terms of physical, emotional and financial demands on informal caregivers and to a lesser extent, on the broader community. The context in which care is provided for people with dementia is one of extended duration, during which caregivers attempt to fulfill the desire of person with dementia to remain at home, while being confronted with a range of behaviors of concern. The palliative care needs of people with end-stage dementia and their caregivers include the diagnosis of dementia so that planning can commence for future care arrangements and services can be obtained. Such services should include assistance with activities of daily living and the provision of equipment required, such as hoists and shower chairs. These services should also be appropriately structured such that the changing needs of people with end-stage dementia and their caregivers can be addressed in a timely manner.

References

Access Economics Pty Ltd (2009) Keeping dementia front of mind: incidence and prevalence 2009-2050.

Alzheimer's Association What is Alzheimer's Accessed 25th May 2010, http://www.alz.org /alzheimers_disease_what_is_alzheimers.asp.

Alzheimer's Association (2008) Tests Used in Diagnosing Dementia. Accessed 26th May 2010 Alzheimer's Association, Canberra, http://www.alzheimers.org.au/ upload/US8June08.pdf.

Anderson B.A., Kralik D., March G. and Briffa M. (2010) "Identification of the palliative care needs of home-based people with late-stage dementia and their caregivers" Project. Royal District Nursing Service SA Inc Research Unit, Adelaide.

Armitage D and Evans J. (2005) Improving end-stage dementia care: A practice development approach. *Geriaction* (Winter), 25-29.

Australian Government Department of Health and Aging (2008) National Initiatives. Department of Health and Ageing. Accessed 6th October, http://www.health.gov.au/internet/main/publishing.nsf/Content/ageing-dementia-resource-guide.htm~ageing dementia-resource-guide-13.htm.

Australian Institute of Health and Welfare (AIHW) (2006) Dementia in Australia: National data analysis and development. *AIHW cat. no. AGE 53.* Accessed 11th August 2009, http://www.aihw.gov.au/publications/index.cfm/title/10368.

Australian Institute of Health and Welfare (AIHW) (2003) Admitted patient palliative care in Australia 1999-00.edn. AIHW. Canberra. Accessed 16th February 2010, http://www.aihw.gov.au/publications/index.cfm/title/9045.

Birch D. and Draper J. (2008) A critical literature review exploring the challenges of delivering effective palliative care to older people with dementia. *Journal of Clinical Nursing* 17, 1144-1163.

Black K., LoGuidice D., Ames D., Barber B. and Smith R. (2001) Diagnosing Dementia. Accessed 26th May 2010 Alzheimer's Association Australia, Higgins, http://www.alzheimers.org.au/upload/DiagnosingDementia.pdf.

Chatterjee J. (2008) End-of-life care for patients with dementia *Gerontological care and practice* 20 (2), 29-34.

Downs M., Clibbens R., Rae C., Cook A. and Woods R. (2002) What do general practitioners tell people with dementia and their families about the condition? *Dementia* 1 (1), 47-58.

Godwin B. and Waters H. (2009) 'In solitary confinement': Planning end-of-life well-being with people with advanced dementia, their family and professional caregivers. *Mortality* 14 (3), 265-285.

Hancock K., Chang E., Johnson A., Harrison K., Daly J., Easterbrook S., Noel M., Luhir-Taylor M. and Davidson P.M. (2006) Palliative Care for People with Advanced Dementia. *Alzheimer's Care Quarterly* 7 (1), 49-57.

Hansen E.C., Hughes C., Routley G. and Robinson A.L. (2008) General practitioners' experiences and understandings of diagnosing dementia: Factors impacting on early diagnosis. *Social Science and Medicine* 67, 1776-1783.

Hughes J.C., Jolley D., Jordan A. and Sampson E.L. (2007) Palliative care in dementia: issues and evidence. *Advances in Psychiatric Treatment* 13, 251-260.

Iliffe S., Manthorpe J. and Eden A. (2003) Sooner or later? Issues in the early diagnosis of dementia in general practice: a qualitative study. *Family Practice* 20 (4), 376-381.

Iliffe S. and Wilcock J. (2005) The identification of barriers to the recognition of, and response to, dementia in primary care using a modified focus group approach. *Dementia* 4 (1), 73-85.

Leifer B.P. (2003) Early Diagnosis of Alzheimer's Disease: Clinical and Economic Benefits. *Journal of the American Geriatrics Society* 51 (No 5, Supplement), S281-S288.

Lunney J.R., Lynn J., Foley D.J., Lipson S. and Guralnik J.M. (2003) Patterns of Functional Decline at the End of Life. *Journal of the American Medical Association* 289 (18), 2387-2392.

Mitchell S.L., Kiely D.K., Miller S.C., Connor S.R., Spence C. and Teno J.M. (2007) Hospice Care for Patients with Dementia. *Journal of Pain and Symptom Management* 34, 7-16.

National Collaborating Centre for Mental Health (2007) Dementia. A NICE-SCIE Guideline on supporting people with dementia and their caregivers in health and social care. The British Psychological Society, Leicester, http://www.nice.org.uk/nicemedia/ pdf/ CG42Dementiafinal.pdf.

NSW Department of Health (2003) Care of Patients with Dementia in General Practice. NSW Department of Health, North Sydney, Accessed 6 October 2009, http://www.he alth.nsw.gov.au.

NSW Department of Health on behalf of Australian Health Ministers' Conference (AHMC) (2006) National Framework for Action on Dementia. Accessed 8th October 2009 NSW Department of Health, North Sydney, http://www.health.gov.au/internet/main/ publishing.nsf/Content/D64BD892C6FDD167CA2572180007E717/$File/nfad.pdf.

Personal Social Services Research Unit (2007) Dementia UK - Summary of Key Findings. Alzheimer's Society. Accessed 25th May, http://www.alzheimers.org.uk/ site/scripts/d ownload_info.php?fileID=1.

Plassman B.L., Langa K.M., Fisher G.G., Heeringa S.G., Weir D.R., Ofstendal M.B., Burke J.R., Hurd M.D., Potter G.G., Rodgers W.L., Steffens D.C., Willis R.J. and Wallace R.B. (2007) Prevalence of Dementia in the United States: the Aging, Demographics, and Memory Study. *Neuroepidemiology* 29, 125-132 Accessed 25th May 2010.

Prince M. (2008) The prevalence of dementia worldwide. Alzheimer's Disease International. Accessed 27th May 2010, http://www.alz.co.uk/adi/pdf/prevalence.pdf.

Robinson A., Emden C., Lea E., Elder J., Turner P. and Vickers J. (2009) Information issues for providers of services to people with dementia living in the community in Australia: breaking the cycle of frustration. *Health and Social Care in the Community* 17 (2), 141-150.

Sachs G.A., Shega J.W. and Cox-Hayley D. (2004) Barriers to Excellent End-of-life Care for Patients with Dementia. *Journal of General Internal Medicine* 19, 1057.

Sampson L., Harrison-Dening K., Greenish W., Mandal U., Holman A. and Jones L. (2009) End-of-life care for people with dementia. Marie Curie Palliative Care Research Unit, London.

Shega J. and Tozer C. (2009) Improving the care of people with dementia at the end of life. *Dementia* 8 (3), 377-389.

Shuster Jr J.L. (2000) Palliative care for advanced dementia. *Clinics in Geriatric Medicine* 16 (2), 373-86.

Treloar A., Crugel M. and Adamis D. (2009) Palliative and end of life care of dementia at home is feasible and rewarding. *Dementia* 8 (3), 335-347.

In: Palliative and Nursing Home Care
Editor: Samuel E. Plunkett

ISBN 978-1-61122-417-7

Chapter 2

Mental Distress in AIDS-Orphaned Children: The Efficacy of Natural Mentoring Palliative Care

Francis N. Onuoha*
Department of Human Care Science
Graduate School of Comprehensive Human Sciences
University of Tsukuba, Tsukuba, Japan

Introduction

Every 2.2 seconds a child tends to lose a parent somewhere around the world to the vagaries of life (CSCV, 2010), particularly war, illicit drug use, traffic accident, famine, hunger, and disease. However, in contemporary times, the probability of parent loss worldwide and in sub-Saharan Africa specifically, has been compounded by the prevalence of HIV/AIDS. Of the world's estimated 17.5 million AIDS-orphaned children, about 75% of them are in sub-Saharan Africa (UNAIDS, 2009).

Orphan children are perceived to be more socially distressed than non-orphans (UNICEF, 2004). Without their biological parents and caregivers, the children are suspects for the varied distress factors from orphaning. These factors may include food insecurity, malnutrition, physiological ill health and poverty. Also, higher experiences of child trafficking, prostitution, organized crime/gangsterism, and child soldiering are not uncommon (CSCV, 2010). Yet other adverse encounters of orphan children may include social discrimination against them in school enrollment and in household resource allocation (Gillespie, 2006; Deininger, Garcia, and Subbarao, 2003). Bereaved children from parental death would show higher emotional distress, hopelessness, unhappiness and frustration than non-orphans. Some may be distressed by their new circumstance that may require them to care not only for themselves but also for their younger siblings (Mbozi, Debit, and Munyati, 2006). Sexual abuse (Pridmore and Yates, 2005) and stigma/discrimination (Cluver, Gardner, and Operario,

*Tel/fax +81-298-53-3971; email: fnonuoha@yahoo.com

2008; Nyblade et al., 2003) against orphans are known but seem to disagree with the social deprivation and distress theses of the orphan child. They argue that these propositions are media-induced stereotyping, which are often orchestrated by research scholars of traditional persuasions. Most orphans have the resilience and agency to positively get on with the challenges of life following parental death (Abebe and Aase, 2007)

If orphans are associated with mental distress, then those orphaned by AIDS may exhibit more distress. Often the misfortune in the death child's parent to AIDS is not a one-snap event. Rather it often entails a chain of lengthy stressors to the child that occur before, during and up to the parent's death owing to the health debilitating consequences of the disease. AIDS-orphaned children would enact unique mental health experiences (Chitiyo, Changara, and Chitiyo, 2007). They may be more vulnerable than *other* orphans to higher distress before and during parental illness owing to the protracted, human-wasting opportunistic sicknesses associated with AIDS (WHO, 2005). The distress of the children may be aggravated by the higher social exclusion often directed at their AIDS-incapacitated parents.

At parent's death, AIDS-orphaned children themselves may become objects of continued social discrimination owing to the public perception that the children may be HIV seropositive and may pass on sooner than later. Their social exclusion experience may manifest in reduced access to schooling and health care for the children. Furthermore, AIDS is more likely than other causes of death to evoke the early double loss of both biological parents by the children (UNAIDS, UNICEF, and USAID, 2004), which factor may provoke vulnerability to lower parental support and higher distress.

To ameliorate distress, orphans would require important adult, non-parent figures in their lives as parent-surrogates. These non-parent adults may range from family-members (such as grandparents, older sisters/brothers, uncles/nieces, etc) to non-family individuals (eg, church ministers, school teachers, neighborhood members, etc). In this article, these social figures are generically referred to as "natural mentors" (Rhodes, Ebert, and Fischer, 1992). Children with important social figure networks in their lives are more likely to show positive behavioral outcomes than those without such figures (Chen *et al.*, 2003). Natural mentors attempt to fill the parental loss gap and in doing so, ameliorate distress symptoms in the orphan child. However, if natural mentors are considered valuable for orphans in general, those orphaned by AIDS (who are more likely to be double-orphaned or to have no parents) would require the palliative care of natural mentors greater. This proposition forms the theoretical thrust of this paper.

The article is presented in two parts. Part I provides definitions for key concepts of the article. These concepts include palliative care, distress, anxiety, child abuse, and social discrimination. Others are social support, self-esteem, foster/parental care, and mentoring. Part II reports findings from the empirical study of the mental health of and effect of natural mentoring on children orphaned by AIDS in two sub-Saharan Africa countries -- South Africa and Uganda. Currently estimated at about 1.4 million, South Africa has the highest AIDS-orphaned children in the African continent, followed by Uganda with about 1.2 million. These unenviable magnitude of AIDS-orphaned children in the two countries informed the choice of the countries for the empirical study. Would children whose parents died of AIDS show higher distress than would *other* orphans? Among AIDS-orphaned children, would a natural mentoring relationship show greater palliative efficacy to moderate distress than it would among *other* orphans? This paper seeks to address these questions after conceptualizing its key concepts.

Part I

Palliative Care

Owing to health crises, some patients may be in the hospital, others may choose the nursing home; still more may prefer the home doctor for receiving medical attention. However, the health crisis confronts the individual with the reality of illness and decision-making about care. The care may be chemo-therapeutic (drug-based) or psychosomatic (imagery based). The first is in the realms of clinical medicine to cure the disease. The second is in the domain of palliative care to ameliorate the discomfort/pains associated with disease and illness. Often, when a clinical/hospital cure fails or is presumed unattainable, there is the recourse to palliative care to provide the required smooth transition between the hospital and other health-seeking services.

Palliative care is interdisciplinary, requiring professionals in the diverse branches of knowledge such as faith medicine, counseling, social work, psychology, nursing, and clinical medicine. The aim is to relieve suffering and improve quality of life for patients with advanced illness and their families. Pain and symptom control through constant communication is central to all stages of palliative care. Palliative care is reported to be different from geriatrics, hospice care, case management, and pain management (CAPC, 2010). In palliative care, patients of any age, at any stage of life-threatening illness are admissible. Throughout the illness course and simultaneously with other treatment forms, palliative care is allowed for comprehensive pain and symptom control, psychological/spiritual care needs, family support, and assistance in the patient's transition to other service facilities (hospice, home care, and nursing homes) and health care settings (geriatrics, case/pain management). In geriatrics, only elderly, frail patients are admitted. Prevention, rehabilitation, disease management, functional assessment, and recovery for elderly patients are the focus of geriatrics. Hospice would cater to dying patients of any age; while case management is the complex care needs of each patient. However, to the extent that palliative care is offered in one form or the other for symptom management at each platform of the care setting, that defines it uniquely interdisciplinary character as already stated.

Distress

To understand distress (depressive symptom), it is important to consider stress. Stress was imported from biology (Selye, 1930) to the psychosocial lexicon. As a biological construct, stress is a condition that depicts bodily responses to environmental threats or stressors. In the three stage alarm-resistance-exhaustion theory, Selye argues that in the event of a threat/stressor, the body autonomously produces *adrenaline* to either fight or escape from the stressor (alarm stage). If the stressor persists, then the body continues the battle to resist or adapt/cope with the stress (resistance stage), whichever is appropriate. But the body's effort to resist the stressor cannot be indefinite. Over time, it begins to give way, leading to the exhaustion state. Here, the body may be unable to maintain normal functioning owing to depleted body chemical resources. The furtherance of this stage precipitates *distress*. Distress may result in the damage/impairment of the gland and immune systems to function appropriately.

Stress may be positive or negative. For example, positive feedbacks, successes, achievements, compliments, sudden good news are positive stressors or "eustress" (Seyle, 1930). Positive stressors are arousals that tend to trigger healthy signals to the brain for optimal body performance. By contrast, negative stressors are "distress" (Seyle, 1930) which tend to enact a wide range of adverse cardiovascular, respiratory, gastrointestinal, renal, and endocrine reactions. These changes manifest in yet varied representations such as poor judgment, excessive worry, moodiness, irritability, agitation, inability to relax, feeling lonely, isolated or depressed, aches and pains, diarrhea or constipation, dizziness, chest pain, and rapid heartbeat. Other stress-induced problems are eating too much or too less, sleeping too much or too less, social withdrawal, procrastination, increased alcohol, nicotine or drug use.

The dynamic nature of cognitive, emotional, physiological, and behavioral manifestations of stress and distress have excited interest in psychologists. For example, sources of stress/distress could be sensory inputs such as pain or bright light. Ill health could be a stressor, so could environmental issues such as food, housing, freedom, and mobility. Others sources of stress include social issues such as relationship conflict, interpersonal struggles, break ups, or the life events of birth, death, marriage and divorce. Yet others could be life experiences such as poverty, unemployment, insufficient sleep, work/exam deadlines, etc. Also, adverse developmental experiences at prenatal and post-birth (Davis et al., 2007; O'Connor et al., 2002), poor child-rearing, and infant sexual-abuse are thought to deplete the stress-fight resourcefulness of individuals.

According to the American Psychiatric Association's Diagnostic and Statistical Manual of Mental Disorder (DSM-IV-TR), the conceptual sources of distress are:

- Problems with primary support group – death of a family member, discord in family, separation, divorce, estrangement, abuse or neglect.
- Problems from the social environment – death or loss of a friend, inadequate social support, living alone, discrimination.
- Educational problems – illiteracy, poor school achievement, school disruption
- Occupational problems – unemployment, potential job loss, difficult work condition
- Housing problems – homelessness, unsafe/inadequate housing
- Economic problems – inadequate income
- Problems with access to health care – inadequate health insurance, transportation problems
- Legal problems – arrest or fear of arrest, use of illegal substances, incarceration
- Other social/environmental problems – no telephone, exposure to natural disaster, violence, no social service agencies.

It is worthy to note that a situation is conceived as stressful only if it is cognitively appraised as such (Lazarus, 1966), and one does not have the coping resources to deal with the situation. These coping resources could be both intrinsic in the individual (positive self-concept) or extrinsic in the environment (availability of social support). Individual differences, therefore, in the cognitive appraisal of stressors present a major challenge in developing test-retest reliable measurement of stress. Also, cognitive stress test outcomes tend to vary with *time* and *space*. What seems constant, however, is the fight-or-flight (or the problem-focused or avoidance-focused) strategies to stress management. In the first, the individual mentally attempts to undermine/dismiss the threat as not serious after it occurs. In the second, the individual may deliberately avoid the threat when it occurs/prevent it from occurring.

Other ways to manage/control stress and distress include setting or defining limits/boundaries in interpersonal relationships early enough; listening to music; doing things you enjoy; spending time in the garden/wilderness.

Anxiety

A major correlate of distress is anxiety. Anxiety is the generalized mood condition that is characterized by uneasiness or worry. Anxiety is considered a future-oriented mood state in that it excites in one the readiness to cope with an upcoming negative event (Barlow, 2002). In this regard, it is different from fear which is a present-oriented state because it occurs in the presence of an observed threat. Also, whereas fear is an avoidance behavior to a threat, anxiety is often a problem-focused behavior to a threat. In positive psychology, anxiety is viewed as a natural response to a challenge for which the subject has insufficient coping. It is also thought to be psychosocially helpful in that it prompts the individual to deal with the threat/challenge. But some psychologists would consider the latter mood state as arousal rather than anxiety.

To illustrate anxiety, Csikszentmihalyi (1997) provided the challenge-skill taxonomy of anxiety. The graph had low-high challenge (on the Y-axis) and low-high skills (on the X). He concluded that the contrasts of worry, anxiety, arousal, and flow in that order were control, relaxation, boredom, and apathy. Thus, the direct opposite of anxiety is relaxation.

Anxiety has both physical and psychological effects. The physical effects include heart palpitations, muscle weakness and tension, fatigue, chest pain, shortness of breath, bowel movement, or headache. As the body prepares to deal with a threat, blood pressure and heart rate are increased, sweating is increased, blood flow to the muscles is increased, while the immune and digestive system functions are inhibited. Other signs of anxiety include sweating and trembling. The emotional symptoms include feelings of apprehension, trouble concentrating, feeling tense, anticipating the worst, and restlessness. Other emotional feelings are nightmares/bad dreams, obsessions, irritability, déjà vu, or being scared . Cognitive effects are the thoughts of suspected danger.

In the brain, amygdale and hippocampus chemicals are thought to underlie anxiety in mammals. Unpleasant and potentially harmful stimuli such as bad odor (Zald and Pardo, 1997) and taste (Zald, Hagen, and Pardo, 2002) are shown to increased blood flow in the amygdale brain region.

Child Abuse

Issues of child abuse are as varied as they are complicated. They are cognitive, physical, emotional or social in nature. The identified forms are:

- Neglect
- Rejection

- Physical abuse
- Sexual abuse
- Psychological maltreatment
- Labor abuse
- Medical abuse
- Others

Approximately 5 children die everyday from child abuse, many of them under 4 years old (childhelp.org, 2010). Child abuse occurs at every socioeconomic level, across cultural lines, within all religions and at all educational levels. For example, 36% of women and 14% of men in prison in the United States were abused as children. Over 60% of persons in drug rehabilitation centers report being abused or neglected as a child. About 30% of abused children will later abuse their own children, thereby continuing the vicious cycle of abuse. About 80% of 21 year olds that were abused as children met criteria for at least one psychological disorder. Sexually abused children are 25% more likely to experience teen pregnancy; three times less likely to practice safe sex, thereby are greater risk of STDs; 2.5 times more likely to abuse alcohol; 3.8 times more likely to develop drug addiction. Nearly 66% of the children in treatment for drug abuse reported being abused children. In the US alone, the estimated annual cost of child abuse and neglect for 2007 was $104 billion.

In agrarian societies, there is a vast under-reporting of child abuse incidents. In these societies, reliable vital statistics or police reports may not exist. In industrialized countries, statistics tend to exist. According to the US Department (2003), an estimated 905,000 children were victims of child abuse and neglect. Although physical injuries may not be common forms of child abuse, physical health, psychological, behavioral, and societal abuses are known (childwelfare.gov):

- Physical health consequences

The consequences of child abuse may range from minor incidents such as physical bruises/cuts to severe ones as broken bones, hemorrhage or death. Whichever, the pain and suffering these abuses may cause should not be underestimated. For example, the injuries caused by vigorously shaking a baby may not be immediately noticeable; they may include bleeding in the eye or brain, damage to the spinal cord, neck, rib or bone (NIH, 2010). Abused and neglected children have shown impaired brain development (DeBellis and Thomas, 2003), language, and academic abilities (Watts-English et al., 2006). The NSCAW (National Survey of Child and Adolescent Well-Being) project found that more than 75% of foster children aged between 1 and 2 years showed medium to high risk of problems associated with impaired brain development, against less than 50% in the control group (ACF/OPRE, 2004a). An association between child abuse and poor health has been reported. Adults who experienced childhood neglect and abuse are more likely to suffer health ailments such as high blood pressure, arthritis, and asthma (Springer et al., 2007).

- Psychological consequences

The psychological impacts of child abuse and neglect would include fear, isolation, and the inability to trust. Others are low self-esteem, depression, and relationship difficulties. Withdrawal and depression symptoms are common among young children who experienced emotional neglect (Dubowitz et al. 2002). As many as 80% of abused young children in the US may meet the diagnostic criterion for at least one psychiatric disorder by age 21. These abused children showed depression, anxiety, eating disorder, and suicide attempts. Other psychological conditions included panic disorder, dissociative disorders, attention-deficit/hyperactivity disorder, anger, posttraumatic stress disorder, and reactive attachment disorder (DeBellis and Thomas, 2003; Springer et al., 2007). Abused children in institutional care scored lower than the general population on cognitive capacity, language development and academic achievement measures (US Dept, 2003). Earlier studies found a relationship between substantiated child maltreatment and poor academic performance, and classroom functioning for school-age children. Rejected or neglected children are more likely to develop anti-social behaviors such as aggression and violent behavior (Schore, 2003).

- Behavioral consequences

Studies have found abused and neglected children to be 25% more likely to experience behavioral problems such as delinquency, teen pregnancy, low academic achievement, drug use, and mental health problems that do the general population (Kelley, Thornberry, and Smith, 1997). Other studies suggest that these children are more likely to engage in sexual risk-taking as they reach adolescence (Johnson, Rew, and Sternglanz, 2006).

Abused and neglected children are 11 times more likely to be arrested for criminal behavior as a juvenile; 2.7 times more likely to be arrested for violent and criminal behavior as an adult; and 3.1 times more likely to be arrested for one of many forms of violent crime reports the National Institute of Justice (English, Widom, and Brandford, 2004).

Research consistently shows an increased likelihood that abused and neglected children will smoke cigarettes, abuse alcohol, or take illicit drugs during their lifetime (Dube et al., 2001). As many as two-thirds of persons in drug treatment programs reported being abused as children (Swan, 1998).

Abusive parents may have experienced abuse during their own childhoods. Thus it is estimated that approx one-third of abused and neglected children will eventually victimize their own children (Prevent Child Abuse New York, 2003).

- Societal consequences

While child abuse and neglect almost always occur within the family, the impact directly or indirectly affects society as a whole. The first costs are expenditures associated with maintaining the child welfare system to enable it to respond to and investigate allegations of child abuse and neglect. Other direct costs are expenditures by the judicial, law enforcement agents, health and mental health systems.

Indirect costs represent the long-term economic consequences of child abuse and neglect. These include juvenile and adult criminal activity, mental illness, substance abuse, and domestic violence. Others are loss of productivity due to unemployment and underemployment, cost of special education services, and increased use of the health care system. Prevent Child Abuse America (2001) estimates these indirect costs at over $69 billion per year, and direct costs at $24 billion per year.

Nevertheless, not all abused and neglected children would experience the short/long term psychosocial consequences. Factors that may influence outcomes include:

- The child's age when the abuse or neglect occurred
- The type of abuse (physical, sexual, neglect, etc.)
- The frequency, duration, and severity of abuse
- The relationship between the child and the abuser

It is not clear why given similar conditions, some children experience long-term consequences of abuse while others may not. A number of protective factors may contribute to the abused child's resilience. These may include individual characteristics such as optimism, intelligence, creativity, humor, independence, and self-esteem. Others are positive individual influences from peers, teachers, mentors, and role models. Community well-being such as neighborhood stability and access to safe schools and adequate health care are some protective factors (Fraser and Terzian, 2005).

In summary, the effects of abuse would vary with the circumstances of the abuse or neglect, the personal characteristics of the child, and the child's environment. The consequences may be mild or severe; disappear after a short time or last a lifetime; and may affect the child physically, psychologically, behaviorally, or a combination of all three ways. Due to related costs to public entities such as the health care, human services, and educational systems, child abuse and neglect impact not just the child and family, but society as a whole.

Social Discrimination

Social discrimination is a form of social behavior *in favor of* or *against* a person or group based on social perceptions of the group's characteristics. It is positive discrimination when *in favor of* the group as in affirmative action; it is negative discrimination when *against* the group as in race or ethnic discrimination. In general, the latter form is the most common meaning of social discrimination

The UN Cyberschool (2001) reports that discriminatory behaviors take many forms, but they all involve some form of exclusion or rejection. Negative social discrimination is generally illegal in most Western societies, while discriminating between people on the grounds of merit (called differentiating) is usually lawful. To understand discrimination, consider that there are over 6 billion people on earth today. What do you have in common with these people? In what ways are you different or unique?

- Similarities and Differences

The earth's 6 billion humans share many similarities and differences. Everyone on earth must eat,, breathe, and drink to stay alive. Everyone has a family, a language, and a culture. All people have hopes, dreams, fears, and feelings of any imaginable things. Humans differ in many ways, too. Some of these differences are physical, such as skin color, hair texture, or sex. Others differences such as language, customs, and beliefs are learned. These similarities and differences are the basis for social groups, a term used to describe common categories of people. Everyone is a member of some social group, even if they don't always realize it.

- Prejudice

Social groups have long been a part of human history. Categorizing people into "us" and "them" helped humans develop tribes, clans, and other early social structures. Deciding who belonged and who didn't also led to conflicts and fighting. "Us" and "them" thinking still continues to permeate human relationships from ancient to the present time. We tend to stick with people who are similar to us while avoiding people who are different. In many ways, this is understandable. It's often comfortable to be among people who are like us, and identifying by similar traits can provide a sense of belonging and community. But when we avoid others who are different, we tend not to learn about them. And when we don't really know what people are like, it's easy to make guesses, fill in the blanks, or make generalizations about "them" based on very limited knowledge. In short, we make judgments about others before we know the full story. These *pre-judgments* are called prejudices. Whether it paints people favorably or not, prejudice is typically based on ignorance, misinformation, and/or and fear of differences.

- Stereotypes

Prejudices are fueled by stereotypes, an exaggerated or distorted belief/image about a person or group. Stereotypes assume that everyone in a group has the same characteristics, leading people to falsely believe that "they" are all alike. Even when the stereotype suggests positive traits (for example, that women are nurturing), everyone is hurt because these images leave no room for individual differences.

No one is born to believe stereotypes; they are learned from media, or parents, peers and many other sources. Social scientists believe that children begin to learn prejudices and stereotypes as early as two or three years old. Even though they don't fully understand what prejudice is, young children may repeat racial slurs or act out stereotypes they see in the media or from their parents. For example, a group of boys may tell a girl that she can't play archery because it's a boy's game. As they are exposed to more stereotypes, young children tend to form attachments to their own group and develop negative attitudes about other groups. As these attitudes deepen over a person's lifetime, they are difficult to change. As they get older, people tend to see the things that support their views and disregard or ignore experiences that challenge them.

Overall, discrimination is an action that treats people unfairly because of their membership in a particular social group. Discriminatory behaviors take many forms, but they all involve some form of exclusion or rejection as with a student who won't let people of a certain race sit with them at lunch. Often, individual actions may point to a larger system of exclusion as when a school won't let girls take the same classes as boys, or a business that doesn't hire people of certain ethnic/racial backgrounds.

On a national scale, discrimination can take the form of official laws and policies. The enslavement of Africans in the United States, the official domination of Blacks by Whites in South Africa, or Hitler's widespread extermination of Jews are some historic examples of systemic, legal discrimination. When discrimination becomes part of a systematic use of power or "just how things are," it is tagged with an "ism." Racism and sexism are a few "isms" you may be familiar with. As to be expected, discrimination is averse to social support.

Social Support

Social support relates to the emotional/material comfort given to one by family, friends, co-workers and significant others. It is the awareness that we are a part of a community of people who value, love, care and think well of us. In its broader sense, social support includes social integration which refers to the *quantity/size* and *frequency/density* of social relations. Social support relates to the *quality* and *function* of social relationships. It occurs in interactive processes and is similar to altruism, obligation, and reciprocity.

The form of social support may be instrumental (assistance with problems), tangible (donate goods), informational (give advice), and emotional (give reassurance), among others. Physical healthiness and well-being are not only the result of medicinal or physical therapy but also derived from the meaningful participation in a social group. Receiving support gives meaning to individuals' lives. It motivates them to give in return, feel obligated, and to develop a sense of attachment.

It must be noted that a communicative experience does not constitute a support unless the receiver views/perceives it as such. Thus, a distinction is made in the literature between *perceived* and *actual* support received. Although closely related, the two must not be confused. Perceived social support is relates to anticipatory or prospective help in times of need. Support actually received is retrospective. It refers to help actually provided at a time of need. Expecting support in the future may be dispositional and laced with optimism; whereas support provided in the past is based on actual experience. To which degree these two distinctions emerge empirically may depend on the specific wordings of the questionnaire items. The more diffuse the questions are, the more general the responses they attract.

Regarding its functional value, social support is known to have a stress-buffering effect to the negative impacts of stressful events (Cassel, 1976). Studies state that social support moderates psychological distresses such as clinical depression (Kendler, Myers, and Prescott, 2005). In their review of 81 studies, Uchino, Cacioppo, and Kiecolt-Glaser (1996) found better cardiovascular regulation (lower blood pressure); better endocrine functioning (lower catecholamines levels); and better immune system functioning from social support. Among Japanese (Sumi, 1997) and Chinese (Jou and Fukada, 1997) college students perceived social support associated with self-reported happiness, physical and psychological well-being. However, in a longitudinal study of more than 3,000 adults, perceived social support did not predict psychological well-being (Emery, Huppert, and Schein, 1996). Social support could not mediate self-reported strains from job stress (Rahim and Psenicka, 1996).

Like stress, there is growing evidence that social support affect humans differently. For example, hardy individuals tend to have a sense of control over events and tend to perceive events as opportunities/challenges rather than stressors. These individuals may experience less strain from stress than non-hardy individuals. Social support is often governed by the exchange or interdependence theory of reciprocity. For example, individuals may give support only to those who either supported them recently, or may support them in the near future. Similarly, individuals may ask for support from persons whom they have either recently supported or to whom they expect to be able to support in the near future.

Old age is often characterized by diminishing reciprocal power and resources. Similarly, very young children may not be in a position to reciprocate social support. Yet there is evidence that these categories of persons are not abandoned by their families and friends (Antonucci and Jackson, 1990). They tend to receive support despite their likely inability to reciprocate. Reasons for this behavior may be explained by the evolutionary theory of kin-selection (the provider-support model). Under this theory, individuals are likely to provide support to persons with whom they are genetically related or share similar genes owing to the necessity to promote the survival of the provider's genes (Brown et al., 2003). The support provider derives intrinsic pleasure in giving rather than receiving, but may give only to persons with whom they are genetically compatible such as kinsmen or friends.

Self-Esteem

Self-esteem is often conceived as similar to self-worth, self-respect, self-regard, self-integrity or self-love. Our self-esteem is the opinion of self-worth we hold of ourselves. It is the judgment we make of our qualities and characteristics. It relates to the individual's overall positive appraisal of him/herself. Psychologists regard self-esteem as an enduring trait. As a trait rather than a state, self-esteem should not be confused with self-confidence. The latter is the knowledge that one can succeed at something; be it a relationship, career or goal. Self-esteem, on the other hand, is the capacity to like and love oneself; feel worthwhile, irrespective of all the ups and downs of life.

Some early theorists conceive self-esteem in terms of one's successes over failures. Others define it to reflect the extent to which we significantly believe ourselves to be capable, successful and worthy. It is a personal judgment of self-worthiness that is expressed in the attitudes we hold of ourselves. But later definitions perceive it as stable sense of personal self-worth, although different from bragging/narcissism. A healthy self-esteem is not contingent on success because there are always failures to contend with. Neither is it a result of comparing ourselves with others because there is always someone better. With a healthy self-esteem, we like ourselves for who we are and not because of what others think of us.

Self-esteem is the foundation of our personality. If you are not happy with yourself for reasons you cannot explain, it is probably because your self-esteem might be in the low phase. Self-esteem defines everything about us. It is something experienced as part of, or background to, all our thoughts, feelings and actions.

Maslow (1987) conceived self-esteem as a basic human motivational need. His popular theory of motivation, has two forms of esteem – respect from others, and respect for self. Respect from others which entails recognition, acceptance, status, and appreciation is believed to be easier lost than self-respect. Without fulfilling the self-esteem need, individuals would not be motivated to seek self-actualization (Maslow, 1987). In this regard, the drive to seek self-esteem would present stress. However, modern theorists who view self-esteem as a trait, state that it has a protective function against stress and anxiety (Greenberg, 2008). Also, although high self-esteem correlates with high self-reported happiness, it is not clear which of the two leads to the other.

Raising our self-esteem is the singular challenge that faces us all. When self-esteem is high, we have a positive and constructive view of ourselves. We tend to believe in our ability to do things. We focus more on our strengths than our weaknesses. We are more likely to set goals, make plans, develop positive relationships, and seek ways to increase our knowledge, skill, and success. Conversely, when self-esteem is low, we have a negative and destructive view of ourselves. Doubt our ability to do things, focus more on our weaknesses. We are unlikely to be interested in goals and plans. Build less rapport with others and increase our knowledge and skills. Self-esteem, therefore, is the battery that powers our belief system about success.

Since self-esteem is not static but dynamic, it is raised when we raise our competence and mastery. There are many techniques to do this. A proven method is to establish a course of positive action that creates a sense of personal success. Personal success is attainable when we set goals, make plans, be disciplined to adopt a great work ethic, then we are on our way to raising our self-esteem through personal successes. The more success we achieve in life, the higher our self-esteem will rise which in turn, leads to more successes. Doubts and frustrations will come, but patience and persistence in refining and renewing our goal plan are essential.

The level and quality of self-esteem, though correlated, may be distinct. For example, while high self-esteem is a desirable characteristic, its quality should also be *stable*. Narcists tend to exhibit high but fragile self-esteem, while humble fellows may show low but stable self-esteem. Quality of self-esteem is measured in terms of its (a) stability over time, (b) non-contingent to a particular situation, and (c) ingrained nature or automaticity in the individual.

Baumeister, Smart, and Boden (1996) report that most hostile groups tend to have high but unstable self-esteem. These people think well of themselves in general, but their self-esteem fluctuates. They are prone to react defensively to ego threats, and they are also more prone to hostility, anger, and aggression than other people. For instance, violent criminals tend to conceive themselves as superior to others or as special, elite persons who deserve special treatment. Many murder and assaults are committed in response to blows (insults and humiliations) to the self-esteem.

Self-esteem has been implicated in domestic violence. Husbands who abuse their wives often had a less-affluent background, poorer education or earned less income than their wives. They use violence to assert their superiority. Also, men who earned high academic qualifications but had poor careers were violent perhaps because they were frustrated their lives didn't reflect their high opinions of themselves. By contrast, individuals who had poor education but very successful careers were six times less likely to be abusive (Baumeister et al., 1996).

Branden (2001) referred to the self-esteem observed in those findings as "pseudo self-esteem" rather than "true self-esteem". The first comes from external validation of the self or from other people's approval. The second comes from internal sources such as self-responsibility and self-competence to deal with challenges regardless of what other people may think. Researchers who agree with Branden argue that "narcissism" (inflated opinion of self) is not "true self-esteem". Violence arises when that false opinion is threatened. Individuals with "true" self-esteem who value themselves and believe wholly in their own competence and self-worth would have no need to resort to violence, or have any need to prove their superiority.

Many authors, including Ellis (2001) have criticized the theoretical foundations of self-esteem. Ellis acknowledged the human propensity for ego as innate, but argues that measures of self-esteem are unrealistic, illogical, and deceptive. He states that self-esteem is based on over-generalized, perfectionist and grandiose premise. A better alternative to self-esteem may be unconditional self-acceptance, leading to unconditional other-acceptance.

Parental/Fostering Care

Parents are arguably one of the most fundamental agents of social stabilization in the lives of young children. As role models, social educators, counselors, and care-givers, parents have a more primary obligation to provide for the spiritual, intellectual, psychosocial, and material needs of their offspring (Turnbull and Turnbull, 2001) than other socialization agents, including peers. Bowlby (1988) alluded to the conceptual difference between intimacy [an affective bond complemented with shared social support] and attachment [an affective bond characterized by social security] (Reis and Patrick, 1996), and argued that dependent children would share both intimacy and attachment to a higher degree with parents for kinship survival (Bowlby,1988) than with other persons. Attachment theorists (Cicchetti, Toth, and Lynch, 1995; Bowlby, 1988) state that children experience in the presence of their parents a sense of security, which empowers them to meaningfully explore their environment. When security is threatened, as when parents are perceived not to be close enough, anxiety arises (Shaver and Hazan, 1993). Because emotional proximity with the caregiver is central in the attachment processes, when denied, the child may adopt a repertoire of social and anti-social behaviors to re-establish proximity, including crying, protest or avoidance behaviors (Reis and Patrick, 1996).

However, the death of one's biological parent inevitably brings about fostering. In Africa and most developing societies, where maternal mortality from child birth are high, orphan prevalence is a historical experience. The prevalence may be confounded by paternal/parental deaths from war, physical accidents, hunger and disease. In Africa, due to a strong extended family system, the left behind children from these deaths are relatively easily adopted by other family members (Preble, 1990) in a fostering arrangement. Fostering may be normative/voluntary; it may be crisis-led fostering. In the first, the biological parents of the child may be living. In some cases, either parent of the child may be deceased. This form of fostering usually takes the form of arrangements between the biological parent of the child and the foster parents based on the mutual socioeconomic benefits to both parties. These benefits include: kinship obligations, trade apprenticeship/education for the child, alliance building, and domestic labor to the foster home (Isiugo-Abanihe, 1985). Social parenting is thought to have advantages over natal parenting in most sub-Saharan Africa countries. The latter lessens the parent-child bond to make the child more independent. Fostered children are thought to be more disciplined, more resilient, and possess more economic values than biological children.

Crisis-led fostering relates to fostering in response to death for severe economic hardship. Usually the death of both parents may precipitate crisis fostering, which is typical for AIDS-orphaned children. Goody (1982) reports that among the Gonja tribe of Ghana, kins who have a right to the child in voluntary fostering are obliged to foster the child in crisis, but do so not as *fathers/mothers* but as *tutors/disciplinarians*. Crisis fostering, therefore, is a normative social obligation, in which the reciprocity of socioeconomic benefits for the child and her natal family are less considered.

Orphaning

Universally, an orphan is defined as a child aged 17 and under who has lost one (single orphan) or both of their parents (double orphan) (UNAIDS, 2004). These children a presumed to be under the universal adult suffrage age of 18 to be eligible for paid job and/or economic independence. They are further presumed to be deprived of the material, social, and psychological support of at least one of their primary caregivers.

While the material deprivation of orphaning may not be in double, the age definition and parental circumstance may vary among countries. In South Africa, for example, only children aged below 15, with a loss of both parents, are officially designated as an orphan. In other words, children whose mother or father is living is not classified to be eligible for government support. Although the government has made a commitment to progressively raise the age bar to below 18 years over time, the parental condition for qualifying as an orphan remains unchanged.

To the extent that a child has no natural parents - whether maternal (loss of mother), paternal (loss of father), or double (loss of both parents), he/she is a "biological" orphan. But there are also "social orphans". These are children with lose family ties. This group includes street children (whose natural parents are living), "missing" parent(s) households (in a war situation as in Uganda), and "absentee" parent(s) households (when one parent deliberately deserts the home, and cut links with the children).

In contemporary times of HIV/AIDS, there is consensus in the anecdotal and empirical literature that the extended family system is becoming increasingly unable to cater for orphan children. Subbarao et al. (2001) identified other care systems, their advantages and demerits to include:

- Formal adoption: Advantages: Family members are most likely to act in the child's best interest. Family integration promotes psychological and intellectual development of the child. Fostered children are integrated into society more readily than in orphanages. Disadvantages: Discrimination in food allocation, workload, education, etc. is possible.
- Government/NGO subsidies distributed through the family. This care is thought to encourage even poor families to foster orphans. But it is difficult to monitor. Subsidies sometimes benefit head of household only rather than the orphan child for whom they are meant. Subsidies may be shared among too many family members, and little to the orphan.
- Government/NGO subsidies distributed through the community. It presumes that communities will better know the needs of families. If distributed by churches, stigma may be reduced. But this care system may not work in urban areas where community living is weak. Also, it may not be feasible in communities where ethnic tension or discrimination exists.

- Government/NGO school meal vouchers/subsidies; government/NGO health vouchers redeemable by clinics. School meal vouchers may be easier to monitor. Most likely to prevent future loss of human capital from hunger and disease. But it may entail horizontal inequity, to the extent that children with parents who live in abject poverty do not receive any subsidy.
- Income-generation schemes for fostering families: Increased short-term incentives for households to take-in children. If successful, may improve the welfare of the orphan. But the program rarely succeeds without training, follow-up, and leadership.
- Family tracing for social orphans: Being reunited with family members brings psychological benefits. It may not be viable in areas where a large percentage of the population has died or missing; or in war-torn economies where family members are unable to care for orphans.
- Orphanages: It is better than child-headed households or being a street-child. If run by religious groups, may reduce stigma and attract donor/charitable funds. But lack of incentive to act in the behalf of orphans may harm the psychological development of orphans. Not cost-effective. Can easily become a commercial venture rather than a welfare one. May not meet the emotional needs of children.

In summary, institutional (such as orphanages) and fostering are the two dominant care systems for orphaned children. The disadvantages of the first seem to outweigh its advantages. Its social milieu is unnatural; it may harm the psychological development of the orphan child. It is not cost-effective, and tends to lack incentives to genuinely act in the behalf of orphans. Other disadvantages is that it can easily become a commercial venture rather than a welfare one. Thus it may not meet the emotional needs of the children. All said, it is presumed to be better than a child-headed household or being a street child. If run by religious groups, it tends to attract charitable funds; and may reduce stigma (Subbarao, Mattimore, and Plangemann, 2001)

Mentoring Programs

In the ancient Greek mythology, Athena (the goddess of wisdom) was referred to as a "mentor" for her role as the teacher and guide of Telemachus (son of the legendary King Odysseus). Mentoring is the structured program that brings together young people and caring adults in a trusting relationship (www.mentoring.org). The caring adults offer guidance, support and encouragement aims at developing the competence and character of the mentee. The mentoring blog describes a mentor as an adult who, along with parents, provides the young with support, counsel, friendship, reinforcement and constructive example. A mentor is not a *foster parent* in that the mentee is not required to live with him/her. Also, a mentor is not a therapist, parole officer, or a peer, but an adult, non-parent person. In the United States and elsewhere, nearly half of the young adult population aged 10-18, live in situations that put them at risk of not living up to their potentials. Without the intervention of caring adults, they could make choices that not only undermine their future, but also the economic and social lives of nations. Constructive mentoring would provide the following values:

- Improving young people's attitudes towards their parents, peers and teachers.
- Encouraging young persons to stay motivated and focused on their education
- Providing a positive way for young people to spend free time
- Helping young people face daily challenges, and
- Offering young people opportunities to consider new career paths, economic skills and knowledge.

As caring adults, a mentor is an adult friend whose ultimate goal is the help the mentee discover their strengths to achieve their potentials. Mentors are not meant to replace a parent, guardian or school teacher. A mentor is not a disciplinarian or decision maker for the child. Rather the mentor echoes the positive values of parents and teachers for the child.

In contemporary times, when traditional family and community linkages to bring younger people and older ones together are becoming loose by the day, the "renaissance of mentoring" is required (Mahoney, 1983), particularly for at-risk children. In the United States, formal mentoring programs are currently very popular. The National Mentoring Database lists more than 4,500 organizations that support mentoring activities (Rhodes, 2002), including Project RAISE, Across Ages, Team-Works, Career Beginning, Sponsor-A-Scholar, Big Brother/Big Sister. These programs show beneficial values for the youth that participated in them. For example, 46% of youths in the BBBS (big brother, big sister) one-on-one mentoring program were less likely than their control counterparts to initiate drug use and 27% less likely to initiate alcohol use. The participants felt more competent to do well in school and received higher school grades then the control. The children (both boys and girls across races) reported more positive relationships with friends and parents (Tierney, Grossman, and Resch, 1995). The Career Beginning, and Support-a-Scholar programs offered academic support and limited financial support for college education. Participants in both programs were more likely to attend college soon after high school than non-participants. The Across Ages mentoring program for substance abuse prevention evaluation had children who participated in all aspects of the program (community service, life-skills curriculum, and one-on-one mentoring by older adults) compared with those who participated in all but the mentoring. There was a third group of children made up of youth who did not participate in any aspects of the programs. Outcomes showed that youth who had mentors had better attitudes toward school, the future, and elders than did those in the other two groups. These youth also used substances less frequently and had better school attendance than did youth who did not participate in the program (Sipe, 2002). But these are formal, programized mentoring.

Natural Mentoring

Parents are arguably one of the most important agents of social stabilization in the lives of children. As role models, counselors, and educators, parents make significant impacts on the belief systems, hopes, and aspirations of their offspring. However, development psychologists would state that as children make the inevitable transition to adolescence, they come into social relationships with a broad array of non-parent adults who make considerable influences on the lives of the children. These adults have been variedly referred to as VIPs (very important persons) (Chen et al., 2003), significant others or natural mentors (Rhodes et al., 1992).

In a national representative US survey of adults, two-thirds of the reported adult-child relationships occurred spontaneously or naturally (MENTOR, 2002). Natural mentors are non-parent/non-peer support figures (Rhodes et al., 1992) whose roles tend to provide comfort, guidance, and inspiration to youth. For instance, Werner and Smith (1982) conducted a longitudinal study of children exposed to poverty and family instability. They found that those who developed into competent, resilient and autonomous young adults had support from a non-parent adult in addition to their parents. Goleman (1987) corroborated the finding when he noted that without exception, all children who thrived had at least one person – a grandparent, clergy, older sister, teacher, after-school providers and neighbor - that provided them consistent emotional support. Among single African American young mothers, Rhodes et al. (1992) found that those who have natural mentors in their lives reported better adjustment.

Children with an extended social network, especially non-parent adults who were important in their lives, were more likely to show positive outcomes than were those without an extended social network (Chen et al., 2003).

We invite the reader to an empirical research that suggests the inverse association of natural mentoring relationship with distress health among AIDS-orphaned children.

Part II

The Literature

Orphan children tend to manifest more depression (Furukawa et al., 1999), personality disorder (Paris, Zweig-Frank, and Guzder, 1994), and anxiety/insomnia (Tweed et al., 1989) tendencies than do non-orphans. These orphan children may present psychosomatic symptoms and health worries (Canetti et al. 2000) that may impede positive mental health. Material and emotional supports from parents during childhood may have enduring psychosocial health benefits (Scroufe et al., 1999). These parental supports, which the orphan child may lack, fulfill the affective function of the family to its members (Turnbull and Turnbull, 2001; UNICEF, 2004). Orphans may encounter hopelessness, and frustration (Mbozi et al., 2006), often owing to their new circumstance that may require them to not only fend for themselves but also for their younger ones, in some cases. However, Abebe and Aase (2007) tend to disagree. They argue that the symptomatic perception of orphans rests on stereotyping: most orphans have shown the resilience to get on with the challenges of life following parental death (Abebe and Aase, 2007). Other authors (Kendler et al., 1992) report higher generalized anxiety disorder from children living in parents' separated homes than from orphans.

Chitiyo et al. (2007) suggest that children orphaned by AIDS may be unique orphans. They tend to grieve long before parental death(s) owing to the debilitating AIDS-defining illnesses that may precede death. Due to the moral shame associated with HIV infection (Chitiyo et al., 2007), AIDS-orphaned children may encounter higher stigma/social discrimination than do other orphan categories (Cluver et al., 2008). According to UNAIDS, UNICEF, and USAID (2004, p.11):

> "An especially important and distinctive characteristic of HIV/AIDS in regard to orphaning is that AIDS is more likely than other causes of death to create double orphans. With HIV/AIDS, if one parent is infected there is a higher probability that the other parent is or will become infected and that both will eventually die .... Surveys consistently show that double orphans are more disadvantaged than single orphans".

Subbarao et al. (2001) identify several care options for the mental health need of the African orphan child. Prominent among them is the "normative" fostering practice (Isiugo-Abanihe, 1985) in which parents may allow their children to be reared elsewhere for kinship or economic gains. For children orphaned by AIDS, "crisis" fostering (Goody, 1982) is the typical, in which moral obligations may compel one to take-in children having no parents. Foster children, however, tend to be unfairly treated in food allocation, domestic chores allocation, and school attendance that may adversely affect mental health (Deininger et al., 2003). What is more, in contemporary times, the magnitude of the AIDS-orphaned crisis seems to overstretch the resources of families in sub-Saharan Africa that the collapse of fostering seems imminent (UNICEF, 2003), necessitating the need for a support/alternative care system.

The present study seeks to estimate the effectiveness of being in a natural mentoring relationship to ameliorate mental distress in children orphaned by AIDS. Natural mentorship is different from organizational mentoring (Sipe, 2002) which is common in the workplace. Natural mentoring is provided in homes and communities (DuBois and Silverthorn, 2005) by adult figures (Rhodes et al., 1992), such as the local school teacher, local elders, the church pastor, neighbors, etc, and extended family members who may exert influences on children as surrogate-parents (Beam, Chen, and Greenberger, 2002). Natural mentoring care is also different from fostering care, in which the child tends to emigrate from her biological home to the fosterer's. In natural mentorship such dislocation is not required. The dyad relationship may not be conflict-free, but a range of its psychosocial benefits such as risk behavior control (Beier et al., 2000), personality adjustment (Rhodes, Contreras, and Mangelsdorf, 1994), and social resilience (Zimmerman, Bingenheimer, Notaro, 2002) have been reported, suggesting its usefulness for orphan population.

Method

Procedure

There was a pilot research before the present study. The purpose was to validate the study instruments in the pilot with the selected African countries before using them for the present study. In keeping with the *UN Convention on the Rights of the Child: its relevance for social scientists* (Limber and Flekkoy, 1995), the study protocols satisfied the ethical requirements of confidentiality, anonymity, and voluntary participation. We visited nine community schools, and six NGO child support centers at Mafikeng/Klerksdorp areas (North-West Province, South Africa) and Kampala district (Uganda) to conduct the survey. The UN definition of orphanhood as the loss of one or both parents (UNAIDS, UNICEF, USAID, 2004) is adopted; so the UN definition of a child as persons aged below 18 is used. Local interviewers are Luganda (Uganda) and Setswana/Afrikaans (South Africa) speaking research collaborators. The interviewer-administered questionnaire method is adopted for low education children; otherwise, the self-report method was dominantly used. The interview duration lasts approximately 45 minutes per session at the end of which the child receives a ball pen.

Assigning the Participants

HIV-awareness questions: Have you ever heard about HIV/AIDS (Yes/No)? Do you know that contacting HIV/AIDS can cause death (Yes/No)? *Social questions:* Is your father living (Yes/No)? Is your mother living (Yes/No)? Children who responded "yes" to both questions were grouped as non-orphans (n=290). Those who answered "no", to either were considered orphans. This group was asked what was the reported cause of parental death (1. HIV/AIDS, 2. Others, 3. Don't know)? Children who checked *"1"* and answered "yes" to the HIV-awareness questions, were classified as AIDS-orphaned (n = 373). Those who checked "2" were grouped as other-causes orphaned children. Owing to the shame associated with HIV infection, children may feign ignorance of HIV-related cause of parent's death (Chitiyo et al., 2007; Gillespie et al., 2005). We added to the other-causes orphaned group children who answered "don't know" to the cause of parent's death, if both parents were deceased (UNAIDS et al., 2004). A negligible few children are also assigned to the group utilizing the "verbal autopsy" (Hosegood, Vanneste, Timaeus, 2004) accounts of the community school/child support center heads, as explained elsewhere. Total *other-causes orphaned children* = 289.

Measures

Mental Health Variables

Anxiety. The renowned General Health Questionnaire (GHQ-28) Anxiety Subscale (Goldberg and Hillier, 1979) measured anxiety. The 6-item Scale (alpha = .81) negatively correlated with self-esteem ($r = -.34$, $p < .01$), and positively with depression ($r = .40$, $p < .01$), suggesting its construct validity. Typical items were; I felt nervous all the time; I lost sleep because of worry; I had been getting a fast heart beat.

Depression. The CES-DC (Center for Epidemiological Studies, Depression Scale for Children; Weissman et al. 1980) was used to measure depression. The test-retest reliability and concurrent validity of the CES-DC are adequate (Faulstich et al., 1986). We utilized the first 10 items (somatic complaints: 5 items; negative affects: 3 items; positive affects: 2 items) of the 20-item CES-DC. Sample items on the CES-DC (alpha= 77) included: I was bothered by things that usually don't bother me; I didn't feel like eating, I wasn't very hungry; I wasn't able to feel happy, even when friends tried to make me feel good; I felt like I was too tired to do things.

Social support. The Schwarzer and Schulz (2000) Received Social Support Scale, as adapt, estimated the construct. The measure (alpha=.83), which positively associated with self-esteem ($r = .36$, $p < .01$) and negatively with anxiety ($r = -.38$, $p < .01$) required the respondent to "think about person(s) that is closest to you - your friend(s), guardian(s) or parent(s)/foster parent(s) - how does this person treat you?" Sample responses are: S/he "is there when I need her/him; shows love to me; takes care of my financial needs; in general, I am satisfied with the way s/he treats me."

Self-esteem. Translated into 28 languages in 53 countries (Schmit and Allik, 2005), the Rosenberg (1965) Self-esteem Scale, which evaluates one's positive/negative perceptions of his/her self-worth, is the most utilized measure of self-esteem (Blascovich and Tomaka, 1991). In the present study, the alpha coefficient for the Scale was .60, which favorably compared with the value found by Lorenzo-Hernandez and Ouellette (1998). The measure showed admissible discriminant validity against anxiety ($r = -.34$, $p < .01$), and social discrimination ($r = -.40$, $p < .01$). Typical items are; I have a lot of good qualities; I am satisfied with myself, more-or-less; I think I'm a good guy, on the whole [positive items]; I've nothing about myself to be proud of; I think I'm good at nothing (negative items).

Discrimination. The 1995 Detroit Area Study Measure of Social Discrimination (alpha = .78) had the following question samples: In your daily life, *compared to other people around you,* do you: Feel differently treated? Feel unfairly treated? Made to feel inferior? Prevented from doing things others are allowed to do? People behave as though they are afraid of you? The measure appreciably correlated with depression ($r = .38$, $p < .01$), child abuse ($r = .30$, $p < .01$), and social support ($r = -.25$, $p < .01$).

The *child abuse* measure estimated the physical, verbal, sexual, and labor dimensions of child abuse (Bagley and King, 1990) thus: Are you physically beaten in a manner you consider unfair; verbally abused in a manner you consider unfair; forced to "sleep"with/have sex with anyone; forced against your will to work on the farm for someone? The alpha reliability for the measure, which discriminated depression ($r = .21$, $p < .01$) and social support ($r = -.36$, $p < .01$) was .76.

We utilized the "Care" dimension of the Parker, Tupling, and Brown (1979) Parental Bonding Instrument (PBI) to estimate *parental/foster care.* The Subscale (alpha = .86) measured parental empathy, affection, warmth, and independence. Support for the reliability and validity of the PBI as a measure of actual and perceived parenting has been reported (Neale et al., 1994). Typical items included; parents/foster parents were affectionate to me; understood my problems and worries; let me do things I enjoy doing; enjoyed discussing things with me; gave me as much freedom as I want.

Distress health factors (alpha = .87) was the sum of the child abuse, depression, social discrimination, and anxiety scores. *Positive health factors* (alpha = .86) comprised the parental/foster care, perceived social support, and self-esteem scores. Responses to all items on the study measures were scored from 0 (never) to 3 (always) and reverse scored as appropriate, such that high scores denoted high prevalence of the measured construct.

Natural Mentoring Relationship

In consonance with the operational definition of natural mentoring (Rhodes et al., 1992; Zimmerman et al., 2002), we ask the participants: Other than your parent(s) or foster parent(s) is there any adult person(s) in the neighborhood you go to for support and guidance for most things you do (Yes/No)? If "Yes," how often do you meet this person (0=rarely,

1=sometimes, 2=often, 3=very often)? Children who answer "Yes", and check any of *1—3* meeting frequencies are classified as being in a mentoring relationship. These children (n=714) rate the Ragins' Mentor Role Instrument (MRI) that estimates parental, modeling, counseling, friendship, and support roles by mentors to mentees. Children not in a mentoring relationship form the control group. The 33-item MRI (Ragins and McFarlin, 1990) measure has 11 mentor roles of 3 items each on a 7-point likert response of 1 (strongly disagree) to 7 (strongly agree). We exclude the 6 workplace-related *formal* mentor roles (ie, job sponsorship, coaching, protection, challenge, exposure and socialization), and utilize the 5 *informal* roles (ie, parenting, counseling, modeling, acceptance, and friendship) each of which is estimated with 2 items on a 4-point likert response score of 0 (never) to 3 (always). The internal stability of the adapted MRI is alpha=.91, which is similar to the value found by Ragins and Cotton (1999). The instrument, which shows discriminant validity against anxiety (r = -.158, p<.01) and social support (r = .379, p< .01), has the following sample items: Treats me as a son/daughter (parental role); represents who I want to be (modeling role); guides me to choose the career I want (counseling role); provides me support and encouragement (friendship); acts as a leader to me (acceptance). Expected score range is 0-30, higher scores suggest higher impact of mentorship on the child.

Analysis

The Pearson's measure of association shows admissible discriminant validity of the study measures. The Chronbach alpha shows sufficient reliability. We separated children who report being in mentoring relationships (n=714) from those who do not (n=234) to perform the ANOVA of distress mental health between them in each of the 3 groups (Figure 1). To examine the association of mentoring relationship with distress mental health factors, we ranked scores of the perceived impact of mentoring relationship as *low (scores 0-10), moderate (11-20)*, and *high (21-30)* and examined their performance on mental health in the 3 groups (Table 1). To estimate performance by orphan-types (ie no parents versus single-parents), we performed the ANOVA of having and not having a natural mentor in the two orphan types (Table 2).

Results, Discussion, and Conclusions

Demographic outcome: 373 AIDS-orphaned, 285 other-causes orphaned and 290 non-orphaned children validly participate in the study. The majority (94%) of the children are aged 10 to 17 years. Grand mean age is 13.59 years (SD=2.34). There are no significant difference (F=.259(2), p=.77) of age in the groups: Mean = 13.54 (SD=2.52), 13.55 (SD=2.11), and 13.67 (SD=2.32) for AIDS-, other-causes, and non-orphaned children, respectively. No significant educational level variance (F=1.96(2), p=.14) in the 3 groups is observed. There is no gender influence on mental health outcomes. Male and female children scored similar levels of distress/positive mental health outcomes in the study and control groups.

Mental health outcomes: AIDS-orphaned children in a natural mentoring relationship show significant lower distress mental health factors (child abuse, social discrimination, anxiety, and depression) than did their counterparts not in a mentoring relationship. Similar significant associations are unobserved in the control groups (Figure 1). Also, natural mentoring relationships show inverse relationships to distress mental health: AIDS-orphaned children who score *low* mentoring relationship show significant high distress mental health factors than do *moderate* and *high* mentoring AIDS-orphaned children (Table 1). In the control groups, variances in the relationship are not significant. The association of having a mentor or not with mental health does not vary by orphan types (Table 2). In both orphan types, single-parent and no-parent orphans having a natural mentor have lower distress mental health factors, suggesting the psychosocial usefulness of mentoring to both AIDS- and other-causes induced orphaning.

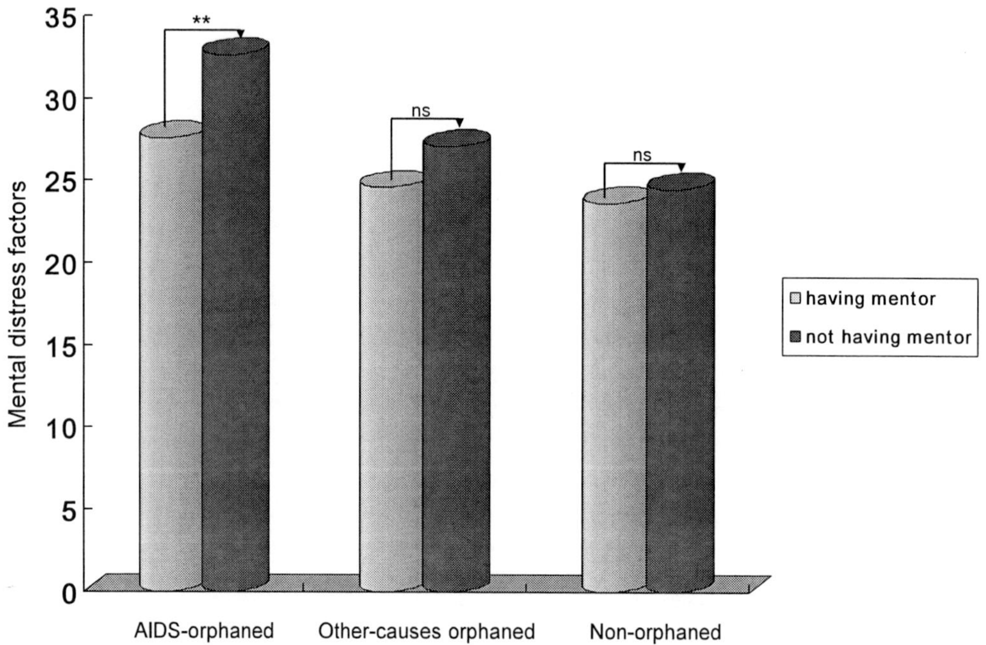

** p <.01, ns=not significant.

Figure 1. ANOVA of having/not having a natural mentor for each of the 3 groups showing significant higher distress mental health factors in AIDS-orphaned children without natural mentors.

Children who receive parental social support (caring, acceptance, and assistance) would show fewer psychosomatic symptoms (Wickrama, Lorenz, and Conger, 1997). For AIDS-orphaned children, who are more likely than other-causes orphaned children to encounter double parental loss (or double loss of parental support), the consequence of orphaning may be graver.

Table 1. ANOVA showing significant inverse asociation of natural mentoring relationship with mental distress in the AIDS-orphaned group

		AIDS-orphaned			Other-causes orphaned			Non-orphaned		
Factors	MR	*n*	*M(SD)*	Posthoc	*n*	*M(SD)*	Posthoc	*n*	*M(SD)*	Posthoc
Child abuse	1	113	3.57(2.95)		98	3.28(3.10)		13	2.23(2.77)	
	2	101	2.91(2.88)		68	2.87(3.05)		54	2.13(2.41)	
	3	157	2.32(2.47)	$1>2^{d}, 1>3^{*}, 2>3^{d}$	117	2.14(2.57)	$1>2^{d}, 1>3^{*}, 2>3^{d}$	141	1.67(2.42)	$1>2^{d}, 1>3^{d}, 2>3^{d}$
Depression	1	113	11.33(5.64)		98	9.59(5.15)		13	7.38(4.15)	
	2	102	10.42(4.21)		69	9.67(4.60)		54	8.48(4.13)	
	3	158	9.93(4.71)	$1>2^{d}, 1>3^{d}, 2>3^{d}$	118	9.80(5.01)	$1<2^{d}, 1<3^{*}, 2<3^{d}$	141	9.76(5.74)	$1<2^{d}, 1<3^{d}, 2<3^{d}$
Social discrimination	1	113	7.01(4.63)		98	5.51(3.79)		13	4.62(4.81)	
	2	101	6.10(3.40)		68	5.57(3.77)		54	4.98(3.35)	
	3	157	5.64(3.65)	$1>2^{d,} 1>3^{*}, 2>3^{d}$	118	4.83(3.85)	$1<2^{d}, 1>3^{d}, 2>3^{d}$	141	6.43(4.84)	$1<2^{d} 1<3^{d}, 2<3^{d}$
Anxiety	1	113	9.15(5.28)		98	6.55(4.50)		13	4.85(3.05)	
	2	101	7.70(4.56)		68	6.69(4.11)		54	6.04(3.25)	
	3	157	6.80(4.31)	$1>2^{d}, 1>3^{*}, 2>3^{d}$	117	5.50(3.77)	$1<2^{d}, 1>3^{d}, 2>3^{d}$	141	5.14(3.79)	$1<2^{d}, 1<3^{d}, 2>3^{d}$
Parental/foster care	1	113	8.37(5.53)		98	11.20(6.66)		13	11.77(5.67)	
	2	101	10.79(5.27)		68	12.00(4.91)		54	11.87(4.51)	
	3	157	13.75(6.03)	$1<2, 1<3^{*}, 2<3^{*}$	118	14.10(5.63)	$1<2^{d}, 1<3^{*}, 2<3^{d}$	141	15.60(5.36)	$1<2^{d}, 1<3^{d}, 1<3^{*}$

Table 1 (Continued)

		AIDS-orphaned			Other-causes orphaned			Non-orphaned		
Self-esteem	1	113	13.93(4.75)		98	15.90(5.18)		13	17.38(4.81)	
	2	102	14.96(4.88)		69	15.50(4.14)		54	16.94(4.56)	
	3	158	16.51(4.58)	$1<2^{d}$, 1<3*, 2<3*	118	17.10(4.57)	$1<2^{d}$, $1<3^{d}$, $2<3^{d}$	141	17.98(4.41)	$1>2^{d}$, $1<3^{d}$, $2<3^{d}$
Social support	1	113	6.08(4.08)		98	8.12(4.53)		13	8.77(3.75)	
	2	101	7.60(3.89)		66	8.98(3.23)		53	8.49(4.01)	
	3	157	9.92(4.24)	1<2*, 1<3*, 2<3*	118	11.00(3.76)	$1<2^{d}$, 1<3*, 2<3*	141	11.45(3.29)	$1>2^{d}$, $1<3^{d}$, 2<3*
Distress mental health	1	113	32.73(13.40)		98	26.40(12.58)		13	21.31(8.77)	
	2	102	28.51(10.20)		69	25.90(11.66)		54	23.13(8.58)	
	3	158	25.96(10.80)	1>2*, 1>3*, 2>3*	118	23.70(11.21)	$1>2^{d}$, $1>3^{d}$, $2>3^{d}$	141	24.23(11.80)	$1<2^{d}$, $1<3^{d}$, $2<3^{d}$
Positive mental health	1	113	32.73(13.40)		98	26.40(12.58)		13	21.31(8.77)	
	2	102	33.16(11.50)		69	35.80(10.17)		54	37.31(10.30)	
	3	158	39.77(11.70)	1<2*, 1<3*, 2<3*	118	42.10(10.26)	$1<2^{d}$, $1<3^{d}$, 2<3*	141	44.78(8.83)	$1>2^{d}$, $1<3^{d}$, 2<3*

[d] not significant, * $p < .05$, MR=ranked mentoring relationship: 1=low, 2=moderate, 3=high.

Table 2. ANOVA showing difference in effects of having and not having a natural mentor on mental health by orphan-types

Orphan-types											
	No parents							Single-parents			
	Having natural mentor		Not having natural mentor			Having natural mentor		Not having natural mentor			
Variables	*n*	*M (SD)*	*n*	M (SD)	*F*	*n*	*M (SD)*	*n*	*M (SD)*		*F*
Child abuse	258	2.76 (2.75)	61	3.57 (3.15)	4.12*	242	2.45(2.65)	100	3.62(3.18)		12.16**
Depression	260	9.99 (4.80)	61	10.59 (6.01)	0.7[d]	244	10.00(4.77)	100	10.86(4.95)		2.23[d]
Social discrimination	258	5.86 (3.55)	61	6.67 (5.04)	2.19[d]	243	5.35(3.93)	100	6.38(3.89)		4.86*
Anxiety	258	7.17 (4.37)	61	8.70 (5.78)	5.29*	242	6.40(4.30)	100	7.66(4.70)		5.75*
Parental/foster care	258	11.87 (6.19)	61	9.67 (6.17)	6.22*	243	12.60(5.59)	100	10.66(6.51)		7.77**
Self-esteem	260	15.50 (4.55)	61	13.89 (4.75)	6.12*	244	16.48(4.78)	100	15.35(5.01)		3.87*
Social support	258	8.53 (4.39)	61	6.85 (4.35)	7.23**	241	9.66(4.06)	100	7.51(4.44)		18.82**
Mental distress factors	260	27.07 (10.92)	61	31.15 (14.91)	5.93*	244	25.60(11.52)	100	30.12(12.64)		10.30*
Positive health factors	260	35.72 (12.27)	61	30.33 (11.45)	9.77**	244	38.38(11.47)	100	33.38(12.33)		12.88**

[d] not significant, *p < .05 **p < .01.

Children orphaned by AIDS, in the present study, show significant higher anxiety, lower self-esteem, lower social support, and lower positive mental health factors than do those in the control groups. Reasons for the situation may be ascribed to double orphaning. Double orphans in this study, whether by AIDS- or other-causes show similar levels of psychological health. Their levels of high child abuse, depression, social discrimination, anxiety, and low foster parental care, self-esteem, social support seem statistically the same, suggesting that they share common psychosocial circumstance. Double-orphaned children in the present study show significantly lower self-esteem, social support, and positive mental health factors than do single-orphaned.

In most domains of the distress mental health construct, having a natural mentor significantly ameliorated distress among the AIDS-orphaned children: natural mentoring relationship inversely associated with distress mental health factors in the group. Children orphaned by AIDS who score *high* impact of mentoring relationships score significant *lower* distress mental health factors than do AIDS-orphans who score *moderate* and *low* mentorship. In the control groups, the variances are weak, suggesting that natural mentoring relationships may be stronger to ameliorate distress mental health factors in AIDS-orphaned children, many of whom have no parents.

Natural mentoring relationships seem more psychosocially beneficial to orphans than to non-orphans. For example, whereas an inverse association of mentoring and distress health is seen in the two orphan groups, the reverse seems the case for non-orphaned children. In this group, high mentoring shows tendencies to elicit high distress mental health factors (Table 1). The reason for the outcome is not clear, although parental censorship of children's mentoring relationship may be likely. In orphans, whether double- or single-orphaned, having a natural mentor show beneficial effects to reduce distress and increase positive mental health factors in them. Age shows an inverse relationship to natural mentorship in all the groups. Younger children significantly engage in higher mentoring relationship than do older children. These younger children significantly regarded their mentors as a father, mother or role model than do older children.

Ideally, natural mentors should be biologically unrelated, non-parent others. But in the traditional African social environment, a thin line may exist between natural mentors and extended family kins. Most of the natural mentors in the present study are extended family kins rather than non-family members. Natural mentorship does not require the mentee to live with the mentor as is the case in fostering. The scenario may mean greater independence for the protégé and lesser social burden for the mentor. Natural mentors have been used to strengthen psychosocial well-being in child-headed households, who are victims of intra-state genocide (Lisanne, Thurman, and Snider, 2005). In children orphaned by AIDS, a natural mentoring relationship seems beneficial to reduce distress mental health factors.

The study method raises some methodology concerns. For example, the design is cross-sectional. Perhaps an anthropological design that participatorily investigates the mentoring behaviors of the mentee and mentor *over a time* may produce a more meaningful result. We are unable to absolutely vouch for the AIDS-orphaned category. Death certificates are unreliable medical data (Cluver et al., 2008) in most AIDS-stigmatizing African countries. Cluver and colleagues review the "verbal autopsy" method validated in several sub-Saharan African studies (Hosegood et al., 2004) to determine the cause of parental death. The method requires the presence of observable AIDS-defining illnesses such as oral candidiasis, Kaposi's sarcoma and the HIV wasting syndrome (WHO, 2005). However, the distinctive characteristic of HIV/AIDS in regard to orphaning is that AIDS is more likely than other causes of death to create double orphans (UNAIDS, 2004). We combined the UN double orphan criterion, the children's self-report, and verbal autopsy reports from the local school/child support center heads to construct the AIDS-orphaned group. The natural mentors in the study are not interviewed. We posit that the omission may not adversely affect the study outcome. If the child rates the social milieu between her and her natural mentor as positive, it seems likely that the natural mentor would positively perceive the social environment in like manner.

References

Abebe, T., and Aase, A. (2007). Children, AIDS and the politics of orphans care in Ethiopia: The extended family revisited. *Social Science and Medicine, 64*: 2058-2069.

ACF/OPRE. (2004a). Administration for children and families, office of planning, research and evaluation. *Who are the children in foster care?* NSCAW Research Brief No. 1.

Antonucci, T.C., and Jackson, J.S. (1990). The role of reciprocity in social support. In B.R. Sarason, I.G. Sarason, and G.R. Pierce (Eds.), *Social support: An interactional view* (pp. 173-189). New York: Wiley.

Bagley, C., and King, K. (1990). *Child sexual abuse: The search for healing*. London: Routledge.

Barlow, D.H. (2002). Unraveling the mysteries of anxiety and its disorders from the perspective of emotion theory. *American Psychologists*, 1247-63.

Baumeister, R., Smart, L., and Boden, J. (1996). Relation of threatened egotism to violence and aggression: The dark side of self-esteem. *Psychological Review, 103*, 5-33.

Beam, M. R., Chen, C., and Greenberger, E. (2002). The nature of adolescents' relationships with their 'very important' non-parental adults. *American Journal of Community Psychology, Vol 32 (2):* 305-325.

Beier, S. R., Rosenfeld, W. D., Spitalny, K. C., Zansky, S. M., and Bontempo, A. N. (2000). The potential role of an adult mentor in influencing high-risk behaviors in adolescents. *Archives of Pediatric Adolescent Medicine, 154*: 327-331.

Blascovich, J., and Tomaka, J. (1991). Measures of self-esteem. In J.P. Robinson, P.R. Shaver, and L.S. Wrightsman (Eds.). *Measures of personality and social psychological attitudes, Volume I.* San Diego, CA: Academic Press.

Bowlby, J. (1988). *A secure base*. New York: Basic Books.

Bradford, E., and Lyddon, W.J. (1993). Current parental attachment: Its relation to perceived psychological distress and relationship satisfaction in college students. *Journal of College Student Development, 34*, 256-260.

Branden, N. (2001). *The psychology of self-esteem: a revolutionary approach to self-understanding that launched a new era in modern psychology*. San Francisco: Jossey-Bass, 2001. ISBN 0787945269.

Brown, S.L., Nesse, R.M., Vinokur, A.D., Smith, D.M. (2003). Providing social support may be more beneficial than receiving it: Results from a prospective study of mortality. *Psychological Science, 14* (4) 320-327.

Childhelp.org. (2010). *Prevention and treatment of child abuse.* Retrieved March 2010 from http://www.childhelp.org.

Childwelfare.gov. (2010). *Child Welfare Information Gateway*. Retrieved March 2010 from http://www.childwelfare.gov/.

CSCV. (2010). *Canadian SOS Children Villages.* Retrieved March 2010 from http://www.soschildrensvillages.ca/Pages/default.aspx.

CAPC. (2010). *Defining Palliative Care.* Retrieved from www.capc.org/building-a-hospital-based-palliative-care-program/case/definingpc/.

Cassel, J. (1976). The contribution of the social environment to host resistance. Journal of epidemiology.

Canetti, L., Bachar, E., Bonne, O., Agid, O., Lerer, B., De-Nour, A. K., and Shalev, A. Y. (2000). The impact of parental death versus separation from parents on the mental health of Israeli adolescents. *Comprehensive Psychiatry, Vol. 41, No. 5*: 360-368.

Chen, C., Greenberger, E., and Farruggia, S. (2003). Beyond parents and peers: the role of important non-parental adults (VIPs) in adolescent development in China and the United States. *Psychology in the Schools, 40* (1), doi: 10.1002/pits.10068.

Cicchetti, D., Toth, S.L., and Lynch, M. (1995). Bowlby's dream comes full circle: The application of attachment theory to risk and psychopathology. *Advances in Clinical Child Psychology*, 17, 1-75.

Chitiyo, M., Changara, D. M., and Chitiyo, G. (2007). Providing psychosocial support to special needs children: A case of orphans and vulnerable children in Zimbabwe. *International Journal of Educational Development* (in press).

Cluver, L. D., Gardner, F., and Operario, D. (2008). Effects of stigma on the mental health of adolescents orphaned by AIDS. *Journal of Adolescent Health*, 42 (4): 410.

Csikszentmihalyi, M. (1997). Flow: the psychology of optimal experience. New York: Harper and Row. Retrieved from http://en.wikipedia.org/wiki/Anxiety

Davis et al. (June 2007). Prenatal exposure to maternal depression and cortisol influences infant temperament. Journal of the American Academy of Child and Adolescent Psychiatry, 46 (6), 737.

DeBellis, M., and Thomas, L. (2003). Biologic findings of post-traumatic stress disorder and child maltreatment. Current Psychiatry Reports, 5, 108-117.

Deininger, K., Garcia, M., and Subbarao, K. (2003). AIDS-induced orphanhood as a systemic shock: magnitude, impact, and program interventions in Africa. *World Development, Vol. 321, No 7*: 1201-1220.

Detroit Area Study (1995). Measure of Discrimination. Retrieved from <http://www.macses.ucsf.edu/Research/Psychosocial/notebook/detroit.html>.

Dube, S.R., Anda, R.F., Felitti, V.J., Chapman, D., Williamson, D.F., and Giles, W.H. (2001). Childhood abuse, household dysfunction and the risk of attempted suicide throughout the life span: Findings from the Adverse Childhood Experiences Study. Journal of the American Medical Association, 286, 3089-3096.

DuBois, D. L. and Silverthorn, N. (2005). Natural mentoring relationships and adolescent health: Evidence from a national study. *American Journal of Public Health, Vol. 95(*3): 518-524.

Dubowitz, H., Papas, M. A., Black, M. M., and Starr, R. H., Jr. (2002). Child neglect: Outcomes in high-risk urban preschoolers. *Pediatrics, 109*, 1100-1107.

Ellis, A. (2001). *Feeling better, getting better, staying better.* Impact Publishers.

Emery, C.F., Huppert, F.A., and Schein, R.L. (1996). Health and personality predictors of psychological functioning in a 7-year longitudinal study. *Personality Individual Differences, 20*, 567-573.

English, D.J., Widom, C.S., and Brandford, C. (2004). Another look at the effects of child abuse. *NIJ Journal*, 251, 23-24.

Faulstich, M. E., Carey, M. P., Ruggiero, L., Enyart, P., and Gresham, F. (1986). Assessment of depression in childhood and adolescence: A evaluation of the Center for Epidemiological Studies Depression Scale for Children (CES-DC). *American Journal of Psychiatry, 143(8)*: 1024-1027.

Fraser, M.W., and Terzian, M.A. (2005). Risk and resilience in child development: principles and strategies of practice. In G.P. Mallon and P.M. Hess (Eds.), *Child welfare for the 21st century: A handbook of practices, policies, and programs* (pp. 55-71). New York, NY: Columbia University Press.

Furukawa, T., Yokouchi, T., Hirai, T., Kitamura, T, and Takahashi, K. (1999). Parental loss in childhood and social support in adulthood among psychiatric patients. *Journal of Psychiatric Research, 33*: 165-169.

Gillespie, S., Norman, A., and Finley, B. (2005). Child vulnerability and HIV/AIDS in sub-Saharan Africa: What We Know and What Can Be Done. Retrieved from <http://www.ifpri.org/publication/child-vulnerability-and-hivaids-sub-saharan-africa>.

Goldberg, D. P., Hillier, V. F. (1979). A scaled version of the General Health Questionnaire. *Psychological Medicine, 9*: 139-145.

Goleman, D. (1987, October). Thriving despite hardship: key childhood traits identified. *The New York Times*, p. C1, 11.

Goody, E. (1982). *Parenthood and social reproduction: Fostering and occupational roles in West Africa*. Cambridge, UK: Cambridge University Press.

Greenberg, J. (2008). Understanding the vital human question for self-esteem. *Perspectives on Psychological Science, 3,* 48-55.

Hosegood, V., Vanneste, A., and Timaeus, I. (2004). Levels and causes of adult mortality in rural South Africa: the impact of AIDS. *AIDS, 5 (18)*: 663-71.

Isiugo-Abanihe, C. U. (1985). Child fosterage in West Africa. *Population and Development Review, 11*: 53-73.

Johnson, R., Rew, L., and Sternglanz, R.W. (2006). The relationship between childhood sexual abuse and sexual health practices of homeless adolescents. *Adolescence, 41* (162), 221-234.

Jou Y.H., and Fukada, H. (1997). Stress and social support in mental and physical health of Chinese students in Japan. Psychological Report, 81, 1303-1312.

Kelley, B.T., Thornberry, T.P., and Smith, C.A. (1997). In the wake of childhood maltreatment. Washington, DC: National Institute of Justice. Retrieved from www.ncjrs.gov/pdffiles1/165257.pdf.

Kendler, K. S., Neale, M. C., Kessler, R. C., Heath, A. C., and Eaves, L. J. (1992). Childhood parental loss and adult psychopathology in women: a twin study perspective. *Archives of General Psychiatry, 49*: 109-116.

Kendler, K.S., Myers, J., and Prescott, C.A. (2005, Feb). Sex differences in the relationship between social support and risk for major depression: a longitudinal study of opposite-sex twin pairs. American *Journal of Psychiatry.* Retrieved March 2010 from http://ajp.psychiatryonline.org/cgi/content/abstract/162/2/250/.

Lazarus, R.S. (1966). *Psychological stress and the coping process*. New York: McGraw-Hill.

Limber, S., and Flekkoy, S. (1995). The UN convention on the rights of the child: Its relevance for social scientists. *Social Policy Report 9 (2)*. Ann Arbor, Michigan: Society for Research in Child Development.

Lisanne, B., Thurman, T. R., and Snider, L. (2005). Strengthening the psychosocial well-being of youth-headed households in Rwanda: Baseline findings from an intervention trial. *Horizons Research Update*. Washington, DC: Population Council.

Lorenzo-Hernandez, J., and Oullette, S. C. (1998). Ethnic identity, self-esteem, and values in Dominicans, Puerto Ricans, and African Americans. *Journal of Applied Social Psychology, 28*: 2007-2024.

MENTOR (2002). National mentoring partnership. Mentoring in America. Alexandria, Va. Retrieved from http://mentoring.web.aol.com/common/one_report/national_ poll_report_ final.pdf.

Maslow, A.H. (1987). *Motivation and Personality* (3rd ed.). New York: Harper and Row.

Mbozi, P. S., Debit, M. B., and Munyati, S. (Eds) (2006). *Psychosocial conditions of orphans and vulnerable children in two Zimbabwean Districts*. HSRC Press, Cape Town, South Africa.

Neale, M. C., Walters, E., Heath, A. C., Kessler, R. C., Perusse, D., Eaves, L. J., Kendler, K. S. (1994). Depression and parental bonding: cause, consequence, or genetic covariance? *Genetic Epidemiology, 11*: 503-522.

NIH. (2010). *Reducing the burden of neurological disease.* Retrieved March 2010 from http://www.ninds.nih.gov/.

Nyblade, L., Pande, R., Mathur, S., MacQuarrie, K., Kidd, R., and Banteyerga, H. (2003). Disentangling HIV and AIDS stigma in Ethiopia, Tanzania, and Zambia. Retrieved from http://www.icrw.org/docs/stigmareport093003.pdf.

O'Connor, Heron, Golding, Beveridge and Glover (June 2002). Maternal antenatal anxiety and children's behavioral/emotional problems at 4 years. British Journal of Psychiatry, 180: 478-9.

Parker, G., Tupling, H., and Brown, L. B. (1979). A parental bonding instrument. *British Journal of Medical Psychology, 52*: 1-10.

Paris, J., Zweig-Frank, H., and Guzder, J. (1994). Risk factors for borderline personality in male outpatients. *Journal of Nervous and Mental Disease, 182*: 375-380.

Preble, E.A. (1990). Impact of HIV/AIDS on African children. Social Science and Medicine, 31 (6), 671-680.

Prevent Child Abuse America. (2001). Total estimated cost of child abuse and neglect in the United States. Retrieved from http://member.preventchildbuase.org/site/DocServer/ cost_analysis.pdf?docID=144/

Prevent Child Abuse New York. (2003). The costs of child abuse and the urgent need for prevention. Retrieved on March 2010 from http://pca-ny.org/pdf/cancost.pdf

Pridmore, P., and Yates, C. (2005). Combating AIDS in South Africa and Mozambique: The role of open, distance, and flexible learning (ODFL). *Comparative Education Review, 49* (4), 490-511. Doi: 10.1086/454371.

Ragins, B. R., and McFarlin, D. (1990). Perception of mentor roles in cross-gender mentoring relationships. *Journal of Vocational Behavior, 37*: 321-339.

Ragins, B. R. and Cotton, J. L. (1999). Mentor functions and outcomes: a comparison of men and women in formal and informal mentoring relationships. *Journal of Applied Psychology, Vol. 84, No.4*: 529-550.

Rahim, M.A., and Psenicka, C. (1996). A structural equation model of stress, locus of control, social support, psychiatric symptoms, and propensity to leave a job. *Journal of Social Psychology, 41,* 171-180.

Reis, H.T., and Patrick, B.C. (1996). Attachment and intimacy: Component Processes. In E. T. Higgins and A. W. Kruglanski (Eds.), *Social Psychology Handbook of Basic Principles* (pp 523-563). New York: The Guilford Press.

Rhodes, J.E. (2002). Stand by Me: The Risks and Rewards of Mentoring Today's Youth. Cambridge, Mass: Harvard University Press.

Rhodes, J. E., Contreras, J. M., and Mangelsdorf, S. C. (1994). Natural mentor relationships among Latina adolescent mothers: psychological adjustment, moderating processes, and the role of early parental acceptance. *American Journal of Community Psychology, 22*: 211-227.

Rhodes, J. E., Ebert, L., and Fischer, K. (1992). Natural mentors: an overlooked resource in the social networks of young, African American mothers. *American Journal of Community Psychology, Vol. 20(4):* 445-460.

Rosenberg, M. (1965). *Society and the Adolescent Self-Image.* Princeton, NJ: Princeton University Press.

Schore, A.N. (2003). Early relational trauma, disorganized attachment, and the development of a predisposition to violence. In M.F. Solomon and D.J. Siegel (Eds.), *Healing trauma: Attachment, mind, body, and brain.* New York, NY: Norton.

Schmitt, D.P., and Allik, J. (2005). Simultaneous administration of the Rosenberg self-esteem scale in 53 nations: Exploring the universal and culture-specific features of global self-esteem. *Journal of Personality and Social Psychology, Vol. 89 (4)*, 623-642.

Schwarzer, R. and Schulz, U. (2000). Berlins Social Support Scales. Retrieved from <http://userpage.fu-berlin.de/~health/soc_e.htm>.

Scroufe, L. A., Carlson, E. A., Levy, A. K., and Egeland, B. (1999). Implications of attachment theory for developmental psychopathology. *Development and Psychopathology, 11*: 1-13.

Selye, H. (1930). History of the stress concept. In Leo Goldberger and Shlomo Breznit Handbook of Stress: Theoretical and Clinical Aspects. Free Press, 1982.

Shaver, P.R., and Hazan, C. (1993). Adult romantic attachment: Theory and evidence. In W.H. Jones and D. Perlman (Eds.), *Advances in personal relationships* (Vol. 4, pp. 29-70). London: Jessica Kingsley.

Sipe, C. L. (2002). Mentoring programs for adolescents: A research summary. *Journal of Adolescent Health, 31*: 251-260.

Springer, K.W., Sheridan, J., Kuo, D., and Carnes, M. (2007). Long-term physical and mental health consequences of childhood physical abuse: Results from a large population-based sample of men and women. *Child Abuse and Neglect, 31*, 517-530.

Subbarao, K., Mattimore, A., and Plangemann, K. (2001). Social protection of Africa's orphans and other vulnerable children: issues and good practice program options. AFR HD working paper.

Sumi, K. (1997). Optimism, social support, stress, and physical and psychological well-being in Japanese women. Psychological Report, 81, 299-306.

Tierney, J.P., Grossman, J.B., Resch, N.L. (1995). Making a difference: An impact study of big brothers/big sisters. Philadelphia: Public/Private Ventures.

Turnbull, A. P., and Turnbull, H. R. (2001). *Families, Professionals, and Exceptionality: Collaborating for Empowerment.* Marrill, Prentice-Hall, Columbus, Upper Saddle River, New Jersey.

Tweed, J. L., Schoenbach, V. J., George, L. K., and Blazer, D. G. (1989). The effects of childhood parental death and divorce on six-month history of anxiety disorders. *British Journal of Psychiatry, 154:* 823-828.

Uchino, B.N., Cacioppo, J.T., and Kiecolt-Glaser, J.K. (1996). The relationship between social support and physiological processes: a review with emphasis on underlying mechanisms and implications for health. *Psychological Bulletin, 119* (3), 488-531.

US Department (2003). US Department of Health and Human Services. National Survey of Child and Adolescent Well-Being: One year in foster care wave 1 data analysis report. Retrieved from www.acf.hhs.gov/programs/opre/abuse_neglect/nscaw/reports/ nscaw_oyfc/oyfc_title.html.

UN Cyberschool. (2010). *Understanding Discrimination. Retrieved August 2010 from* http://cyberschoolbus.un.org/discrim/id_8_ud_print.asp.

UNAIDS. (2009). *AIDS Epidemic Update 2009.* Retrieved from http://www.unaids.org/en/KnowledgeCentre/HIVData/EpiUpdate/EpiUpdArchive/2009/default.asp.

UNAIDS, UNICEF, USAID. (2004). *Children on the Brink 2004. A Joint Report on New Orphan Estimates and a Framework for Action.* UNAIDS, UNICEF, and USAID, 1-42.

UNICEF. (2004). *The framework for the protection, care and support of orphans and vulnerable children: living in a world with HIV and AIDS.* Retrieved on March 2010 from <http://one.wfp.org/food_aid/doc/Framework_English.pdf>.

UNICEF. (2003). *Africa's orphaned generations.* New York: UNICEF.

Watts-English, T., Fortson, B.L., Gibler, N., Hooper, S.R., and De Bellis, M. (2006). The psychobiology of maltreatment in childhood. Journal of Social Sciences, 62 (4), 717-736.

Weissman, N. M., Orvaschel, H., and Padian, N. (1980). Children's symptom and social functioning self-report scales: comparison of mothers' and children's reports. *Journal of Nervous Mental Disorder, 168(12)*: 736-40.

Werner, E.E., and Smith, S. (1982). *Vulnerable but invincible: A study of resilient children.* New York; McGraw-Hill.

Wickrama, K. A. S., Lorenz, F. O., and Conger, R. D. (1997). Parental support and adolescent physical health status: A latent growth curve analysis. *Journal of Health and Social Behavior, 38:* 149-163.

WHO. (2005). *World Health Organization/Euro Report of the Technical Consultation on Clinical Staging of HIV/AIDS and HIV/AIDS Case Definitions for Surveillance.* Copenhagen.

Zald, D.H., Pardo, J.V. (1997). Emotion, olfaction, and the human amygdala: amygdale activation during aversive olfactory stimulation. Proc National Academy of Science (USA), 94 (8): 4119-24.

Zald, D.H., Hagen, M.C., and Pardo, J.V. (Feb 2002). Neural correlates of tasting concentrated quinine and sugar solutions. Journal of Neurophysiology, 87 (2): 1068-75.

Zimmerman, M. A., Bingenheimer, J. B., and Notaro, P. C. (2002). Natural mentors and adolescent resiliency: A study with urban youth. *American Journal of Community Psychology, 30*: 221-243.

In: Palliative and Nursing Home Care
Editor: Samuel E. Plunkett

ISBN 978-1-61122-417-7

Chapter 3

Quality of Sexual Life of Nursing Home Residents

André Dupras*
Department of sexology, Université du Québec à Montréal,
BO 8888, Downtown Station, Montreal (Quebec) Canada H3C 3P8

Abstract

The goal of this review article is to discuss the meanings and the functions of sexuality of older adults living in nursing homes and to increase awareness of staff and family members to these issues. Although nursing homes are increasingly recognized as provider of sexual health services, there is evidence that a majority of residents do not receive the services.

The article tackles the subject of the sexual well-being of nursing home residents by proposing theoretic and practical tools in order to guide professional interventions. Sexology may contributes to enhance quality of sexual life by helping nursing homes to ensure the physical, psychological and social well-being of their residents with regards to sexuality. They can achieve this goal by integrating sexual rights in the cultural change movement of nursing homes.

The sexual modernization of nursing homes is described first by specifying the project's purpose with the presentation of the historical and social context, second by observing the present situation with a description of the attitudes and behaviors of residents and staff, third by choosing strategies for change such as *setting a general goal that must be clarified in a sexuality policy and a staff training program, preserving sexual identity of residents entering institution, and finally establishing a research structure. It is concluded that listening to sexual needs of residents is necessary for the enhancement of their quality of sexual life.*

* E-mail: dupras.andre@uqam.ca

Introduction

At first glance, taking interest in the sexual lives of nursing home residents may seems surprising and may causes discomfort. People residing in nursing homes are affected both physically and mentally, resulting in a deterioration of their sex lives. Social imaginary suggests that nursing home residents do not care to live anymore and wish to prepare themselves for death. They become disinterested in sexuality for they are looking for tranquility and detachment. The exercise of sexuality strikes fear because it is perceived as dangerous for individuals as well as for the institution (Dupras and Poissant, 1987). Sexuality would trouble the peaceful lifestyle sought out by residents. In light of this, it is not surprising that some nursing homes do not consider the quality of the sexual lives of residents to be a priority. Added to these obstacles is the general lack of privacy in nursing homes as well as the poorly trained staff with regards to meeting the residents' sexual needs.

The fact remains however that residents are still alive, although they may be sick and fragile. And like all living creatures, they are sexual beings with desires and sexual pleasures that help them hold on to life and maintain mental stability. They continue to be people who have sexual needs on the psychological, physical and social levels. Their physical condition doesn't encourage them to intensely live out their sexual needs because of a lack of vitality, but this doesn't mean the end of their sexual life. The exercise of sexuality does not only have negative repercussions that should be minimized, but also has positive effects for their physical and mental health. Nursing home staff thus have the duty to take care of the sexual well-being of the people under their care.

But what can be done to improve the quality of the sexual lives of residents? How can their needs be grasped? What goals should be set? What means should be used? What professional abilities should be possessed? How can sexual autonomy be developed in residents who are progressively more and more dependant? How can interventions be individualized in the context of collective environment where personnel is cruelly lacking? The question of the sexual lives of the elderly is linked to the idea of complexity advocated in gerontology and sexology (Dupras and Ribes, 2008). It requires a global approach of sexual life, as well as consideration of its multiple components. Ultimately, it is important to reflect on the place of sexuality in the lives of the elderly in nursing homes. In order to fuel this reflection, we must refer to observations reported in scientific literature. The objective of this paper is thus to draw information from scientific writings in order to better comprehend the sexual life of residents, as well as conceive appropriate interventions.

The sexogerontology model is based on the view that aging is another stage of sexual life and older people's sexuality is still developing. A cultural change is necessary to transform nursing homes from restrictive institutions to permissive communities regarding sexuality. The focus of this culture change is to reinvent the nursing home so that the deterioration of the sexual identity after admission is replaced by the improvement in quality of sexual life (QOSL). Managing change in organization requires four steps: specifying the project's purpose, observing the present situation, choosing strategies for change and evaluating the results of their implementation (Cummings, 2008). This text will adopt this pattern starting with the presentation of the historical and social context in which the change can be located and defined, followed by a description of the attitudes and behaviors of residents and staff in the interest of assessing the current situation, and finally end with the selection of the most appropriate ways of realizing a favorable transformations for the betterment of the residents' quality of sexual life.

Historical and Social Context

In the context of social transformations, it is essential to remember how nursing homes' gerontology field came to be historically. Engaging oneself in an act for change requires knowing in which context sits the organization of nursing homes in the United-States. It is important to decipher the evolutions at work in this area of activity in order to graft innovations to it, aiming for the improvement of residents' sexual well-being.

Toward Quality of Life

Special homes for the elderly were established in the beginning of the nineteenth century (Haber, 2002). Before that, old people who needed shelter were placed in an almshouse. New asylums for the aged were created in order to give appropriate care for the elderly. The access to special homes was limited, since fees were required which caused a rising proportion of elderly in almshouses. Old people became the majority of residents in public almshouses, where they could not find happiness and experienced degradation. The Social Security Act (1935) was proposed to avoid indigence for the aged who had taken refuge in poorhouses. But the majority of residents of almshouses required nursing and medical attention. Trained nurses were invited to provide care for the unfortunate people who lived there (Zinn, 1999). The 1965 federal legislation that created Medicare and Medical stimulated the growth of nursing homes, but the industry's rapid expansion did not equate into the advancement of adequate services. In 1971, government regulation began to control the quality of long-term care. Another legislation in 1987 (ORBA) introduced changes in nursing home organizations in favor residents' rights and their quality of life. In the 1990s, a culture change was proposed to focus on resident-centered care, a homelike environment, staff/resident relationships, staff empowerment, nursing home leaderships and quality improvement (Doty *et al.*, 2008).

In recent decades, there has been the recognition that the primary outcome of care and services provided by long-term facilities should be quality of life oriented for its residents. In 1986, the Institute of Medicine Report on Quality of Care in Nursing Homes, and subsequent legislative reforms in 1987, placed high priority on quality of life (QOL). A variety of theoretical models describe the QOL in long-term care settings. Bennett (1980) defined long-term care quality of life in terms of satisfaction of basic human needs: physiological, safety and security, social, self-esteem, and accomplishment. More recently, Kane *et al.* (2003) identified the following domains of long-term care QOL: emotional health, physical health, functional status, comfort and security, social function, and self-worth or personal agency. Sexuality and its expression contribute significantly to a person's quality of life. Robinson and Molzahn (2007) found that satisfaction with personal relationships, followed by health status and sexual activity, explained older adults' rating of their quality of life. The authors invited gerontological nurses to discuss sexuality with older adults. In this context, the improvement of residents' sexual well-being can be conceptualized using the QOL perspective.

Toward the Sexualization of the Elderly

For a long time in our western societies, the elderly were considered as asexual beings (Gott, 2005). Among our conceptions of sexuality, someone is sexual if his/her sexual behaviors have the potential to result in reproduction: older people don't give life; they are at the end of life. Someone is sexual if his/her physical appearance causes sexual attraction: older people's physical changes cause more repulsion than attraction. Someone is sexual if their physical and psychological conditions permit them to be motivated by sexuality and to achieve orgasm: older people are in a process of physical and mental decline that introduces a loss of interest in sexuality and difficulties reaching orgasm. Someone is sexual if he/she has a sexual intelligence that permits the development of a good understanding of their sexual self and a clear idea about his/her motives for engaging in sexual activity (Conrad and Milburn, 2001): older people can have cognitive impairments that involve misunderstanding sexuality. These thoughts exclude the elderly from having normal sex lives. During the last forty years, studies challenged sexual myths and prejudices regarding the asexuality of aging individuals. In her annoted bibliography, Walker (1997) compiled 457 references concerning the sexuality of the elderly. In his preface of this document, Palmore, the author of the Duke Longitudinal Studies on Aging (1981), stated that « It has become more and more evident that most elders are not asexual, but have sexual interests just as other ages do, even though various sexual problems may develop in later years. There is also evidence that many of these problems may be prevented and/or ameliorated with better understanding, counseling, and medical care » (p. x). If, previously, the expression of sexuality by older people was a sign of morbidity, it is now, in contrast, considered a sign of good health.

In the past, nursing homes adopted the values and religious beliefs of a society that did not permit sexual activity outside the context of marriage and procreation. Because of society's sexual myths and stereotypes, the elderly residing in institutions had little freedom of expression of their sexuality and could have be considered as « sexually oppressed » (Gochros, 1972). Sexuality was a taboo in institutions for the elderly: they were forbidden to practice it or even talk about it. Residents who faulted in this regard were looked down upon and punished. Up until recently, it was possible to note that in numerous nursing homes, sexual behavior was seen as problematic and was often restricted (Brown, 1989). Consequently, Kane (2003) decided to omit sexual functioning as a factor of QOL since many nursing homes prohibited the expression of sexuality among their residents.

Meanwhile, we are witnessing a sociocultural shift in attitudes towards the sexuality of the elderly living in nursing homes. Research on staff attitudes with regards to the sexual expression of the elderly in nursing homes began in the second half of the 1970s (Kass, 1978 ; La Torre and Kear, 1977 ; Wasow and Loeb, 1975). This interest in the sexuality of nursing home residents was conceded within a desire to understand the affect of nursing implication on human sexuality in the early 1970s (Watherhouse, 1996). The modernization of nursing homes manifested itself by introducing heterosexual living spaces which improved residents' behavior, self-care and satisfaction (Silverstone and Wynter, 1975). More and more publications approach the question of nursing home residents' sexual lives. A systematic literary search of material pertaining to sexuality in adult long-term care facilities made possible a review of 214 documents by a group of guideline developers (Wright, 2008). Many documents invited staff and nursing home managers « to work together towards developing a home environment that is supportive of residents' sexuality rights and permits sexual expression, and a culture where all people concerned are comfortable with sexuality issues » (Roach, 2004, p. 379). This change in the culture and philosophy of nursing homes brings new attention to residents' rights to sexual expression. The movement to humanize nursing homes includes the recognition of geriatric sexuality.

State of the Situation

The second step in a process of change is to make observations in order to make a diagnosis of the causes and consequences of the problematic situation that we want to change. To clarify the situation, an inventory of data from various studies on the sex lives of residents and on barriers to the expression of sexuality in nursing homes will be presented.

Residents' Sexual Lives

But what is it we are referring to? How can our subject of interest be described? It is necessary to define sexuality not only to determine its characteristics, but also to provide a frame of reference. First of all, several meanings are assigned to sexuality. For some people, sexuality is limited to genitalia and sex corresponds to penetrative intercourse for the purpose of reproduction. For others, however, everything is sexual and sex is everywhere. If the first definition is too narrow, the second is too broad. Thus, it is important to define more accurately our field of study. Secondly, the definition of sexuality refers to concepts, representations, and ideas on its organization and actualization in different expressions. This vision reflects the philosophical, scientific, and sociocultural affiliations of an author, allowing him to define his point of view. Our way of thinking about sexuality falls under a sexological perspective that studies the multiple components of sexual life in an interdisciplinary approach (Dupras, 2010).

In our view, the concept of sexual life seems most appropriate to define the object of study of sexology. The choice of this concept is both strategic and scientific. The word "life" allows to put forward the positive nature of sexuality, because it evokes the idea of something good and desirable. This optimistic connotation of the concept of life counterbalances the pessimistic view of sexuality that has intensified with the spread of AIDS (Johnson, 2000). Let us add that the concept of "life" evokes a set of components used to define sexuality (Walker, 2006). Human life is (a) a complex system involving various systems, notably biological, psychological and sociological; (b) a structure incorporating a set of elements forming a whole; (c) an evolving process that grows and changes over the years; (d) a project to carry out from a projection of oneself in a desired future. Sexual life can be conceived as an essential human characteristic that includes a complex set of components and evolves from birth to death by performing procreational and recreational functions. Sexual life includes biological factors (such as hormones and genitals), psychological factors (such as desires and fantasies), spiritual factors (such as beliefs and values), and social factors (such as norms and roles). These multiple factors are in constant interaction and form a whole which is expressed as a personal sexual identity.

Many older adults have an active sexual life (Lindau *et al.*, 2007). Aging leads to losses, but sexual needs persist as long as life continues. These needs are answered in different ways: looking nice; getting dressed up and feeling pampered; spending time with the opposite sex; talking « dirty »; enjoying sexually stimulating material; masturbating; kissing; cuddling with a partner in bed; intercourse with a long-time partner or a sex worker (Nay, 2004). In their literature scan, McAuliffe *et al.* (2007) found that barriers to sexual expression in older adults can be physiological (such as illness or sexual dysfunction), psychological (such as negative attitudes or body image disturbances) or sociological (such as loss of a partner or lack of privacy).

A conceptual apparatus is necessary to acknowledge the full range and complexity of human sexual expression and its particular determinants in nursing home residents. The ecological systems theory can be helpful in examining residents' sexual life (Bronfenbrenner, 1979). This theory states that an individual's thoughts and actions can be described accurately in reference to the microsystem and macrosystem of the person's environment. Therefore, the sexual development of elderly individuals living in nursing homes can be explained by incorporating the interactions within individuals, between other individuals, and between the social structures of society. The microsystem includes sexual attitudes and activities, whereas the macrosystem includes the organizational culture of nursing homes that might influence the expression of sexuality.

The social image of older people as asexual beings fuels the prejudice that they necessarily adopt a negative view of sexuality. However, studies report that older residents have positive attitudes towards sexuality and are more open about the subject than expected (Aizenberg *et al.*, 2002; Walker et Ephross, 1999; Wasow and Loeb, 1975). These data confirm the role played by values and social norms in the construction of the perception of sexuality. Some elderly residents were born and lived out their youth in an era of sexual conservatism (D'Emilio et Freedman, 1988) and some of them retain the more restrictive attitudes that were in force in their young age towards specific sexual behaviors such as masturbation and sex outside marriage (Story, 1989). However, they have also been influenced by the more liberal ideas that were prevalent in American society during the 1960s and thereafter. Residents in nursing homes can be cleaved into three distinct attitudinal clusters: traditional (guiding by religious belief), relational (guiding by romantic values), and recreational (guiding by sex for pleasure) (Laumann *et al.*, 1994). It is important to study and work on the sexual attitudes of residents, because they influence their sexual behavior. The research undertaken by White (1982) indicates that sexual activity in the institutionalized age is linked to their attitudes and behavior toward sexuality and also to their sexual interest level and prior frequency of sexual activity. Some nursing homes have already held sex education sessions for users in order to clarify their sexual attitudes (Guarino et Knowlton, 1980; Tunstull et Henry, 1996).

Interest for sexuality can be seen as a continuum, ranging from hyposexuality to hypersexuality, where some residents show little interest in sexuality. In fact, popular belief conveys the idea that the elderly manifest a natural disinterest with regard to sexuality that accompanies aging. Studies contradict this myth by reporting that older residents maintain an interest in sexuality (Mulligan et Palguta, 1991; Wasow et Loeb, 1975). However, this interest in sex does not always translate into actions and practices. Older people living in nursing homes are less sexually active than their community peers (Spector and Fremeth, 1996). Among obstacles to sexual expression, Hajjar and Kamel (2003), as well as Parker (2006), identified the following barriers to sexual activity for nursing home residents: physical changes and limitations, illnesses and adverse effects of medications, erectile dysfunction in men, dyspareunia in women, feeling of being unattractive, lack of willing and able partner, lack of partner, attitudes of staff and family members, design of care home and lack of privacy. Added to this, residents often prefer expressing their interest in sexuality in non sexual interactions, such as physical attractiveness and flirtation (Hubbard *et al.*, 2003). Ehrenfeld *et al.* (1999) have defined three types of sexual behaviors among institutionalized elderly patients: loving/caring, romance, and eroticism. Furthermore, it is well known that the gender of residents has a crucial influence on the sexual behavior. Gendered expression of sexuality continues to apply in later life: sexual expression is more often reported by men than by women (Ward *et al.*, 2005; White, 1982).

Residents' sexual behaviors can be classified into two general categories: acceptable and unacceptable. This classification is not universal but depends on personal and cultural values. For some caregivers, acceptable sexual behaviors are limited to hugging and kissing on the cheek (Szasz, 1983). Unacceptable behaviors may be sex talk (such as using foul language), sexual acts (such as touching or grabbing, exposing genitalia), and implied sexual behavior (such as openly reading pornographic magazines). Inappropriate sexual behavior is often observed among inhibited cognitively impaired residents (De Medeiros *et al.*, 2008; Nagaratnam and Gayagay, 2002). Sexual misbehavior is often investigated and behavioral management or medication may be used to stop or modify the inappropriate behavior (Harris et Wier, 1998; Kettl, 2008). Inappropriate sexual behavior has legal and ethical outcomes, especially when a resident does not have the competency to consent to a sexual activity (Kamel and Hajjar, 2003). The resident may not only be the author of inappropriate sexual behavior, but can also be the victim. Ramsey-Klawsnik *et al.* (2008) reported cases of sexual perpetrators abusing elderly individuals residing in care facilities.

For some people, homosexual behavior is inappropriate in nursing homes. Residents and caregivers may adopt a « heteronormative » discourses that disapproves of homosexual behavior. Lesbian and gay residents may experience homophobia from caregivers and other residents (Hubbard *et al.*, 2003). Homosexual transgression can provoke a punishing response, including discharge from a home. For these reasons, non-heterosexual residents may decide to veil their sexuality, therefore homosexual populations within residential care are largely invisible (Harrison, 2001). The marginalization of lesbians and gay residents can compromise their quality of care and consequently their quality of life (Cohen *et al.*, 2008).

Before ending this section, it is important to mention that the sexuality of residents in nursing homes is socially constructed by the culture in which it evolves. Cultural scripts guide what is considered to be appropriate sexual behavior within the nursing home (Simon and Gagnon, 2003). Cultural norms of sexual behavior are applied in sexual scripts that reflect the sexual lifestyles adopted by residents in order to meet their sexual needs. Added to this is the fact that sexual behavior is also influenced by intrapsychic scripts that represent images about the sexual self, fantasies, and expectations of residents. Staff perceptions and reactions regarding the sexual behavior of residents also contribute to the construction of their sexual life.

Staff Perceptions and Reactions

Long-term geriatric nursing must respond appropriately to the significant needs of elderly residents in order to promote quality of care. Identifying these needs is crucial to their quality of life. If, for nurses, providing skilled physical care is considered a primary need, for residents, the most significant need is access to mental and emotional support (Natan, 2008). Clinical staff members often view nursing home residents more as patients than as people, focusing primarily on their medical needs rather than their emotional and relational needs. Cahill and Diaz (2010) reported that « nursing home staff and interactions with staff were also identified as a key factors that positively influence the quality of life of interviewed resident » (p. 4). Nursing home residents expect their need for adequate communication to be fulfilled (Santo-Novak, 1997). In conversations with caregivers, do residents have the opportunity to talk about sexuality? At first glance, it seems that they rarely address the topic of sexuality with health professionals. Aizenberg *et al.* (2002) confirm this observation by reporting that few elderly residents were interviewed about sexuality by a doctor.

Very often professionals don't want to intervene regarding the expression of sexuality of residents. Ehrenfeld *et al.* (1999) found that most of the sexual interactions recorded were between residents, rather than towards staff members. Their reaction can be explained by the theory of planned behavior (Ajzen, 1991). This theory postulates that intention to perform a given behavior are function of (a) attitudes toward the behavior that refer to beliefs about the outcomes associated with performing a particular behavior, (b) subjective norms that refer to perceptions about how others would judge a person for performing the behavior, (c) perceived control which refers to self-assessment of both the capability or skill and the opportunity to perform the behavior. To illustrate this theory, a practitioner may hesitate in beginning a discussion about sexuality with a resident because the elderly are often perceived as conservative with regards to their view about sexuality: the practitioner might misunderstand the resident's point of view and may offend him or her (Gott *et al.*, 2004). Furthermore, staff members may be concerned that other colleagues might disapprove and blame them for being too sympathetic to the sexual needs of residents (Archibald, 2002). Finally, staff members are usually ill-equipped to cope with sexual relationships between residents, especially among practitioners of a younger age or that have less than five years of experience working with older people, because they often have more negative and restrictive attitudes towards later life sexuality (Bouman *et al.*, 2007). The theory of planned behavior provides not only a model to predict the reactions of professionals towards the expression of sexuality of residents but also to organize continuing education in nursing homes. Casper (2007) found that significantly more mental health practitioners in the theory-guided class than in the standard class had applied a tool for the assessment of needs by the three-month follow-up. However, the theory of planned behavior is based on cognitive processing and overlooks emotion variables. Moreover, members of nursing home staff have fears and negative feeling when residents express sexuality. Experiencing feelings of discomfort with sexuality issues may induce restrictive and controlling practices among nursing home staff (Roach, 2004). It is thus important for them to develop their emotional intelligence skills by managing their own emotions and helping residents manage theirs as well. Considering the emotions produced by sexual situations, it is suggested that caregivers' education should address emotional intelligence skills. A workshop may be helpful in recognizing and responding to caregivers' and residents' emotional manifestations (Ruckdeschel and Van Haitsma, 2004).

Despite the taboo to talk about it, staff might gossip about residents sexual behavior (Archibald, 2002 ; Bauer, 1999 ; Ward *et al.*, 2005). A privileged way to talk about sexuality is to spread rumors. Faced with difficulties in understanding the sexuality of residents and in speaking about it in an articulated fashion, it is tempting to fall back on this. Caregivers recount sexual situations they heard about, and the stories spread within the facility. These stories will probably continue to circulate because they offer the opportunity to talk about sexuality, to express concerns and aspirations, values and normative frameworks (DiFonzo and Bordia, 2007). Furthermore, the chatter is used to control the expression of sexuality, as residents may fear being ridiculed by staff members. Therefore, residents may not trust the nursing staff when speaking with them about their sexual needs. If they distrust their caregivers, they may be not confident that they will help them to fulfill their need for sexual wellbeing.

Some caregivers are willing to talk seriously about sex with residents; however, they rarely take the initiative to start conversations on the topic. They wait for residents to address the issue themselves and this approach seems to appeal to residents as well. In the study lead by Walker and Ephross (1999), elderly respondents were divided on the initiative taken by caregivers to want to talk about sexuality with residents. Many wanted the process to be initiated by residents themselves. Like many family environments, initiatives come from residents (children) and caregivers (parents) are ready to listen to them and make a decision. This way of beginning a conversation about sexuality has the advantage of being sure not to disturb the resident. However, there are also disadvantages, including the fact that a resident may hesitate to speak because of feeling too embarrassed to begin the conversation or because he or she do not know how. It also happens that the residents have already heard too much to speak: what's done is done, whether it had a positive or a negative effect.

Staff attitudes towards the sexual expression of elderly individuals may have a significant impact on the beliefs and behaviors of residents. In their literature review, Bouman *et al.* (2006) report both restrictive and permissive attitudes of care staff regarding sexuality in older residents, with a tendency towards some positive changes occurring more recently. Among factors predictive of negative attitudes, they mentioned strong religious beliefs and past negative interactions with residents; positive attitudes were predicted by higher educational levels and socio-economic background, as well as having more work experience. In addition to individual variables, socio-cultural factors influence attitudes. Therefore, social attitudes regarding the expression of sexuality in nursing homes may be different among countries. Roach (2004) found that Swedish nursing homes adopt a more accepting attitudes towards the sexual behaviors of residents than homes in Australia. This should also be the case in American nursing homes. In fact, Weinberg *et al.* (2000) found that sexual attitudes are more permissive in Sweden comparatively to the United States because of several reasons, notably: (a) a lower level of religiosity, (b) a more widespread naturalistic conception of sexuality, and (c) a more private-autonomous non-regulatory view of sexuality that is reflected in legal and social policy. Finally, it should also be mentioned that a seminar named Sexual Attitude Reassessment (SAR) can promote participants' awareness of their attitudes related to sexuality and understanding on how these attitudes influence their personal and professional lives (Sitron and Dyson, 2009).

More often than not, practitioners see residents' sexual expression as a problem (Ward *et al.*, 2005). In fact, its expression constitutes a situation that prevents the normal course of business activities. Caregivers can be thrown off when accomplishing their roles and daily tasks and, from there follows a search for a solution to overcome this disrupting barrier to the normal functioning of health services. The upside to this perception is that it is likely to raise questions, reflections and discussions. In this sense, an opportunity arises to develop ideas and practices by putting in place strategies that could improve the quality of sexual life of residents.

Strategies to Enhance Quality of Sexual Life

The third step of a process of change consists in choosing the way to carry out the project. What strong elements should nursing homes rely on in order to pursue their evolutions towards support focused on increasing the sexual well-being of residents? It seems that five strategies that combine reflection and action must be undertaken. First, we must set a general goal that will guide accompanying modes of sexual life by professionals. Following this, the goal must be clarified in a sexuality policy that includes the guidelines of the establishment concerning the expression of sexuality, sexual life conditions, and operating processes of services aiming the sexual well-being of residents. Implementing the sexual policy includes preserving sexual identity of residents entering institution and staff training in order to develop their skills when accompanying the sexual lives of residents. Finally, it is necessary to establish a research structure so as to instrument and professionalize caregivers.

Defining a Sexological Goal

Many professionals deal with sexuality in their clinical practice. Every mental health worker aims to achieve specific goals that fit their disciplinary expertise and professional practice. It is therefore important to find the common goal that links and unifies them. Depending on the context and state of the situation as described earlier, the general and ultimate purpose of the interventions on residents' sexuality should be the quality of sexual life, which is defined as follows: the perception of a person to live a state of sexual well-being expressed through the adoption of an individual and relational lifestyle that will satisfy his or her sexual needs on the physical, mental and social levels, in a fulfilling manner. This goal adopts a global view of sexuality and is inspired by the holistic biopsychosocial intervention model. It takes into account all aspects of sexual well-being which are interdependent and constantly interacting.

Caregivers' response to biosexual needs can take many forms. Physicians may proactively address the sexual health of residents by questioning on sexual infection and dysfunction (Nusbaum and Hamilton, 2002). An occupational therapist can facilitate sexual activity, such as finding sexual positions appropriate to their physical condition and obtain technical aids (Sakellariou and Simo Algado, 2006). Residents may experience body image disturbance. They are likely to refuse to look at, touch or show the affected body parts for fear of feeling different or of being rejected. Body image can impact sexuality: poor body image is related to a reduction in sexual desire and sexual activity (Koch *et al.*, 2005). Residents can work out their problems by participating in different therapies: "Physical therapy, occupational therapy, speech therapy, pharmacy, and other departments may get involved in the case of individuals who have experienced significant changes in body function. Nurses spend the most time with the individuals and are aware of the total effect of various therapies. Nurses should coordinate these activities in the care plan to insure that all groups are working toward the same goals" (Wold, 2004, p. 154).

On the psychosocial level, quality of sexual life manifests itself by a feeling of appreciation towards sexuality, of being able to satisfy ones sexual needs, of being a good sexual partner and of considering one's self as a man or a woman. These components of psychosexual well-being may be altered by emotional problems. The prevalence of depression in the nursing home population is very high (Jongenelis *et al.*, 2004). Functional limitations, negative life events, loneliness and lack of social support are risk indicators for depression. It is known that depression has a profound negative impact on sexuality, especially decreased sexual desire (Balon, 2007). Psychiatric nurses, psychologists and social workers can help residents overcome their mental health problems and better appreciate sexuality. Most of the time, a clinical intervention is not necessary to enhance the quality of sexual life. In this sense, everyday actions can contribute to sexual self-esteem: listening to demands and meeting sexual needs, seeking advice and obtaining agreement regarding interventions that can affect sex life, taking interest in romantic feelings and sexual desires towards another resident, approving and commending an affectionate gesture towards a spouse.

The nursing home should be a place of life conductive to the fulfillment of residents' sociosexual needs. Therefore, social activities should allow residents to network, develop close relationships, even form couples (Hubbard *et al.*, 2003). The cultural and structural context of the nursing home must frame the social interaction in a way that residents may express sexuality. Management must recognize the sexual rights of residents. It must educate residents, staff and families in order for them to develop a positive vision of sexuality. For example, the Center on Aging of Kansas State University designed a training program for caregivers and another for families (Jankowiak and Doll, 2008a,b). Caregivers must acknowledge residents' needs and rights to privacy in order to express and fulfill their sexual desires (Bauer, 1999). They need to provide them with space and opportunities for sexual intimacy, the must respect residents' intimacy, by knocking on the door and waiting for an answer before entering a room. Nursing home inspectors should verify if installations have been made to ensure sexual intimacy (Dessel, 2010).

Developing a Sexuality Policy

In their professional practice, caregivers sometimes find themselves in situations where residents engage in sexual activities. The expression of sexuality bothers them and raises unease. They do not always know how to react. A framework helps to guide interventions, to give them meaning and consistency. For the leaders of an establishment, it is important to develop a policy so as to define the principles and guidelines that promote a consensus on how to intervene with respect to the expression of sexuality among residents. The policy gathers the orientations of the establishment concerning the expression of sexuality, the conditions of sexual life, and the operating processes of the services aiming the sexual wellbeing of the residents. It is a basis for attitudes and behaviors of caregivers.

Some establishments have sought to enshrine the sexual rights of residents in an institutional policy on sexuality. In 1995, The Hebrew Home for the aged at Riverdale, New York, devised a set of policies and procedures which served as a reference for dealing with sexual expression at the Home (Holmes, 1995). In 1997, Shalom Village Nursing Home in Hamilton, Ontario, followed suit by drawing up guideline on sexuality as well. Two years later, Providence Centre in Scarborough, Ontario, announces that it has executed a similar project (Doyle *et al.*, 1999). Facilities may decide to develop an intimacy and sexuality practice guideline drawing on a document already prepared by another institution. For example, the guidelines of Shalom Village served as a template for Lanark, Leeds and Grenville Long-Term Care Liaison Network, Ontario (Steele, 2007).

Because they may not have the resources and expertise to do so, many facilities need practical guidance to develop their own fully articulated written policies, procedures, and guidelines to support sexual expression for adults living in long-term residence. A group of professionals in Hamilton, Ontario, have developed a responsive and effective policy regarding sexuality and dementia (Schindel Martin, 2002). The Center for Practical Bioethics (Reeder, 2006) have written a document that provides practical guidance to help long-term care facilities address their residents' needs and desires for intimate relationships and sexual activities. This document provides working definitions, principles of ethics, conceptual frameworks, procedurals considerations and methodology. The Vancouver Coastal Health Authority (Breen *et al.*, 2009) suggests eight guidelines : supporting freedom and autonomy of sexual expression, determining sexual consent capability, intervening to reduce risk of harm, providing sexual health information and assistance with sexual expression, informing clients and their family of sexual activity policies, providing clients' rights for privacy and protection of confidentiality, providing procedures and addressing concerns regarding sexual expression, as well as training staff for sexual health care.

Sometimes, the policy remains a statement of intent for a long period without being put into effect in everyday life. Discourse and statements of principle are often ahead of practice. Ideas may take time to translate into concrete actions. It is essential to create conditions favoring an implementation project that engages and empowers all concerned around common goals. The qualitative change aiming the sexual well-being of residents is not decreed in a policy: it is realized through the work of a team of professionals who have the desire to shape and share its expertise.

Training for Staff

Accompanying the sex lives of residents requires the execution of complex and delicate tasks. To help residents improve their quality of sexual life, caregivers need to develop personal and professional skills through training. Caregiver must prepare for their guidance role by working on themselves, which will help them to exorcise their fears, and examine their ideas, attitudes, and values with regards to sexuality, as well as reflect on their own sexuality. Furthermore, they must also acquire theoretical knowledge on sexuality, as well as be familiar with practical and effective interventions. Finally, caregivers must be able to work in teams in order to engage in collective projects for the sexual emancipation of residents.

Some general training programs can be used to develop these skills. For example, Annon's (1976) *PLISSIT* model is often used to organize sexological interventions. This model requires knowing and applying the four stages of sexological action: *P*ermission, *L*imited *I*nformation, *S*pecific *S*uggestions and *I*ntensive *T*herapy.

The *BETTER* model was developed by Mick *et al.* (2004) to assist health care providers to include sexuality assessment in the care of patients with cancer. The six levels of intervention involves bringing up the topic (*B*), explaining (*E*) that sexuality is part of quality of life, telling (*T*) the patient that appropriate resources will be found to address their concerns, and that while the timing (*T*) may not be appropriate now, they can ask for information later, educating (*E*) the patients about the sexual side effects of their treatment, and finally, recording (*R*) in the patient chart that this topic has been discussed.

Furthermore, it is also possible to have recourse to specific training programs. In this sense, Mayers and McBride (1998) have developed a training program pertaining to the sexuality of geriatric residents for caretakers and administrators in a long term facility. This training is focused on: attitudes toward sexuality and the elderly; terminology and communication; residents' rights and abilities to make decisions about their sexuality; information sharing and handouts. Steinke (1997) have experimented with an educational intervention whose aim was the following learning objectives: explore attitudes about the sexuality of aging individuals; identify the components of a sexual health assessment; describe physiological, sociocultural, and psychological variables that influence sexuality in aging; identify approaches for dealing with sexual issues in nursing facilities; describe strategies for helping older adults maintain sexual wellness in light of chronic diseases and medication. Authors found that the educational intervention increased nursing facility staff knowledge about sexuality in aging. For their part, Walker *et al.* (1998) have constructed a curriculum pertaining to elder adult sexuality in nursing facilities to be used by staff members. This curriculum focuses on three areas: increasing knowledge about the sexuality of elders; encouraging a more positive, tolerant outlook toward elderly sexuality; and educating staff about appropriate responses toward elderly sexuality. This training program appears to bring about positive changes in knowledge and attitudes surrounding sexuality and aging (Walker et Harrington, 2002). Finally, Menzel (2005) reported a significant difference in attitudes toward geriatric sexuality after staff training in a nursing home setting.

However, we must ask ourselves: do trainees *apply* the skills they gain while learning to do their jobs? It is known that professional training programs in gerontology have problems when it comes to transferring knowledge into practice (Aylward *et al.*, 2003). Individual factors affect skill and knowledge transfer: motivation, goal orientation and perception of self-efficacy. Contextual factors contribute also to this transfer, such as supervision, team meetings and peer support (Baldwin and Ford, 1988). If we discount the actual effects of training in practice, it is important to articulate training with the situations encountered on the field. Ehrenfeld *et al.* (1997) therefore decided to work with nursing home staff by using case studies in order to help them in selecting ways of coping with sexual relationships among elderly patients suffering from dementia. In the same vein, a training-action model was tested with a group of health workers by proposing to examine their professional practices to better identify ways to improve and resolve their shared problems (Dupras and Rousseau, 2007). Action training of staff has four major steps as instrumental objectives: identify and describe problem situations; analyze and explain problematic sexual behaviors; inventory and choose sexological intervention strategies; experiment these strategies and observe the results. This formative approach allows a close link between theory and practice in the sense of applying the acquired knowledge and understanding the chosen interventions. It also allows the reunification of caregivers around common goals. The training should enable interdisciplinary team work, thus facilitating the inclusion of medical, psychological, social and spiritual aspects of the sexual lives of residents.

During training, we must introduce the idea of complexity in sexological interventions. For many people, sexuality is simplified by reducing it to genitalia. When faced with the sexual behavior of residents, it is tempting to seek a quick and easy reassuring answer. For example, a male resident of 75 years of age requests the services of a sexual escort. The establishment manager rejects his request and threatens to expel him if he insists. For the sake of efficiency, a sexual problem is simplified, decomposed and isolated. The desire to tame and control the expression of sexuality of residents often leads to a reductive and disjunctive reading of a problematic situation. Working to improve the quality of the sexual life of residents requires taking into account several individual and collective components of sexuality. To find a solution that takes into account the multiple dimensions of a sexual problem, we must complicate the situation. It is a matter of connecting the elements while focusing on the interactions in order to try to understand the multidimensionality of sexuality and to develop an integrated intervention. To take the example cited previously, it is essential to adopt multiple approaches, notably legal, clinical, ethical and political, to resolve the problem of the escort in a nursing home (Dionne and Dupras, 2008). In facilities where significant changes were noticed, a willingness to work together was found, as well as environmental modifications, respect for sexual rights and freedoms, development of sexual life projects, improvement of the quality of sexual life and implementation of a training plan. An example is the approach undertaken by The Hebrew Home for the Aged at Riverdale, as described in a paper by Reingold and Burros (2004). Under the leadership of their Executive Vice President, the Hebrew Home conducted a survey with their staff, created a formal policy, developed a staff education program, modified the physical environment and implemented a family orientation service. Training sessions with staff focused on the policy concerning sexual expression first and then case studies were discussed. The Hebrew Home also developed a video to be used for staff training. In summary, this establishment has managed to develop a comprehensive strategy to change attitudes and practices related to the sexuality of residents.

Facilitating the transfer of new learning is not just trainers and trainees responsabilitity but also organizations. For Stolee *et al.* (2005), management support was identified as the most important factor impacting the effectiveness of continuing education in long term care. Other factors included resources (staff, funding, space) and the need for ongoing expert support. Management and organizational support is central to the development of a nursing home that fosters innovation and change in the area of sexuality. According to Ross *et al.* (2002), relationship between staff training and quality of care is mediated by the quality of the organization. In this prospect, nursing homes that provide adequate sexological care have to pay attention to staff motivation, to develop adequate planning, to make available many resources to implement new programs, to value lower-level care providers, to improve staff cohesion, and to focus staff on better models of care.

Preserving Sexual Identity

The entry of the elderly person in a nursing home is marked by breaches with the environment. Pace of life, habits, usual reference points are overturned. There exists an important risk of identity loss, thus it is of importance to recognize the person in their identity. As early as the arrival in the establishment, members of the personnel make an effort to get to know the life story, family situation, life style of their new residents. Following this, they must tune in to their desires and interests in order to help them articulate a life project within the institution. Personal and collective organized activities serve to meet their needs, develop self-esteem, and put them in contact with what makes sense to them. These moments of discussion have the merit of considering the resident as a desiring subject rather than an object of care.

Entry in the institution potentially jeopardizes the stability and continuity of the sexual identity· The notion of sexual identity usually refers to the feeling of belonging to the male or female sex. Separation from the spouse can disturb sexual identity and entering the institution often forces one to re-arrange marital roles. This is why some establishments allow couples to spend the night with each other in order to perpetuate an emotional presence, which insures a marital sense of belonging, self definition as a spouse, as well as maintaining sexual identity through dialogue and exchanges with their partner. Maintaining marital habits supports sexual identity. Consequently, it is necessary to reduce the gap between the couple's prior life and life in the institution in order to facilitate consistency with habits by using intimate accommodations and objects which place the elderly person in a familiar arrangement. Admittance to the institution underlines the importance of the marital relationship in the construction of the personal and sexual identity. In their life narratives, the elderly describe their past sources of reassurance, fixe their identities and define themselves as married or widowed by articulating past and present identities.

The institution can be a legitimate actor in helping with the reconstruction of sexual identity. Discussing sexuality with members of the medical staff and with other residents may help in perceiving themselves as sexuated beings and in developing sexual self-esteem. Identity continuity is facilitated when one can maintain an affective and sexual life. Knowledge of the sexual lives of the residents gives the health care professional the opportunity to recognize the residents in their identity, to talk about their past sexual experience and of their current aspirations. We must put into place a process of accompaniment as soon as the realization is made that sexual desire is legitimate and compatible with available means. This accompaniment is often necessary because the resident has been through a great deal of losses and fears of finding him or herself risking failure if he or she tries to satisfy sexual needs. Furthermore, the shortening of life expectation will cause hesitation with regards to pursuing a sexual life project, not knowing if he or she will have time to realize it before death. At the institutional level, it is essential that animation activities favor appearance of sexual interest and expression of sexual roles.

In order to illustrate this, we should mention an initiative undertaken in a nursing home that had the goal of enhancing the sexual identities of residents (Citron and Levy Kartman, 1982). On Fathers's Day, an activity director invited six Belly Dancers which resulted in awakening the sexual interest of residents: « The writers noticed more flirting and many men commenting about the opposite sex in a way they had not talked for many years » (p. 58). This activity demonstrates that residents are still alive and have indeed sexual desires. For example, two residents, Mrs. A and Mr. B, practically never leave their room anymore, but they frequently discuss their passion for classical music. One caregiver offers them to meet in order to listen to music together. These two residents share a common interest that opens the door to exchange and communication. It is important to propose activities oriented towards identity continuity, development of bonds with peers, and sexual resocialisation of relationships. We must offer residents a chance to renew sexuated and sexual relationships similar to those they had prior to entering the institution in order for them to continue to feel like men or women. Aged care institutions should address the question of intimacy and sexuality in their information documents, available for current and prospective residents and their families. Bauer *et al.* (2009) reported that, among participating establishments, sixty-four percent of facilities in Australia indicated that they had no information available on the topic.

We mustn't forget that nursing homes can limit the identity expression of older gay, lesbian, bisexual and transgendered individuals (GLBT). Some residents may be insulted and isolated because of their sexual orientation. Administration, care staff, and residents of nursing homes themselves are all potential sources of discrimination. Aged care providers and workers need to construct relatively safe environments that enable older GLBT to disclose and express their sexual identity (Hughes, 2004). A survey sample of older GLBT adults in large metropolitan areas indicated a strong desire for the development of GLBT-exclusive or GLBT-friendly retirement care facilities (Johnson *et al.*, 2005). In 2008, Europe's first gay nursing home opened in Berlin (GenerationQ, 2008).

Conducting Research

Training programs are putting more and more emphasis on the acquisition of practical knowledge, as caregivers are often not interested in the appropriation of theoretical knowledge. To develop their skills, they want useful knowledge that enables them to solve the problematic situations they encounter in their daily work. The lack of theoretical knowledge is compensated by intuition and improvisation. The preferential use of empirical knowledge has the potential risk of being guided by emotional reactions, personal values and popular belief (Commons *et al.*, 1992). Although a large amount of professional work requires the use of practical knowledge, the fact remains that health workers must make choices as a team and unify their efforts. They must adopt a systematic, rigorous approach to obtain valid observational and evaluation data as well as analyze and theorize them. It thus becomes essential to engage in a process that is both scientific and empirical in order to articulate theoretical and practical knowledge.

This vision of sexology research in nursing homes encourages us to privilege the production of knowledge about the sex lives of residents without ignoring other matters discussed in this essay. The life history technique is a tool for gathering information to better understand the needs and aspirations of residents in matters of sexuality. The autobiographical narrative can put into words the resident's personal history in relation to attitudes, interests, past and present sexual experiences, and how sexual identity is built (Rosenfeld, 2009). This research practice invites to resist the temptation of essentially considering the sexuality of residents like unambiguous and unchanging structures. Rather, it allows to better understand the sexual life of residents in their uniqueness, built and modifiable according to their biological, psychological and social evolution. Caregivers can engage in a support mode of residents by considering them like subjects who want to maintain an emotional and sexual life, whatever their level of physical and mental deterioration. Residents remain actors of their sex life by clarifying and expressing their interests and wishes. Knowledge of sexual life history of residents allows us to recognize them in their identity, to explore what might make sense for them in their sexual desires and support their efforts to achieve them.

Significant change in nursing homes will occur if caregivers modify their attitudes and behaviors towards sexuality in a context of self-managed work teams and cross-training. A way to empower the staff is to conduct a Participary Action Research (PAR). A PAR is an approach that invites caregivers to work together to identify problems in clinical practice and to generate solutions to improve practice. Staff members discuss potentially difficult sexual issues and set priorities for actions. In a PAR conducted by Osborne *et al.* (2002), it was found that the approach "produced practical and useful resources, such as a sexual health policy contextualized for the particular setting, guidelines and helpsheets, and client behavior profile proformas for documentation of a psychosocial profile" (p. ix). These actions can help resolve the conflict between protecting residents from the negative effects of expressing sexuality and respecting their right to express themselves sexually (Ehrenfeld *et al.*, 1997; Tabak and Shemesh-Kigli, 2006).

The present literature review has allowed the tabulation of a certain number of studies which in turn allowed the current situation to be gauged and future orientations to be guided. Additional research is needed in all areas of sexuality considered in the present paper. Some research problems need to be expanded while others need to be initiated. In QOSL perspectives, instruments must be developed and validated for the assessment of sexual needs. If steps have been made toward culture changes in nursing homes so that quality of sexual life can be improved, research is necessary to proceed to formal testing of residents' QOSL, in order to assess if it has been affected.

Conclusion

Gerontology has participated in a humanizing movement in nursing homes by inviting them to listen to the needs of their residents and by individualizing services. Elderly care facilities are trying to create an environment that allows residents to lead a life akin to the one they had home. This new institutional culture recognizes the sexual rights of residents. Rather than being an environment where the death of sexuality is favored, the nursing home should privilege its pursuit by offering support and a way of living that are suitable for its expression. The nursing home is an environment where people live and grow old, which implies sacrifice, suffering and nostalgia. These losses are made up by adjustment and the taking on of new roles. Residents do not have to abandon their sexual lives at the entrance door of the establishment. Training of the health care personnel can help in identity reconstruction as well as in the refitting of sexual life styles. Life in the institution requires that they reformulate their identity and their needs, and that they adjust the course of their sex lives, without having to end it. The nursing home has the duty of respecting the diversity with which sexuality is lived out in the lives of residents. We mustn't wait for tragic consequences to prompt furthering our reflection and action on this subject. Too often, professionals demonstrate interest in this issue following unfortunate incidents. This reactive attitude has the inconvenient consequence of favoring correction instead of prevention and feeds into the bias that the expression of sexuality is necessarily problematic when residents are concerned. A proactive attitude allows the establishment of a positive approach that promotes quality of sexual life for residents.

The idea of sexuality in nursing homes is progressively becoming more acceptable. Since the beginning of the 1990s, there has been a steady increase in the publication of articles and commentaries in which authors discuss the necessity to respect and support the sexual needs of the elderly residing in nursing homes and other care facilities. However, much work is still needed in these establishments in order to make them into true living quarters where the sexual rights of residents are recognized. Changing of the institutional culture of nursing homes with regards to sexuality must rely on the evolution of representations and mentalities, which requires investing time, money, and energy. Cultural development is no longer limited to statements of intent and improvement policies related to the quality of sexual life, but now requires providing effective means of engaging in real and concrete change. If this new culture is simple to understand, it remains nonetheless difficult to implement and requires time. Each and every establishment must take into account its history, organization, hosted individuals, environment, obstacles to change, and available resources. The slow changes in certain establishments should not discourage the most confident, but should be used to ensure the quality of a deep-rooted change. This will allow the nursing homes to no longer be viewed as death row, but as a warm place to live where sexuality continues to develop and exist for the greater well-being of residents.

In any case, it will be difficult for caregivers in nursing homes to ignore the sexuality of residents in the near future. Two key factors will produce a sociocultural shift: a new cohort of resident, and the medicalization of sexuality (Gott, 2006). The baby-boomer generation will come to reside in nursing homes and their sexual attitudes and practices are more liberal than the previous generations. They may demand that the nursing home accommodate their sexual needs. Furthermore, medical treatments such as Viagra can help them to pursue their sexual activities in old age.

Finally, this text does not pretend to have approached all the subjects relating to sexuality in nursing homes, for they are too numerous to be condensed in a single article. However, this review has hopefully provided some useful insight into the current practice of residential aged care to enhance the quality of sexual life of their residents.

References

Aizenberg, D., Weizman, A., and Barak, Y. (2002). Attitudes toward sexuality among nursing home residents. *Sexuality and Disability*, 20 (3), 185-189.

Ajzen, I. (1991). The theory of planned behavior. *Organizational Behavior and Human Decision Processes*, 50 (2), 179–211.

Annon, J. S. (1976). The PLISSIT model : A proposed conceptual scheme for the behavioral treatment of sexual problems. *Journal of Sex Education and Therapy*, 2 (2), 1-15.

Archibald, C. (2002). Sexuality and dementia in residential care—whose responsibility? *Sexual and Relationship Therapy*, 17 (3), 301-309.

Aylward, S., Stolee, P., Keat, N., and Johncox, V. (2003). Effectiveness of continuing education in long-term care : a literature review. *Gerontologist*, 43 (2), 259-271.

Balon, R. (2007). Depression, antidepressants, and human sexuality. *Primary Psychiatry*, 14 (2), 42-50.

Baldwin, T. T., and Ford, J. K. (1988). Transfer of training : A review and directions for future research. *Personnel Psychology*, 41 (1), 63-105.

Bauer, M. (1999). Global aging : their only privacy is between their sheets : Privacy and the sexuality of elderly nursing home residents. *Journal of Gerontological Nursing*, 25 (8), 37-41.

Bauer, M., Nay, R., and McAuliffe, L. (2009). Catering to love, sex and intimacy in residential aged care : What information is provided to consumers? *Sexuality and Disability*, 27 (1), 3-9.

Bennett, C. (1980). *Nursing home life: What it is and what it could be*. New York, NY: Tiresias Press.

Bouman, W. P., Arcelus, J., and Benbow, S. M. (2006). Nottingham study of sexuality and ageing (NoASSA I). Attitudes regarding sexuality and older people : A review of the literature. *Sexual and Relationship Therapy*, 21 (2), 149-161.

Bouman, W. P., Arcelus, J., and Benbow, S. M. (2007). Nottingham study of sexuality and ageing (NoSSA II). Attitudes of care staff regarding sexuality and residents : A study in residential and nursing homes. *Sexual and Relationship Therapy*, 22 (1), 45-61.

Breen, S., Carlson, M., Clements, G., Everett, B., and Young, J. (2009). *Supporting sexual health and intimacy in care facilities : Guidelines for supporting adults living in long-term care facilites and group homes in British Columbia, Canada*. Vancouver, BC: Vancouver Coastal Health Authority.

Bronfenbrenner, U. (1979). *The Ecology of Human Development: Experiments by Nature and Design*. Cambridge, MA : Harvard University Press.

Brown, L. (1989). Is there sexual freedom for our aging populations in long-term care institutions? *Journal of Gerontological Social Work*, 13 (3/4), 75-90.

Cahill, S., and Diaz, A. (2010). *Living in a nursing home. Quality of life : The priorities of older people with a cognitive impairment*. Dublin, Ireland : Trinity College Dublin, School of Social Work and Social policy, Living with Dementia program.

Casper, E. S. (2007). The theory of planned behavior applied to continuing education for mental health professionals. *Psychiatric Services*, 58 (10), 1324-1329.

Citron, H., and Levy Kartman, L. (1982). Preserving sexual identity in the institutionalized aged through activities. *Activities, Adaptation and Aging*, 3 (1), 55- 63.

Cohen, H. L., Curry, L. C., Jenkins, D., Walker, C. A., and Hogstel, M. O. (2008). Older lesbians and gay men: Long-term care issues. *Annals of Long-Term Care*, 16 (2), 33-38.

Commons, M. L., Bohn, J. T., Godon, L. T., Hauser, M. J., and Gutheil, T. G. (1992). Professionals' attitudes towards sex between institutionalized patients. *American Journal of Psychotherapy*, 46 (4), 571-580.

Conrad, S. D., and Milburn, M. A. (2001). *Sexual intelligence*. New York, NY: Random House.

Cummings, T .G. (2008). *Handbook of organization development*. Los Angeles, CA: Sage Publications.

D'Emilio, J., and Freedman, E. B. (1988). *Intimate matters : A history of sexuality in America*. New York, NY: Harper and Row.

De Medeiros, K., Rosenberg, P. B., Baker, A. S., and Onyike, C. U. (2008). Improper sexual behaviors in elders with dementia living in residential care. *Dementia and Geriatric Cognitive Disorders*, 26 (4), 370-377.

Dessel, R. (2010), director of Memory Care Services at the Hebrew Home for the Aged at Riverdale (NY). Personal communication when visiting the Home in avril 2010.

DiFonzo, N., and Bordia, P. (2007). *Rumor psychology : Social and organizational approaches*. Washington, DC: American Psychological Association.

Dionne, H., Dupras, A. (2008). Sexological opinion : A reflection and action tool for care staff of nursing homes. *Sexologies*, 17 (3), 127-134.

Doty, M. M., Koren, M. J., and Sturla, E. L. (2008). *Culture change in nursing homes : How far have we come ? Finding form The Commonwealth Fund 2007 National Survey of Nursing Homes*. Vol. 91. New York (NY) : The Commonwealth Fund.

Doyle, D., Bisson, D., Janes, N., Lynch, H., and Martin, C. (1999). Human sexuality in long-term care. *The Canadian Nurse*, 95 (1), 26-29.

Dupras, A. (2010). The future of sexology. *Sexologies*, 19 (2), 69-73.

Dupras, A., and Poissant, M.-S. (1987). The fear of sexuality in residents of a long-term care hospital. *Sexuality and Disability*, 8 (4), 203-215.

Dupras, A., and Ribes, G. (2008). Sexual gerontology. *Sexologies*, 17 (3), 124-126.

Dupras, A., and Rousseau, P. (2007). A training-action program in sexual education. *Sexologies*, 16 (2), 102-111.

Ehrenfeld, M., Tabak, N., Bronner, G., and Bergman, R. (1997). Ethical dilemmas concerning sexuality ol elderly patients suffering from dementia. *International Journal of Nursing Practice*, 3 (4), 255-259.

Ehrenfeld, M., Bronner, G., Tabak, N., Alpert, R., and Bergman, R. (1999). Sexuality among institutionalized elderly patients with dementia. *Nursing Ethics*, 6 (2), 144-149.

GenerationQ (2008). Europe's First Gay Nursing Home Opens. http://www.generationq.net/news/GLBT/europe-first-gay-nursing-home-1818.shtml. Consulted July 13th 2010.

Gochros, H. L. (1972). The sexually oppressed. *Social Work*, 17 (2), 16-23.

Gott, M. (2005). *Sexuality, sexual health and aging*. Buckingham, UK: Open University Press.

Gott, M. (2006). Sexual health and the new ageing. *Age and Ageing*, 35 (2), 106-107.

Gott, M., Hinchliff, S., and Galena, E. (2004). General practitioner attitudes to discussing sexual health issues with older people. *Social Science and Medecine*, 58 (11), 2093-2103.

Guarino, S. C., and Knowlton, C. N. (1980). Planning and implementing a group health program on sexuality for the elderly. *Journal of Gerontological Nursing*, 6 (10), 600-603.

Haber, C. (2002). « Nursing Homes: History », *Encyclopedia of Aging*. <http://www.encyclopedia.com>. Consulted July 13th 2010.

Hajjar, R. R., and Kamel, H. K. (2003). Sexuality in the nursing home, Part 1 : Attitudes and barriers to sexual expression. *Journal of the American Medical Directors Association*, 4 (3), 152-156.

Harris, L., and Wier, M. (1998). Inappropriate sexual behavior in dementia : A review of the treatment literature. *Sexuality and Disability*, 16 (3), 205-217.

Harrison, J. (2001). 'Its none of my business'. Gay and lesbian invisibility in aged care. *Australian Occupational Therapy Journal*, 48 (3), 142-145.

Holmes, D. (Chair) (1995). *Policies and procedures concerning sexual expression*. Riverdale, NY: The Hebrew Home for the Aged at Riverdale.

Hubbard, G., Tester, S., and Downs, M. G. (2003). Meaningful social interactions between older people in institutional care settings. *Ageing and Society*, 23 (1), 99-114.

Hughes, M. (2004). Privacy, sexual identity and aged care. *Australian Journal of Social Issues,* 39 (4), 381-392.

Institute of Medicine. (1986). *Improving the quality of care in nursing homes*. Washington, DC: National Academy Press.

Jankowiak, M.; Doll, G. (2008a). *A guide for families of long-term care residents. Addressing residents' sexual needs in long-term care*. Manhattan, KS: Kansas State University, Center on Aging.

Jankowiak, M.; Doll, G. (2008b). *Pioneering change. Sexuality in nursing home. Education module to promote excellent alternatives in Kansas nursing homes*. Manhattan, KS: Kansas State University, Center on Aging.

Jongenelis, K., Pot, A. M., Eisses, A. M. H., Beekman, A. T. F., Kluiter, H., and Ribbe, M.W. (2004). Prevalence and risk indicators of depression in elderly nursing home patients : the AGED study. *Journal of Affective Disorders*, 83 (2/3) 135-142.

Johnson, B. (2000). *Positive thinking : A sex positive approach to HIV/AIDS education*. Ottawa. CAN : Planned Parenthood Federation of Canada.

Johnson, M. J., Jackson, N. C., Arnette, J. K., and Koffman, S. D. (2005). Gay and lesbian perceptions of discrimination in retirement care facilities. *Journal of Homosexuality*, 49 (2), 83-102.

Kamel, H. K., Hajjar, R. R. (2003). Sexuality in the nursing home, Part 2 : Managing abnormal behavior – legal and ethical issues. *Journal of the American Medical Directors Association*, 4 (4), 203-206.

Kane, R. A. (2003). Definition, measurement, and correlates of quality of life in nursing homes : Toward a reasonable practice, research, and policy agenda. *The Gerontologist*, 43, Special issue II, 28-36.

Kane, R. A., Kling, K. C., Bershadsky, B., Kane, R. L., Giles, K., Degenholtz, H. B., Liu, J., and Cutler, J. (2003). Quality of life measures for nursing home residents. *Journal of Gerontology: Medical Sciences*, 58A (3), 240–248.

Kass, M. J. (1978). Sexual expression of the elderly in nursing homes. *The Gerontologist*, 18 (4), 372-378.

Kettl, P. (2008). Inappropriate sexual behavior in long-term care. *Annals of Long-Term Care*, 16 (12), 29-35.

Koch, P. B., Mansfield, P. K., Thurau, D., and Carey, M. (2005). "Feeling Frumpy": The relationships between body image and sexual response changes in midlife women. *The Journal of Sex Research,* 42 (3), 215-223.

La Torre, R. , and Kear, K. (1977). Attitudes toward sex in the aged. *Archives of Sexual Behavior*, 6 (3), 203-213.

Laumann, E. O., Gagnon, J. H., Michael, R. T., and Michaels, S. (1994). *The social organization of sexuality. Sexual practices in the United States*. Chicago, IL: The University of Chicago Press.

Lindau, S. T., Schumm, L. P., Laumann, E. O., Levinson, W., O'Muircheataigh, C. A., and Waite, L. J. (2007). A study of sexuality and health among older adults in United States. *New England Journal of Medicine*, 357 (8), 762-774.

Mayers, K. S., and McBride, D. (1998). Sexuality training for caretakers of geriatric residents in long term care facilities. *Sexuality and Disability*, 16 (3), 227-236.

McAuliffe, L., Bauer, M., and Nay, R. (2007). Barriers to the expression of sexuality in the older person : the role to the health professional. *International Journal of Older People Nursing*, 2 (1), 69-75.

Menzel, J. C. (2005). The impact of staff training in a nursing home setting on knowledge of and attitudes toward sexuality in the elderly. *Dissertation Abstracts International : Section B. The Sciences and Engineering*, 65 (12-B), 6664.

Mick, J., Hughes, M., and Cohen. M. Z. (2004). Using the BETTER model to assess sexuality. *Clinical Journal of Oncology Nursing,* 8 (1), 84-86.

Mulligan, T., and Palguta, R. F. (1991). Sexual interest, activity and satisfaction among male nursing home residents. *Archives of Sexual Behavior*, 20 (2), 199-204.

Nagaratnam, N., and Gayagay, G. (2002). Hypersexuality in nursing care facilities : A descriptive study. *Archives of Gerontology and Geriatrics*, 35 (3), 195-203.

Natan, M. B. (2008). Perceptions of nurses, families, and residents in nursing homes concerning residents' needs. *International Journal of Nursing Practice*, 14 (3), 195-199.

Nay, R. (2004). « Sexuality and older people ». In R. Nay, R.; and S. Garratt (Eds): *Nursing Older People : Issues and innovations* (p. 276-288). Sydney, Australia : Churchill Livingstone.

Nusbaum, M. R. H., and Hamilton, C. D. (2002). The proactive sexual health history. *American Family Physician*, 66 (9), 1705-1713.

Osborne, D., Barrett, C., Hetzel, C., Nankervis, J., and Smith, R. (2002). *The wellness project : Promoting older peoples' sexual health*. Melbourne, Australia: The National Ageing Research Institute (NARI), Melbourne Extended Care and Rehabilitation Service (MECERS).

Palmore, E. (1981). *Social patterns in normal aging : Findings from the Duke Longitudinal Study*. Durham, NC: Duke University Press.

Parker, S. (2006). What barriers to sexual expression are experiences by older people in 24-hour care facilities. *Reviews in Clinical Gerontology*, 16 (4), 275-279.

Ramsey-Klawsnik, H., Teaster, P. B., Mendiondo, M. S., Marcum, J. L., and Abner, E. L. (2008). Sexual predators who target elders: findings from the first national study of sexual abuse in care facilities. *Journal of Elder Abuse and Neglect*, 20 (4), 353-376.

Reeder, R. (Ed.) (2006). *Considerations regarding the needs of long-term care residents for intimate relationships and sexual activity*. Kansas City, MO: Center for Practical Bioethics.

Reingold, D., and Burros, N. (2004). Sexuality in the nursing home. *Journal of Gerontological Social Work*, 43 (2/3), 175-186.

Roach, S. M. (2004). Sexual behaviour of nursing home residents : staff perceptions and responses. *Journal of Advance Nursing*, 48 (4), 371-379.

Robinson, J. G., and Molzahn, A. E. (2007). Sexuality and quality of life . *Journal of Gerontological Nursing*, 33 (3), 19-27.

Rosenfeld, D. (2009). From same-sex desire to homosexual identity : History, biography, and the production of the sexual self in lesbian and gay elders' narratives. In P. L.Hammack, and B. J. Cohler (Eds.): *The story of sexual identity : Narrative perspectives on the gay and lesbian life course* (p. 425-450). New York, NY: Oxford University Press.

Ross, M. M., Carswell, A., and Dalziel, W. B. (2002). Quality of workplace environments in long-term care facilities. *Geriatrics Today : Journal of the Canadian Geriatrics Society*, 5 (1), 29–33.

Ruckdeschel, K., and Van Haitsma, K. (2004). A workshop for nursing home staff : Recognizing and responding to their own and resident's emotions. *Gerontology and Geriatric Education*, 24 (3), 39-51.

Sakellariou, D., and Simo Algado, S. (2006). Sexuality and occupational therapy : exploring the link. *British Journal of Occuptional Therapy*, 69 (8), 350-356.

Santo-Novak, D. A. (1997). Older adults' descriptions of their role expectations of nursing. *Journal of Gerontology Nursing*, 23 (1), 32-40.

Schindel Martin, L. (Ed.) (2002). Intimacy, sexuality and sexual behaviour in dementia. How to develop practice guidelines and policy for long term care facilities. www.fhs.mcmaster.ca/mcah/cgec/toolkit.pdf. Consulted July 13th 2010.

Shalom Village (1997). *Intimacy and sexuality practice guidelines*. Hamilton, ONT.

Silverstone, B., and Wynter, L. (1975). The effect of introducing a heterosexual living space. *The Gerontologist*, 15 (1), 83-87.

Simon, W., and Gagnon, J. H. (2003). Sexual scripts : Origins, influences and changes. *Qualitative Sociology*, 26 (4), 491-497.

Sitron, J. A., and Dyson, D. A. (2009). « Sexuality attitudes reassessment (SAR) : Historical and new considerations for measuring its effectiveness », *American Journal of Sexuality Education*, 4 (2), 158-177.

Spector, I. P., and Fremeth, S. M. (1996). Sexual behaviors and attitudes of geriatric residents in long-term care facilities . *Journal of Sex and Marital Therapy*, 22 (4), 235-246.

Steele, D. (2007). *A best practice approach to intimacy and sexuality. A guide to practice and resource tools for assessment and documentation*. Lanark, Leeds and Grenville Long-term care working group.

Steinke, E. E. (1997). Sexuality in aging : implications for nursing facility staff. *Journal of Continuing Education in Nursing*, 28 (2), 59-63.

Stolee, P., Esbaugh, J., Aylward, S., Cathers, T., Harvey, D. P., Hillier, L. M., Keat, N., and Feightner, J. W. (2005). Factors associated with the effectiveness of continuing education in long term care. *Gerontologist*, 45 (3), 399-409.

Story, M. D. (1989). Knowledge and attitudes about the sexuality of older adults among retirement home residents. *Educational Gerontology*, 15 (5), 515-526.

Szasz, G. (1983). Sexual incidents in an extended care unit for aged men. *Journal of the American Geriatrics Society,* 31 (7), 407-411.

Tabak, N., and Shemesh-Kigli, R. (2006). Sexuality and Alzheimer's disease : can the two go together? *Nursing Forum*, 41 (4), 158-166.

Tunstull, P., and Henry, M. E. (1996). Approaches to resident sexuality. *Journal of Gerontological Nursing*, 22 (6), 37-42.

Walker, B. L. (1997). *Sexuality and the elderly. A research guide*. Westport,CO: Greenwood Press.

Walker, B .L., and Ephross, P. H. (1999). Knowledge and attitudes toward sexuality of a group of elderly. *Journal of Gerontological Social Work*, 31 (1/2), 85-107.

Walker, B. L., and Harrington, D. (2002). Effects of staff training on staff knowledge and attitudes about sexuality. *Educational Gerontology*, 28 (8), 639-654.

Walker, B. L., Osgood, N. J., Ephross, P. H., Richardson, J. P., Farrar, B., and Cole, C. (1998). Developing a training curriculum on elderly sexuality for long term care facility staff. *Gerontology and Geriatrics Education*, 19 (1), 3-22.

Walker, M. G. (2006). *LIFE ! Why we exist... and what we must do to survive*. Indianapolis, IN: Dog Earl Publishing.

Ward, R., Vass, A. A., Aggarwal, N., Garfield, C., and Cybyk, B. (2005). A kiss is still a kiss? The construction of sexuality in dementia care. *Dementia*, 4 (1). 49-72.

Wasow, M. ; and Loeb, M. (1975). « Sexuality in nursing homes », In Burnside, I. (Ed.) : *Sexuality and aging* (p. 35-41). Los Angeles, CA: University Southern California Press.

Watherhouse, J. (1996). Nursing practice related to sexuality: A review and recommendations . *Nursing Times Research*, 1 (6), 412-418.

Weinberg, M. S., Lottes, I., and Shaver, F. M. (2000). Sociocultural correlates of permissive sexual attitudes : A test of Reiss's hypotheses about Sweden and the United States. *The Journal of Sex Research*, 37 (1), 44-52.

White, C. B. (1982). Sexual interest, attitudes, knowledge and sexual history in relation to sexual behavior in the institutionalized aged. *Archives of Sexual Behavior*, 11 (1), 11-21.

Wold, G. (2004). *Basic geriatric nursing*. St. Louis, MO: Mosby.

Wright, M.-D. (2008). *Literature Search. Supporting sexual health and intimacy in care facilities*. Vancouver, BC: Apex Information.

Zinn, L. (1999). A good look back over our shoulders. The first nursing homes often provided no nursing and could hardly be classified as 'homes'. Long-term care has come a long way! *Nursing Homes Long-Term Care Management*, 48 (12), 20-54.

In: Palliative and Nursing Home Care
Editor: Samuel E. Plunkett

ISBN 978-1-61122-417-7

Chapter 4

Back to the Future: A Research Journey in Haematology and Palliative Care

Pam McGrath
International Program of Psycho-Social Health Research (IPP-SHR),
Central Queensland University, Kenmore, Brisbane, Australia

Abstract

For many years, increasing research evidence has indicated that the discipline of palliative care, recognised as best practice in end-of-life care, is not integrated adequately into adult haematology. Research indicates that most haematology patients are likely to die in acute care health care settings, exposed to an escalation of invasive technology, aware that they are dying but with no knowledge of or referral to palliative care, in hospital situations that are not designed to be responsive to the support or spiritual needs of terminally ill patients or their families. This chapter provides an overview of a program of psycho-social research that for over a decade has not only increased awareness of the problem by documenting the end-of-life experience of haematology patients and their families, but has also contributed to a solution through the development of a model for the integration of palliative care in haematology. The discussion will follow the program's journey of research starting with consumer work directly related to end-of-life concerns in haematology including work on post-traumatic stress, spiritual pain, bereavement, relocation for specialist treatment, informed consent, supportive care and carers' issues.

The journey concludes with the description of a research-*based* model for health professionals developed to inform the integration of palliative care and haematology that is now disseminated and informing practice both nationally and internationally. In short, the reader is taken on a journey back to the future to see what was, what is and what can be in relation to the provision of appropriate supportive and palliative care for haematology patients, their families and the health professionals who care for them.

Introduction

In recent years, there have been major advances in haematology that are the cause for much celebration for haematologists and their patients (Joske and McGrath, 2007). The overall survival for younger patients with multiple myeloma eligible for dose-intensified therapy has significantly improved (Kyle and Rajkumar 2004). Another important example is the success of Imatinib for chronic myeloid leukaemia where it is now estimated that responding patients have a prognosis of over twenty years (Anstrom, et al., 2004). Treatments for the common types of non-Hodgkin's lymphoma have also improved with the addition of rituximab to CHOP chemotherapy. The event-free survival at 3 years for diffuse large cell lymphoma is now approaching 80% in those under 65 years of age (Pfreundschuh, et al., 2006) and 60% in the elderly (Feugier, et al., 2005). There has been a positive shift in the survival curve in follicular low grade NHL (van Oers, et al., 2006). All of these advances need to be set in the context of the continuing outstanding curative success of Hodgkin's lymphoma and paediatric acute lymphoblastic leukaemia. The present discussion applauds and honours these advances.

As brilliant as these advances are, however, they can never avoid the fact that all haematology patients will inevitably reach a terminal or palliative phase of their illness. Yet for many years, increasing research evidence has indicated that the discipline of palliative care, recognised as best practice in end-of-life care, is not integrated adequately into adult haematology (Hunt and McCaul, 1998; Maddocks, Bentley and Sheedy, 1994; Mander, 1997; Shapiro, et al., 1997; McGrath, 1999a; 2001a; 2001b; 2002a; 2002b; 2002f; 2002g). It is this lack of integration of palliative care and haematology that is the focus of this chapter. Research indicates that most haematology patients are likely to die in an acute care health care setting, exposed to an escalation of invasive technology, aware that they are dying but with no knowledge of or referral to palliative care, in hospital situations that are not designed to be responsive to the support or spiritual needs of terminally ill patients or their families (McGrath 1999a; 2001a; 2001b; 2002a; 2002b; 2002f; 2002g). This chapter provides an overview of an established program of psycho-social research that has not only increased awareness of the problem by documenting the end-of-life experience of haematology patients and their families, but has also contributed to a solution through the development of a model for the integration of palliative care in haematology.

The discussion will follow the program's journey of research starting with consumer work directly related to end-of-life concerns in haematology, including work on post-traumatic stress, spiritual pain, bereavement, relocation for specialist treatment, informed consent, supportive care and carers' issues. The journey concludes with the description of a research-based model for health professionals developed to inform the integration of palliative care and haematology that is now disseminated and informing practice both nationally and internationally. In short, the reader is taken on a journey back to the future to see what was, what is and what can be in relation to the provision of appropriate supportive and palliative care for haematology patients, their families and the health professionals who care for them.

For the following discussion the World Health Organisation (WHO) definition of palliative care will be the starting point for considerations of best practice. According to the WHO (2010): 'Palliative care is an approach that improves the quality of life of patients and their families facing the problems associated with life-threatening illness, through the prevention and relief of suffering by means of early identification and impeccable assessment and treatment of pain and other problems, physical, psychosocial and spiritual. Palliative care:

- Provides relief from pain and other distressing symptoms;
- Affirms life and regards dying as a normal process;
- Intends neither to hasten or postpone death;
- Integrates the psychological and spiritual aspects of patient care;
- Offers a support system to help the family cope during the patient's illness and in their bereavement;
- Uses a team approach to address the needs of patients and their families, including bereavement counselling, if indicated;
- Will enhance quality of life, and may also positively influence the course of illness;
- Is applicable early in the course of illness, in conjunction with other therapies that are intended to prolong life, such as chemotherapy or radiatin therapy, and includes those investigations needed to better understand and manage distressing clinical complications.'

In short, palliative care is about living. It is a compassionate humane response to providing services to those who are confronted by a terminal illness, to ensure that the focus is on their quality of life. This holistic, multi-disciplinary response ensures that patients with a serious illness are able to live life according to their own choices and to their fullest ability.

From the Consumer Perspective

The initial work from the program of psycho-social research completed on this topic was from the consumers' perspective (McGrath, ; 1999a; 2001a; 2001b; 2002a; 2002b; 2002f; 2002g). This body of research points to the fact that during the dying trajectory haematology patients are exposed to escalating technological and invasive treatments within the curative system and are not referred to palliative care. The families and significant others who care for the patients enter the bereavement stage in a debilitated state from the regret, exhaustion and spiritual pain associated with coping with such a difficult situation. A high proportion of the carers of these patients suffer post-traumatic stress related to the experience and are left, unsupported, to deal with bereavement (McGrath, 1999b; 2002c; 2002d; 2002e).

The research completed (McGrath, 2002a) indicates that, for haematology patients and their carers, the fact of the terminal trajectory is obvious to some degree by the state of physical deterioration of the patient's body and the sequence of confronting life-threatening events through treatment. However, the naming and acknowledgement of the fact of dying in the curative ward is described as an emotionally complex and ineffectively handled process. According to this consumer research, with few exceptions health professionals did not indicate that death was imminent and there were few honest statements and scant useful information provided to prepare the individual for dying. At best, the patient and their family relied on non-verbal or situational clues in an environment that rewarded them for a positive and stoic determination based on unrealistic hope. The ever-present expectation of a 'breakthrough' in treatment and the acceptance of experimentation in haematological malignancy exacerbated this situation, sometimes allowing the continuation of treatment past acceptable boundaries.

Importantly, it was reported by the participants in this consumer research that patients and their families need help coming to terms with the possibility of the finality of the prognosis. The available research (McGrath, 2002b) indicates that patients and their carers are struggling with issues of dying, even though the medical system is not providing the opportunity for them to 'name' and deal with this process. There is evidence that discussion at an earlier point in the dying trajectory could help families to prepare for the event of death. Without such preparation, families are left with unresolved concerns and deep regrets.

Importantly, the insights provided by the carer research (McGrath, 2002b) highlights the contraction that individuals can simultaneously hold the two seemingly incompatible notions of acceptance of death and hope for a miracle. To base medical interventions on the belief that haematology patients will be exclusively hoping for a cure is only recognizing part of the story. The powerful emotion of hope combined with the technological imperative in this cure-oriented area of medicine is a potent mix that will deflect any possibility of appropriate and timely referrals to the palliative system. However, the indications are that involvement in palliative care support would be welcome by haematology patients and their families.

There are a range of special difficulties for patients who have to relocate from regional, rural and remote areas for specialist haematological treatments, as they are often separated from their support network of family and friends and have to re-establish contact with this support network when they return home after treatment (McGrath, 1999c; 1999d; 2001c; 2001d; 2001e). The impact of relocation for specialist treatment creates many major challenges during end-of-life care when the patient wishes to return home to die.

Research by Bertero and associates (1993; 1997) on quality of life for haematology patients affirms the consumer concerns by highlighting the serious psycho-social impact of the demands and complications of what can be quite invasive and difficult therapies. Similarly, the work of Baker and associates (1991) in relation to bone marrow transplantation posits that, if consideration is given to the stress of being near death, the strain of hospitalization, the physical complication of aggressive cancer treatments and the burden imposed on the carer and family, assessment of quality of life become central to the question of whether stressful therapeutic interventions are actually worth it. As Escalante and associates (1997) point out, it is important to give patients appropriate supportive care and assist them to understand and accept end-of-life issues.

From an ethical perspective, the accumulated consumer evidence points to the fact that giving priority to the palliative perspective is an essential imperative during end-of-life decision-making in haematology (McGrath and Kearsley, 1995). As research indicates that haematology patients are likely to accept treatments offered, there is a significant ethical responsibility on the part of haematologists in offering aggressive curative, rather than palliative, treatments (McGrath, 2000).

From the health professionals' Perspective

In order to respond professionally to the increasing evidence of consumer problems at the interface of cure and palliation in haematology, the research focus turned to exploring end-of-life care from the perspective of the health professionals who provide care for haematology patients. The program's first research effort in this regard was a case study approach to identify and document instances where palliative care was successfully integrated into the treatment of patients with haematological malignancies. The case study (McGrath and Joske, 2002) shows that it is possible for patients with haematological malignancies to experience all of the satisfactions of dying at home that are usually associated with hospice care, including the intimate sharing with close family and friends and the respect and dignity that can be afforded to a patient in their own home. The positive outcomes that were documented through the case study include a strong sense of satisfaction and closure for consumers, where the family is left with a sense of rightness about their decision-making and a deep-felt sense of having made every effort to fulfil the needs of the dying patient. An orientation to living rather than dying pervades such experiences. Post-traumatic stress, regrets and spiritual pain, documented as more expected outcomes of terminal care in haematology, are not evident. The carer is left well supported and nourished by the experience - a firm foundation for coping with the challenges of bereavement. The positive outcomes from the pilot pointed to the possibility of effective integration of palliative care.

The Model for Integration of Haematology and Palliative Care

The next step was to develop a service delivery model that would provide health professionals with best practice insight for the integration of haematology and palliative care. The two-year study, funded by the Australian National Health and Medical Research Council, developed the model within the context of the experience and insights of the multi-disciplinary range of Australian health and allied professionals involved in adult haematology.

The phenomenological descriptive methodology used open-ended interviews (n=90), audio-taped, transcribed verbatim and thematically analysed. The national study was based on interviews with a wide representation of health professionals (haematologists: n=20; haematology nurses: n=19; allied health professionals: n=8) from public and private hospital haematology units, palliative care units (palliative care doctors: n=8; palliative care nurses: n=7; pastoral care workers: n=1), hospices (n=2), general practitioners (n=2) and support organizations (n=8) throughout Australia. The information was enriched by individuals (n=15) who shared their experience of caring for a loved one who died of a haematological condition.

The three-stage process for model development was based on the National Cancer Control Initiative's methodology for Optimising Cancer Care in Australia. The trilogy of models developed by the research were subject to rigorous peer review by a national panel of haematology and palliative care experts. In addition, the model was peer-reviewed nationally by expert audiences in haematology, oncology, social work, palliative care and acute medical care. The model was enthusiastically affirmed by all groups who indicated that the insights resonate with the reality of health professionals' experience in haematology.

As practical research informed by both consumers and health professionals at the coalface of service provision, the work begins to explore strategies to ensure that haematology patients receive best practice end-of-life care. A booklet for health professionals has been developed from the study, titled: 'Haematology and Palliative Care: Towards an

Integrated Practice' (available by request from www.ipp-shr.cqu.edu.au) and widely distributed both nationally and internationally.

The findings indicate that there are three distinct models in end-of-life care in haematology in Australia: (a) the 'functional' model; (b) the 'evolving' model; and (c) the 'refractory' model. The following discussion details the characteristics of each model of service delivery from the perspective of the consumer and each disciplinary group within the multi-disciplinary team of health professionals who provide the care.

At one end of the continuum is the 'functional' model that provides satisfying care from diagnosis to bereavement for patients and their families. At the other end is the 'refractory' or death denying model which is resistant to palliative care resulting in unnecessary hardship for patient and families. A transitional or 'evolving' model links the two.

It is important to note that the trilogy of overlapping models (labelled 'functional', 'evolving' and 'refractory') that addresses the complexity of issues associated with the integration of haematology and palliative care is set within the notion of professional and hospital culture. Leininger (1991) defines culture as the learned common and transmitted values, convictions, norms and ways of life that direct people's patterns of thinking, decision-making and actions. For example, hospice culture is described as a specific care culture with a humanistic base and set of values reflecting the meaning of life and death while the cure-oriented biomedical culture usually does not take existential or spiritual issues into consideration (Andersson-Segesten, 2001; Hermansson and Ternestedt, 2000; Ternestedt, et al., 2002). The research findings from which the model(s) were developed clearly indicated that different team and hospital cultures create different attitudinal, behavioural and knowledge environments in which health professionals can engage with patients and their families during end-of-life care in haematology. The individual can influence the culture, but ultimate the pre-existing culture is the most powerful determination of action.

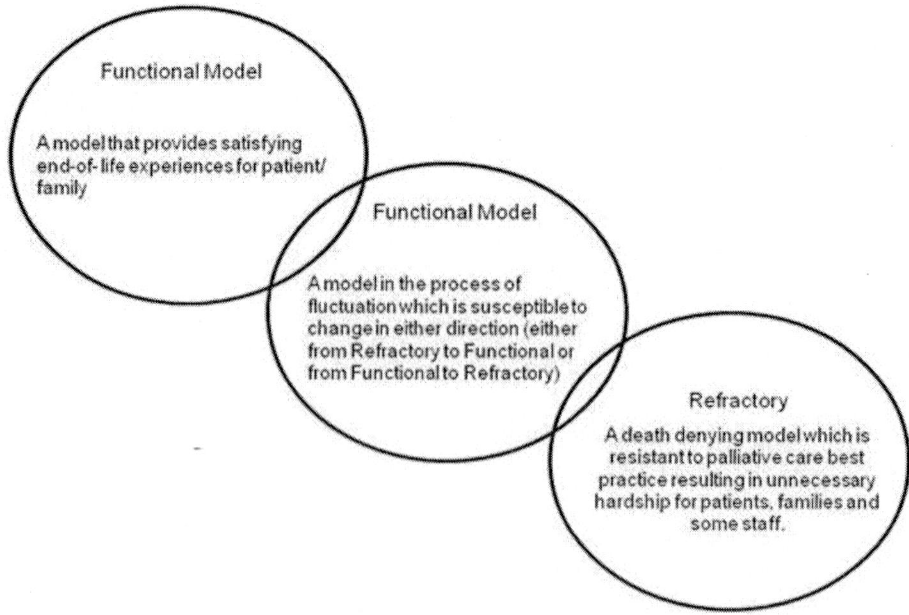

Diagram 1. Models of care (mcgrath and holewa, 2007).

The statements made by participants for the 'functional' and 'refractory' models are akin to a mirror image of each other, created by a distorted mirror that reflects the image of the same issue but is accompanied by the opposite attitudes or practice. For example, as outlined in Table 1, haematology nurses from different setting made opposing statements about the same issue. The same was true for all the other health professionals interviewed. The important point is that the factors influencing the integration (or not) of palliative care in haematology are not inherently clinical in relation to these specific diagnostic groups, but rather correlate with the attitudinal approach of the health professionals. Any haematological clinical issue can be seen as either a reason for or against palliative care depending on whether the professional has a 'functional' or 'refractory' perspective. In short, the integration of palliative care in haematology has more to do with the thoughts and attitudes of health professionals than any unique clinical feature.

Table 1. Same Theme But Opposite Beliefs And Practices

Reference: McGrath and Holewa (2007)	
FUNCTIONAL MODEL	*REFRACTORY MODEL*
Issue and representative statement	*Issue and representative statement*
Issues of death and dying addressed openly and sensitively "All you can do is give them all the options and give them all the information, be honest." "Yeah, I just think let's starting talking about it, and most people when you do, are actually fine with it."	Issues of death and dying denied "So it is really a cure culture even though the writing's on the wall." "What we do is cruel, but it's not nice put it that way. And then you try and make an 80 year old go through that..."
Leadership – positive attitudes to palliative care "And most of the doctors acknowledge the fact that you have that knowledge [of palliative care] and if you ring them and if you're concerned they'll let you go with it. So I think we're lucky in that respect where we work."	Leadership – negative attitudes to palliative care "... and so you have a system where you can't have palliative care coming in because they don't want to stand on the haematologist's toes so um trying to get the lamb and the lion together is very, very hard."
Positive experience with palliative care "Our consultants absolutely fantastic - our palliative care one. And he deliverers news in such a way that it is magic. It is like it is beautiful to watch, I have never seen anybody do it in such a way that he has been able to do it. I think that they need that sort of experience as well, and it is not something that you can just learn, I understand that, but you get better at it the more often you do it."	Lack of positive experience with palliative care "It's really important for the palliative care doctors to educate and educate in the way that they can help the haematologist understand this is a really positive process. It's not giving up or it's not a soft option. It's actually a positive strong option."
Best practice end-of-life care "I think it's important that the nurse very much stays as the patient advocate." "It's all in communication isn't it, everything is communication."	Lack of best practice end-of-life care "I think there are a core number of us who, you know, time and time again think "you know, what are we doing?!" And it is an ethical issue, we're not at ease with it, and it just makes you feel like you're, like you know, you're not doing the best for the patient. And you're just not doing the best for the profession either, it's just all wrong. And you just wish that somebody would listen to you!"

Table 1. (Continued)

Hope – complexity understood "...there's always hope in giving them quality of life." "We are honest about it and not giving false hope." "The hope button that won't actually help them deal with it."	Hope – simplistic, black and white understanding of 'hope equals cure' "You can't do that [introduce palliative care] because you would take away their hope." "They're not offering hope of cure then they are not offering hope."
Organizational issues – democratic, collaborative, inclusive "There has to be a healthy respect between all members of the collaborative team; an acknowledgment that each member has a role to play and no one person is any more important than the next one." "We have a lot of autonomy as nurses we do a lot of referrals." "We are a very well supportive group of people, we support each other quite well, I don't ever feel burnt out."	Organizational issues – medico-centric, paternalistic, hierarchical "But I still think that it's still very much the nurse is seen as the handmaiden and the doctor still as the paternal father." "I've been told that can be a bit of a medical territory issue. It's got to do with the pecking order and palliative care is down on that pecking order, rather than just realising that that's multi disciplinary team approach that's all about patient needs."
Appropriate and timely involvement of palliative care "... to bring palliative care into the forefront early on in everybody's treatment. So suddenly going off to palliative care area is not a death sentence, it is just a continuation of care from day one. Our haematologists actually refer earlier on, than medical oncology. And that just the way it is and it is fantastic."	Lack of appropriate or timely involvement of palliative care "Because we are too busy treating them without actually saying "maybe it is time to pull out", let these die peacefully and without this myriad of machinery and technology and where do they want to die?"
Integration of cure and palliation "I think that the Pall Care Team should be just part and parcel naturally of any of these types of conditions they have a role to play throughout the disease health continuum. They often have valuable input right throughout. And they should be involved right throughout."	Lack of integration of cure and palliation "It's very territorial." "Palliative care are not utilized enough for the knowledge and the experience and skills they have."
Specific issues regarding patients with haematological malignancies addressed "Palliative care would be quite capable of managing Haematological patients. Palliative Care basically are quite capable of doing things like assessing and ordering blood transfusions to help manage fatigue, especially where anaemia is an issue."	Specific issues regarding patients with haematological malignancies seen as an obstacle "I would be reluctant to be giving a blood transfusion at home by myself. And I think a lot of nurses are reluctant to do that."

The 'Functional' Model

In essence the best practice 'functional' model is a patient-centred continuum of care from diagnosis to bereavement. Important factors associated with the provision of such care were found to be an ability to address issues of death and dying openly and sensitively; a democratic, collaborative and inclusive multi-disciplinary unit sub-culture; the provision of honest information and respect for patient choice; an understanding of the changing nature of hope; an understanding and use of palliative care expertise from diagnosis to bereavement; the appropriate and timely integration of palliative care; and an awareness that specific issues regarding patients with haematological malignancies can be addressed.

There are a myriad of strategies for successfully addressing palliative care issues in haematology (McGrath and Holewa, 2007) – honest information-giving, openness to hearing each patient's particular circumstances, an awareness of quality of life issues and adequate timely and sensitive preparation of the patient and their family of the unique circumstances of haematology underpin all interventions. This is an area where forewarned is forearmed; the treating team should have a sound awareness of the wishes of the patient and their family and systems in place to respond to palliative needs (Joske and McGrath, 2007). Evidence of effective community-based clinical services for provision of some blood products is an indication of innovation in this area.

Traditionally, the belief that there were factors associated with the unique biology of blood cancers has been one of the key obstacles to the integration of palliative care. The research for the model development highlighted the fact that it is the varying professional perspectives, rather than the unique biological circumstances of haematology, that will determine whether or not haematology patients receive best practice palliative care. There are special consideration for haematology patients which need to be taken into considerations, such as the high-tech and invasive nature of treatments offered that at times are myeloblative and may involve transient bone marrow failure; the speed of change to a terminal event; the need for blood products; and the possibility of catastrophic bleeds. At times there can be a blurring of the distinction between the curative and palliative phase, however evidence indicates that in the majority of cases there are clear indications that the terminal stage has been reached (McGrath and Holewa, 2007). The important point from a functional perspective is that such factors need not been seen as obstacles to palliative care integration but rather define the uniqueness of services in this area.

An example of a topic where the unique biology of blood cancers creates concern in relation to palliative care and haematology is the provision of clinical and supportive care to haematology patients who are vulnerable to catastrophic bleeds. Catastrophic bleeds are a significant palliative care issue because of their association with immediate death (Pereira and Phan, 2004). Indeed, the very fact of the possibility of catastrophic bleeds for haematology patients, despite their low incidence, is a reason commonly posited by some health professionals for arguing against the possibility of integration of palliative care in haematology and against the possibility of haematology patients dying at home. The literature indicates that catastrophic bleeds only occur in a small proportion of the 6-10% of patients with advanced cancer who experience clinically significant bleeding (Gagnon, et al., 1998; Pereira and Phan, 2004; Prommer, 2005). However, in the 'functional' model, the health professionals have a range of strategies for dealing with the possibility of catastrophic bleeds including the use of dark towels to reduce the distress of the visibility of the bleed, the importance of advance planning for care, accepting the limits of the situation, reassuring family that the patient is likely to lapse into lack of consciousness and will not be suffering and the administration of sedation (McGrath and Leahy, 2009). Nevertheless, it is important to note that the research on this topic is still contradictory and inconclusive especially as regards such issues as whether it is possible to identify individuals likely to be affected, the role of blood products and whether it is wise to warn family or carers (McGrath and Leahy, 2009). Indeed, the insights from Australian haematologists indicate that there is a paucity of literature in this area and health professionals have only broad guidelines (TGL, 2008) on which to base their work with patients and their families.

There is heartening evidence that some haematology departments in Australia are providing leadership through their respect for the expertise of palliative specialists and their willingness to integrate such specialists (usually for psychosocial support, pain and symptom management) from the point of diagnosis (Joske and McGrath, 2007). This is usually achieved by making an early referral under the guise of assistance with symptom control, which allows an introduction to be made between patients, carers and the Palliative Care Team (Joske and McGrath, 2007).

The 'Refractory' Model

The findings on the 'refractory' model resonate with the previous consumer research on end-of-life experience in haematology in that the professionals interviewed similarly indicated that, based on their professional experience, patients from these diagnostic groups typically die in the acute ward dealing with escalating technology and invasive treatments (McGrath and Holewa, 2006). The refractory model was described in terms of a medico-centric sub-culture, informed by negative attitudes to palliative care, driving a curative culture based on 'false signals' of hope and lack of honesty about death and dying. There is a lack of integration of best practice palliative care. Patients in this sub-culture are not aware of, and hence do not request, either palliative care or consideration of the possibility to die at home. Haematology specific issues are seen as an obstacle and used to justify non-provision of palliative care.

As described in detail elsewhere (McGrath and Holewa, 2006), nurses experience stress and a sense of powerlessness in such a refractory system. Nurses indicated that it is stressful to be caught in a cure-oriented medico-centric system having to be witness to the distress of dying patients coping with high-tech and invasive treatments. The situation is exacerbated by their duel role of coping with dying patients on the same ward as those hopeful of a cure. Futterman and Wellisch (1990) also record nursing concern and guilt about being involved in medical treatments that do not respond sensitively to the patient's dying needs.

The research is affirmed by a survey of Australian haematologists (Auret, Bulsara and Joske, 2003) that indicated a widespread lack of consensus about when to refer patients with haematological malignancies to palliative care, and much variation in access to palliative care, for haematologists across the Australian scene. Furthermore, patients with leukaemia, lymphoma and myeloma are documented as unlikely to receive community-based palliative care services (Addington-Hall and Altmann, 2000).

The 'Evolving' Model

Linking the two polarities of the 'functional' model and the 'refractory' model are descriptions of the factors that create the possibility of change that are labelled the 'evolving' model. It is important to note that, depending on the particular factors that come into play in a culture, the evolution can be in either a constructive direction (from the 'refractory' towards 'functional') or can be a negative change (from 'functional' towards 'refractory').

Factors influencing the integration of palliative care into haematology include: recognition of the positive contribution of palliative care by the Head of Haematology; a proactive unit sub-culture; increased participation of all team members in decision processes; the presence of palliative care staff, providing role models for successful service delivery; new staff and graduates who introduce knowledge and practice of the discipline; continuing professional education on best practice; and exposure of staff to satisfying experiences with hospice and palliative care.

Changes between the 'functional' and 'refractory' paradigms can occur relatively quickly as the result of a change in management or culture as can be seen by the following list of factors influencing change:

- Leadership and attitudes of Head of Haematology;
- Unit presence and leadership of hospital palliative care practitioners;
- The experience and attitudes of new graduates and staff with regards to palliative care; and
- Exposure of staff to positive experiences with palliative care cases.

An example of such change (McGrath and Holewa, 2007) would be if a haematology unit appoints a new Head of Department with knowledgeable and respectful attitudes towards palliative care service provision, the leadership may be able to influence a previously 'refractory' hospital culture towards openness to best-practice end-of-life care. Conversely, a change of leadership to a Head of Department who is not comfortable with death and dying issues can undermine the efforts of practitioners committed to palliative care integration.

Conclusion

The outcome of a decade of research on the psycho-social aspects of haematology reported in this chapter is the initiation of a dialogue for palliative care in haematology informed by a trilogy of models developed from the findings of a national research project. The model builds on and shares the wisdom of the health professionals who have successfully identified problems and found solutions. The hope and expectation is that the insights will go some way to ensuring haematology patients and their families are given the benefits of compassionate, best practice palliative care during the difficult time of dealing with the challenges imposed by the diagnosis of a life-threatening illness. For as Michael Barbato (2005:637) reflects:

> Dying is not something we can ignore and the suffering that accompanies it cannot be treated within a biomedical framework. … Dying is the most significant time in any person's life. Its meaning may be lost within a system that has as its solitary goal the need to preserve life. In such a system, the drive to prolong life and maintain homeostasis can become so deeply entrenched that it takes precedence over matters of the soul, casting a pall over those who are dying.

References

Addington-Hall, J., and Altmann, D. (2000). Which terminally ill cancer patients in the UK receive care from community specialist palliative care nurses? *Journal of Advanced Nursing*, 32, 4, 799-806.

Andershed, B., and Ternestedt, B. (2001). Development of a theoretical framework describing. *Journal of Advanced Nursing*, 34, 4, 554-562.

Anstrom, KJ., Reed, SD., Allen, AS., et al. (2004). Long-term survival estimates for Imatinib versus Interferon-Alpha plus Low-Dose Cytarabine for patients with newly diagnosed Chronic-Phase Chromnic Myeloid Leukemia. *Cancer,* 101, 2584-92.

Auret, K., Bulsara, C., and Joske, D. (2003). Australasian haematologist referral patterns to palliative care: lack of consensus on when and why. *Journal of Internal Medicine*, 12, 566-572.

Baker, F., Curbow, B., and Wingard, J. (1991). Role retention and quality of life of bone marrow transplant survivors. *Social Science and Medicine*, 32, 6, 697-704.

Barbato, M. (2005). Personal viewpoint: Caring for the dying patient. *Internal Medicine Journal*, 35, 636-637.

Bertero, C, and Ek, A. (1993). Quality of life of adults with acute leukaemia. *Journal of Advanced Nursing*, 18, 1346-353.

Bertero, C, Eriksson, B., and Ek, A. (1997). A substantive theory of quality of life of adults with chronic leukaemia. *International Journal of Nursing Studies*, 34, 1, 9-16.

Escalante, C., Martin, C., Elting, L., et al. (1997). Medical futility and appropriate medical care in patients whose death is thought to be imminent. *Supportive Care in Cancer*, 5, 4, 274-280.

Feugier, P., Van Hoof, A., Sebban, C., et al. (2005). Long-term results of the R-CHOP study in the treatment of elderly patients with Diffuse Large B-cell Lymphoma: A study by the Groupe d'Etude des Lymphomes d'Adulte. *Journal of Clinical Oncology*, 23, 18, 4117-4126.

Fulton, J. (1998). Public health briefing: Palliative care for cancer patients – current issues. *Medicine and Health Rhode Island*, 81, 8, 276-277.

Futterman, A., and Wellisch, D. (1990). Psychodynamic themes in bone marrow transplantation. *Haematology/Oncology Clinics of North America*, 4, 3, 699-709.

Gagnon, B., Mancini, I., Pereira, J., et al. (1998). Palliative management of bleeding events in advanced cancer patients. *Journal of Palliative Care*, 14, 50-54.

Hermansson, A., and Ternestedt, B. (2000). What do we know about the dying patient? Awareness as a means to improve palliative care. *Journal of Medicine and Law*, 19, 2, 335-344.

Hunt, R., and McCaul, K. (1998). Coverage of cancer patients by hospice services, South Australia, 1990 to 1993. *Australian and New Zealand Journal of Public Health*, 22, 1, 45-48.

Joske, D., and McGrath, P. (2007). Palliative care in haematology. *Internal Medicine Journal*, 37, 589-590.

Kyle, RA., and Rajkumar, VS. (2004). Multiple Myeloma. *New England Journal of Medicine*, 351, 1860-73.

Leninger, M. (1991). Culture care diversity and universality: A theory of nursing. New York: National League for Nursing.

Maddocks, I., Bentley, L., and Sheedy, J. (1994). Quality of life issues in patients dying from haematological diseases. *Annals of Academic Medicine*, Singapore, 23, 2, 244-248.

Mander, T. (1997). Haematology and palliative care: An account of shared care for a patient undergoing bone marrow transplantation for chronic myeloid leukaemia. *International Journal of Nursing Practice*, 3, 1, 62-66.

McGrath, P. (1999a). Palliative care for patients with haematological malignancies. If not, why not? *Journal of Palliative Care*, 15, 3, 24-30.

McGrath, P. (1999b). Posttraumatic stress and the experience of cancer: A literature review of new directions in rehabilitation in oncology. *Journal of Rehabilitation*, 65, 3, 18-24.

McGrath, P. (1999c). Accommodation for patients and carers during relocation for treatment for leukaemia: A descriptive profile. *Supportive Care in Cancer*, 7, 1, 6-10.

McGrath, P. (1999d). The experience of relocation for specialist treatment for haematological malignancies. *Cancer Strategy*, 1, 157-163.

McGrath, P. (2000). Informed consent to peripheral blood stem cell transplantation. *Cancer Strategy*, 2, 44-50.

McGrath, P. (2001a). Dying in the curative system - the haematology/oncology dilemma: Part 1. *The Australian Journal of Holistic Nursing*, 8, 2, 22-30.

McGrath, P. (2001b). Insights on the dying trajectory in haematology-oncology from the carer's perspective. *Cancer Nursing*, 24, 5, 413-21.

McGrath, P. (2001c). Post-treatment support for patients with haematological malignancies: Findings from regional, rural and remote Queensland. *Australian Health Review*, 23, 4, 142-50.

McGrath, P. (2001d). Follow-up of patients with haematological malignancies and their families in regional, rural and remote Queensland: The GPs perspective. *Supportive Care in Cancer*, 9, 199-204.

McGrath, P. (2001e). Returning home after specialist treatment for haematological malignancies: An Australian study. *Family and Community Health*, 24, 36-48.

McGrath, P. (2002a). Are we making progress? Not in haematology! Omega, *Journal of Death and Dying*, 45, 4, 357-374.

McGrath, P. (2002b). End-of-life care for haematological malignancies: The 'technological imperative' and palliative care. *Journal of Palliative Care*, 18, 1, 39-47.

McGrath, P. (2002c). Dying in the curative system - the haematology/oncology dilemma: Part 2. *Australian Journal of Holistic Nursing*, 9, 1, 14-21.

McGrath, P. (2002d). Qualitative findings on the experience of end-of-life care for haematological malignancies. *American Journal of Hospice and Palliative Care*, 19, 2, 1-9.

McGrath, P. (2002e). Creating a language for spiritual pain through research. *Supportive Care in Cancer*, 10, 8, 637-646.

McGrath, P. (2002f). Dying in the curative system - the haematology/oncology dilemma: Part 2. *The Australian Journal of Holistic Nursing*, 9, 1, 14-21.

McGrath, P. (2002g). Qualitative findings on the experience of end-of-life care for haematological malignancies. *American Journal of Hospice and Palliative Care*, 19, 2, 1-9.

McGrath, P., and Holewa, H. (2006). Missed opportunities: Nursing insights on end-of-life care for haematology patients. *International Journal of Nursing Practice*, 12, 295-301.

McGrath, P., and Holewa, H., (2007). A model for end-of-life care in haematology: An Australian nursing perspective. *Oncology Nursing Forum*, 34, 1, 79-85.

McGrath, P., and Joske, D. (2002). Palliative care and haematological malignancy: A case study. *Australian Health Review*, 25, 3, 48-54.

McGrath, P., and Kearsley, J. (1995). Is there a better way? Bioethical reflections on palliative cytotoxic drug use. *Palliative Medicine* (editorial), 9, 4, 269-271.

McGrath, P., and Leahy, M. (2009). Catastrophic bleeds during end-of-life care in haematology: Controversies from Australian research. *Supportive Care in Cancer*, 17, 5, 527-32.

Pereira, J., and Phan, T. (2004). Management of bleeding in patients with advanced cancer. *Oncology,* 9, 561-570.

Pfreundschuh, M., Trümper, L., Österburg, A., et al. (2006). CHOP-like chemotherapy plus rituximab versus CHOP-like chemotherapy alone in younger patients with good-prognosis diffuse large B-cell lymphoma: A randomised controlled trial by the Mabthera International Trial (MinT) Group. *Lancet Oncology*, 7, 379-91.

Prommer, E. (2005). Management of bleeding in the terminally ill patient. *Hematology,* 10, 3, 167-175.

Shapiro, J., Brown, S., Briggs, P., et al. (1997). Adult acute leukaemia – A retrospective study of sixty-six consecutive patients. *Australian and New Zealand Journal of Medicine*, 27, 301-306.

Ternestedt, B., Andershed, B., Eriksson, M., et al. (2002). A good death: Development of a nursing model of care. *Journal of Hospice and Palliative Nursing*, 4, 3, 153-160.

Therapeutic Guidelines Limited (TGL). (2008). Therapeutic guidelines: Guidelines Internat ional Network. North Melbourne, Victoria. (http://www.tg.com.au) accessed 24th March, 2010.

Van Oers, MHJ., Klasa, R., Marcus, RE., et al. (2006). Rituximab maintenance improves clinical outcome of relapsed/resistant follicular non-Hodgkin's lymphoma in patients both with and without rituximab during induction: results of a prospective randomised phase 3 intergroup trial. *Blood,* 108, 3295-3301.

World Health Organisation (WH)). (2010) WHO definition of palliative care (www.who.int/cancer/pallitive/definition/en - accessed 19th April 2010).

In: Palliative and Nursing Home Care
Editor: Samuel E. Plunkett

ISBN 978-1-61122-417-7

Chapter 5

The Changing Role of the Licensed Practical Nurse in Nursing Home Care

Aggie T. G. Paulus [*] ***and Arno J. A. van Raak***
School for Public Health and Primary Care (Caphri)
Maastricht University, Faculty of Health, Medicine and Life Sciences
Department of Health Organisation,
Policy and Economics (HOPE) The Netherlands

Abstract

Traditional care for older people is increasingly being substituted or supplemented by care arrangements such as integrated care. The ageing of the population, economic pressures and social developments are among the primary reasons. To match the emerging range of care arrangements, changes in the traditional role performed by the licensed practical nurse (LPN) are considered both likely and necessary.

To find out if LPNs perform a different role in traditional and emerging care types, the main goal of this chapter is to compare this role in three varieties of care for older people: traditional care, transitional care and integrated care. Between 1999 and 2003, data were assembled in three nursing homes in the Netherlands. Each home represented one type of nursing home care. At three measurement points (each lasting 14 consecutive days), LPNs (on average 177 per measurement) registered the type, frequency and duration of activities delivered to older people with somatic and psycho-social problems. Data-analysis showed that the more nursing home care became integrated, the more (frequently) the LPN became involved in indirect care activities and in activities for psycho-geriatric residents. Some parts of the role of the LPN, however, did not differ between the care types. On the basis of these results it can be concluded that the licensed practical nurse, to a limited extent, performed a different role in different types of care. In all care types, however, the LPN also remained a generalist. In view of these results, the future role of the LPN is not expected to become less important in emerging care types.

[*] Tel: ++31-43-3881706 ; Fax: ++31-43-3670960, E-mail: a.paulus@beoz.unimaas.nl

Introduction

In reaction to the ageing of the population, economic pressures and a growing demand from users, various countries are developing and implementing integrated care, managed care or primary care arrangements for older people. Many of these arrangements supplement or replace traditional care types as they entail changes in the organization of care delivery [Coile 1995, Richardson and Cunliffe 2003, Hay 2004, Jooste 2004, Faithfull and Hunt 2005, Paulus *et al.* 2006]. To match the emerging range of care arrangements, changes in the traditional roles of certain nurses are expected [Valanis 2000, Deutschendorf 2003, Porter-O'Grady 2003a,b, SGNA 2006]. Roles refer to collections of activities commonly conducted by people with a certain function.

The licensed practical nurse (LPN) is one of the roles for which changes are considered both likely and necessary. In traditional care, the LPN is a generalist who participates in the entire nursing process through planning, implementation and evaluation of nursing care [Kelsey 2006]. Emerging care types, however, are expected to lead to less generalization and more specialization in nursing roles [Coile 1995, Reeves 1997, Sherman *et al.* 1998, Barber *et al.* 2000, Williams *et al.* 2001, Perla 2002, Faithfull and Hunt 2005; Kelsey 2006]. If expectations prove to be true, the role of the LPN in traditional care should differ from the role of the LPN in emerging care types.

By comparing the role of the LPN in different types of care (i.e. care arrangements which differ with respect to the organization of care delivery) it can be shown whether these expectations are correct. This is not only important from a scientific point of view, as research on the role of the LPN is generally lacking [Kelsey 2006], but also for practical reasons. If the introduction of certain care types brings about changes in the role of the LPN, additional requirements may be needed to successfully and optimally deliver care to older people. In countries, for instance, in which LPNs all receive the same training, a differentiation or adaptation of general education schemes may be needed to prepare LPNs for their role in particular care types. Furthermore, the role of the LPN in relation to other roles may have to be redefined, especially if certain care types effectuate changes in the activities performed by the LPN which (partly) replace, substitute or complement activities traditionally performed by other roles.

Against this background, the aim of this chapter is to compare the role of the LPN in traditional and emerging care types. We focus on the role of the LPN in the delivery of care to older people in the Netherlands. In this country, in 2006, almost 64% of the main employees working in nursing homes and homes for the elderly were licensed practical nurses [Van der Windt *et al.* 2007]. Because of ongoing economic pressures and the ageing of the population, the organization of the delivery of care to older people, particularly nursing home care, has been changing [Paulus *et al.* 2005, Paulus *et al.* 2008]. One of the major changes encompasses the development and implementation of integrated care [Van Raak *et al.* 2003, Kümpers 2005]. Studies have shown that the period needed to develop and implement integrated care in the Netherlands can be formidable as a pain-staking and time consuming process of change usually precedes the actual introduction of the complete integrated care arrangement [van Raak *et al.* 2008a]. During this transition period, traditional care and integrated care often supplement each other. After this period, integrated care frequently replaces traditional care. Consequently, besides traditional care, there are two emerging care types in this country: transitional care and integrated care [Paulus *et al.* 2003, Paulus *et al.* 2005]. Since the LPN is involved in all three varieties of nursing home care, the Dutch case presents a good example of a (changing) nursing practice that allows a comparison of the role of the LPN in dissimilar types of care. Before we further elaborate on these different types of care, we first provide a general description of the role of the LPN in the Netherlands.

The Role of the LPN

In the Netherlands, in 2006, approximately 152000 LPNs [in Dutch: 'ziekenverzorgende niveau 3'; 'verzorgende IG'] were employed. Almost 86000 of them (i.e. about 56 per cent or the equivalent of 55200 full-timers) worked in nursing homes and homes for the elderly. The remaining LPNs worked in hospitals, institutions for mental health care and care for the disabled, home care, youth and child care and social services [Van der Windt *et al.* 2007]. With a background of intermediate vocational education and usually under the supervision of the head of the nursing ward, LPNs involved in nursing home care conduct direct care activities and indirect care activities. Direct care refers to activities directly conducted for individual patients. They include activities such as basic bedside care, monitoring and changing catheters and treatment of bedsores. Indirect care refers to activities conducted for a group of patients or for a specific ward. These activities are not directly related to individual patients and, among others, encompass some household chores, ensuring a safe living environment, preparing general activities and supporting residents. It follows that the (traditional) role of the LPN in the Netherlands is defined in terms of a generalist who is involved in both direct care and indirect care activities.

Different Types of Care

Table 1 summarizes the main characteristics of the three types of nursing home care in the Netherlands.

The table shows that there are several differences between these care types. Traditional care is marked by a supply-oriented delivery of nursing home care in a large-scale setting in which residents can not influence decisions with respect to their meals or living environment. In other words, the delivery of care is seen from the perspective of the caregivers: they mainly dictate what is delivered, when, how often, how long, by whom, et cetera. The delivery of care is also mono-disciplinary and requires no integrated –i.e. cooperative or coordinated – actions from the caregivers involved. Integrated care, on the contrary, is delivered by caregivers with different disciplinary backgrounds. Caregivers have to cooperate and coordinate – and thus integrate - their provision of services. Integrated care is also demand-oriented (i.e. the delivery of care is mainly seen from the perspective of the residents and what they want, when, from whom et cetera) and delivered in a small-scale setting in which residents are engaged in daily activities such as cooking, cleaning and doing the laundry [Paulus *et al.* 2006; Paulus and van Raak 2008]. Transitional care is a hybrid type of care as it contains elements of both traditional care and integrated care (see Table 1). Transitional care is delivered during the period in which traditional care transforms in to integrated care.

Table 1. Nursing home care types and their characteristics

Characteristics	Traditional care (Nursing home A)			Transitional care (Nursing home B)			Integrated care (Nursing home C)		
	T1	T2	T3	T1	T2	T3	T1	T2	T3
1. Structure of care delivery process									
A. Demand-oriented					X	X	X	X	X
B. Supply oriented	X	X	X	X					
2. Influence of residents on living environment and meals									
A. Yes					X	X	X	X	X
B. No	X	X	X	X					
3. Size of wards									
A. Large scale (approximately 30 per ward; shared bedrooms)	X	X	X	X					
B. Small scale (a maximum of 12 per ward)					X	X	X	X	X
4. Service delivery									
A. Integrated and multi-/interdisciplinary					X	X	X	X	X
B. Not-integrated and mono-disciplinary	X	X	X	X					

T1, T2, T3 = First, second, third measurement point, respectively.

Methods

Design

To compare the role of the LPN in traditional, transitional and integrated care, which is the main purpose of this chapter, we assembled data in three separate nursing homes in the Netherlands. Each home had to represent one type of nursing home care. Other criteria included the drive to contribute to the research, the existence of a stable working environment and comparability of size. We purposefully selected three nursing homes that fulfilled all of the criteria. Since nursing home care in the Netherlands is delivered to somatic residents (i.e. persons with physical limitations) as well as psycho-geriatric residents (i.e. persons with psycho-social problems), we included homes which served both types of residents.

Nursing home A (with 121 beds and four wards) delivered traditional nursing home care during the entire research period. Traditional care had the four characteristics mentioned in table 1. The delivery of services took place by a care team, which was responsible for care activities but not for social activities or for activities such as cooking or cleaning. For these activities other caregivers (e.g. a recreational activity supervisor; nutrition assistant or household assistant) were responsible.

Nursing home B (with 141 beds and five wards) delivered transitional care. At the beginning of the research, this home delivered traditional care. After the first measurement point, which took place in May and June 2000, this nursing home gradually introduced integrated care (see Table 1).

Finally, a nursing home (with 88 beds and three participating wards (with 28 beds in total)) was selected as home 'C'. This nursing home delivered integrated care during the entire research period. Integrated care was introduced in this nursing home in March 1998. In this home, the delivery of services took place by a team of caregivers with different disciplinary backgrounds, who cooperated and coordinated their provision of care.

Data-Collection

Between September 1999 and February 2003, data were collected at three measurement points (hereafter referred to as T1, T2 and T3). Data collection at T2 and T3 took place in January/February 2001 and in May, June and July 2002, respectively. The collection of data regarding the role of the LPN was part of a longitudinal research in which also other research issues were investigated. These issues included the effects and costs of the introduction of integrated care (compared to traditional care), formal and informal care delivery and the process of change (i.e. the transition phase). Approval to conduct the study was obtained from the relevant ethics committees in the nursing homes.

From our background description it became clear that the role of the LPN involves direct and indirect care activities. To assess (changes in) this role, we asked the LPNs in the participating nursing homes to record the activities conducted for individual residents (direct care activities) or for a group of residents or a specific ward (indirect care activities). Actions were recorded on lists that indicated selected activities with respect to direct and indirect care. Selections of activities were made on the basis of a literature study, interviews with caregivers in nursing homes throughout the country and observations in nursing homes that offered traditional or integrated care. The lists of activities that were composed were tested and further enhanced during a pilot study [for a more elaborate description of the composition of the specific lists and their reliability, see Paulus *et al.* 2008]. Table 2 gives an overview of the resulting 22 activities that were recorded by each LPN. Recording took place for each patient (with respect to direct care). Each recording took place immediately after an activity was performed (for both direct care and indirect care).

Roles refer to collections of activities. Correspondingly, if the LPN conducts dissimilar activities in different types of care, this points to different roles of the LPN. To express these differences, we used three indicators: the *type of activity* in which the LPN was involved (which activity was performed?), the *frequency* (how often was a certain activity performed?) and the *duration* (how long did a certain activity last?). Accordingly, at each measurement point (each lasting 14 consecutive days, i.e. 14 * 24 hours); each LPN recorded the type of activity performed and the frequency and duration of each activity.

For residents receiving traditional care, activities were registered at the three measurement points for 84, 89 and 98 residents, respectively. In transitional and integrated care, these numbers were 101, 91, 97 and 25, 23 and 26, respectively. Since research on the role of the LPN was part of a larger longitudinal research (see above), all LPNs who were part of the research population of the latter research were also included in this study. This allowed us to obtain a detailed and elaborate overview of the role of the LPN. At T1, a total of 192 LPNs recorded activities (A: 79; B: 93: C: 20). At T2 and T3, actions were registered by respectively 173 (A: 73; B: 79; C: 21) and 168 (A: 68; B:72; C:28) LPNs.

Table 2. Recorded activities

Activities	Description
Direct care:	
Morning care	Getting residents out of bed, bathing, dressing, shaving, combing hair
Coffee/tea-making	Making and pouring out coffee and tea, doing the dishes, cleaning up
Medication	Recording, distributing and helping with medication
Toileting	Helping residents who need to go to the bathroom, changing incontinence slips, emptying catheters
Afternoon care	Bringing residents to bed (and sometimes getting out of bed), dressing/undressing residents, combing hair
Extra care	Giving extra attention to residents through conversations, walking or shopping, extra pedicure or hair treatment.
Evening care	Bringing residents to bed, bathing, cleaning teeth and dentures
Meal activities	Preparing meals, setting the table, helping residents with eating, do the dishes.
Medical care	Taking care of wounds, catheterize, medical treatments etc.
General activities	Preparing and doing activities such as pottering, singing, playing games with residents and cleaning up afterwards
Club activities	Preparing and doing social activities in groups (e.g. a choir or bridge-club)
Transfer/transport	Bringing residents to or back from a particular social activities meeting ward or room for general activities or appointments
Reacting to incidents	Taking care of residents in case of extra-ordinary events (e.g. a sudden change in health, aggressive behaviour towards staff)
Additional direct activities	Activities other than those mentioned above such as: buying extra food or clothing or doing the laundry for a particular resident.
Indirect care:	
Consultation	Having consultations on and evaluating the course of matters with residents or caregivers during planned or unplanned meetings.
Administration	Keeping and readjusting patient's files; administration
Schooling	Participating in courses, training and schooling sessions and attending meetings relevant for keeping a specific function up to date.
Handling supplies	Ordering, handling and storing durable and non-durable goods (such as towels, incontinence slips, toilet paper, cleaning products)
Handling food	Ordering and taking care of food, shopping to buy food, storing food supplies, etc.
Handling Medication	Ordering and preparing medication
Cleaning	Cleaning/dusting rooms, bathrooms, hallways, beds
Additional indirect activities	Activities other than those mentioned above such as: making rounds on wards, etc.

Source: based on Paulus *et al.* (2003).

Data-Analysis

SPSS 10.0 was used to file and analyze all data. The analysis proceeded in different steps. First, the type of activities in which the LPN was involved was determined. Per measurement point and per care type, the percentage of the total number of registered activities was calculated for each activity. At T1, for instance, LPNs in nursing home A registered 6225 activities. 83 per cent of these activities was related to various direct care activities (e.g. 10.8 per cent was related to morning care). 17 percent was related to different indirect care activities (e.g. 2.2 percent was related to administration, see Table 3). These percentages indicate the degree of involvement of the LPN in particular activities.

Table 3. Type of activities performed by LPNs and degree of involvement (in percentages)

	Traditional care			Transitional care			Integrated care		
	T1	T2	T3	T1	T2	T3	T1	T2	T3
Direct care activities									
Morning care	10.8	10.0	9.9	7.4	8.9	9.7	5.4	5.3	4.9
Coffee/tea-making	1.8	1.6	1.6	1.5	2.0	2.0	1.9	2.5	2.8
Medication	11.1	11.0	9.9	18.0	13.4	11.3	22.9	14.1	17.1
Toileting	16.1	14.3	14.5	11.6	12.1	9.1	20.3	14.9	15.0
Afternoon care	1.3	1.4	1.2	4.5	5.0	4.3	1.4	3.1	3.7
Extra care	2.1	5.1	5.9	3.1	4.4	3.1	1.9	6.5	5.5
Evening care	15.1	14.4	12.5	8.7	7.7	10.0	5.2	5.5	6.4
Meal activities	6.8	8.2	7.5	12.0	13.0	11.3	10.3	9.7	12.4
Medical care	7.3	3.8	5.2	4.5	3.0	1.9	5.6	4.9	3.2
General activities	0.08	0.12	0.1	0.2	0.3	0.3	0.6	0.1	0.7
Club activities	0.0	0.03	0.01	0.0	0.03	0.03	0	0.04	0.05
Transfer/transport	7.4	11.1	13.8	6.8	6.6	6.7	3.3	1.5	2.4
Reacting to incidents	0.4	0.3	0.5	0.8	1.6	1.0	1.5	1.5	1.1
Additional direct activities	2.7	1.7	2.0	2.4	1.5	2.5	1.5	2.7	2.5
Indirect care activities									
Consultation	6.3	6.4	5.7	8.0	8.2	9.4	10.	14.3	10.7
Administration	2.2	2.9	3.9	3.3	3.6	4.2	3.8	5.8	4.7
Schooling	0.06	0.19	0.04	0.2	0.4	0.2	0	0.3	0.05
Handling supplies	0.05	0.04	0.04	0.1	0.1	0.1	0.1	0.3	0.2
Handling food	0.03	0.10	0.04	0.1	0.07	0.07	0.05	0.1	0.1
Handling Medication	0.3	0.2	0.7	0.4	0.6	1.1	0.3	0.8	0.9
Cleaning	1.5	1.3	1.0	1.7	1.62	4.8	1.8	2.1	2.2
Additional indirect activities	6.6	5.7	4.8	4.7	5.8	6.7	2.0	3.9	3.3
Direct care (in total)	83.0	83.1	83.8	81.5	79.6	73.3	81.9	72.3	77.7
Indirect care (in total)	17.0	16.9	16.2	18.5	20.4	26.7	18.1	27.7	22.3

Second, the average frequency per activity (for somatic and psycho-geriatric residents) per LPN per day was determined. At each measurement point, this frequency was calculated by dividing the total number of registrations per activity by the total number of registration days. A one-sample t-test (α= 5 per cent) was performed to determine whether the average frequencies significantly differed from zero. The average frequencies per activity per LPN per day are summarized in Table 4 for traditional, transitional and integrated care.

Third, the average duration of direct and indirect care for somatic and psycho-geriatric residents per LPN per day was determined for each type of nursing home care (see Table 5). The average duration per day was calculated by dividing the total number of registered minutes per activity (for somatic and psycho-geriatric residents) by the total number of registration days.

Table 4. Average frequency per LPN per day

	Traditional care						Transitional care						Integrated care					
Activity	T1 som	T1 pg	T2 som	T2 pg	T3 som	T3 pg	T1 som	T1 pg	T2 som	T2 pg	T3 som	T3 pg	T1 som	T1 pg	T2 som	T2 pg	T3 som	T3 pg
Morning care	1.8	2.3	1.6	1.9	1.3	2.8	1.8	1.9	1.4	2.3	1.1	2.3	0.9	1.3	0.8	0.7	0.9	0.6
Coffee/tea-making	0.5	0.3	0.5	0.4	0.7	0.4	0.6	0.3	0.6	0.5	0.4	0.6	0.7	0.5	0.6	0.8	1.0	0.5
Medication	2.8	1.0	3.1	1.2	4.7	1.7	5.1	2.7	3.6	1.2	2.7^	1.4	2.4	4.8	2.1	2.1	3.3	1.2^
Toileting	4.4	1.4	3.7	1.6	4.4	2.6	2.9	2.5	2.5	2.6	1.7^	2.0	4.1	3.2	2.4	2.4	3.2	1.6
Afternoon care	0.2	0.3	0.3	0.2	0.5	0.1	1.1	0.8	1.0	0.7	0.8	0.8	0.2	*0.2*	0.4	0.3	0.7	*0.1*
Extra care	0.6	0.2	1.2	0.5	1.5	1.5	1.0	0.4	1.3	0.7	0.8	0.5	0.4	0.2	1.5^	0.7	1.0	0.5
Evening care	2.6	2.7	2.6	2.9	4.3	3.3	1.6	2.8	1.4	1.8	1.2	3.4	0.8	0.9	1.0	0.6	1.7	0.7
Meal activities*	1.5	1.2	1.5	1.7	2.9	1.9	3.6	2.4	3.0	2.1	2.1^	2.7	2.0	2.8	1.6	1.8	2.4	2.0
Medical care	1.5	1.0	0.5^	0.9	1.5	1.2	1.2	1.1	0.7	0.4^	0.4^	0.2^	1.0	0.5	0.8	1.1	0.7	0.2
General activities	*0.0*	*0.0*	*0.0*	0.0	*0.0*	0.0	0.1	0.0	0.1	*0.0*	0.0	*0.0*	*0.1*	*0.2*	0.0	*0.0*	*0.0*	0.3
Club activities	0.0	0.0	*0.0*	*0.0*	*0.0*	0.0	0.0	0.0	*0.0*	0.0	*0.0*	0.0	0.0	0.0	0.0	*0.0*	*0.0*	*0.0*
Transfer/transport	1.6	1.5	2.0	2.2	2.9	4.7^	1.5	2.0	0.8	2.0	0.6^	2.1	0.5	0.8	0.1	0.5	0.3	0.7
Reacting to incidents	0.0	*0.0*	0.0	0.1	0.4	0.1	0.3	0.1	0.3	0.1	0.2	0.2	*0.3*	*0.4*	0.3	*0.4*	0.1	*0.4*
Additional direct activities	0.2	*0.5*	0.1	*0.6*	0.2	0.8	*1.2*	0.3	0.3	0.3	0.6	0.3	0.4	*0.2*	0.4	0.5	0.6	0.3
Total frequency direct care	17.8	12.5	17	14.1	25.2	21.3	22.0	17.4	17.0	14.7	12.8	16.7	13.7	16.0	12.2	12.2	16.0	9.2
Consultation*	1.5	1.3	1.4	1.6	1.6	1.9	2.8	1.6	2.1	1.7	2.0	1.9	1.8	2.1	2.4	2.8	2.9	2.1
Administration	0.3	0.5	0.3	0.7	0.4	1.3	0.7	1.0	0.5	1.1	0.4	1.1	0.3	1.2	0.8	1.0	0.7	1.0

Table 4. Continued

	Traditional care						Transitional care						Integrated care					
Activity	T1 som	T1 pg	T2 som	T2 pg	T3 som	T3 pg	T1 som	T1 pg	T2 som	T2 pg	T3 som	T3 pg	T1 som	T1 pg	T2 som	T2 pg	T3 som	T3 pg
Schooling	*0.0*	*0.0*	*0.1*	*0.0*	0.0	*0.0*	0.1	*0.0*	0.1	*0.0*	0.0	*0.0*	0.0	0.0	*0.1*	*0.0*	*0.0*	0.0
Handling supplies	*0.0*	0.0	*0.0*	*0.0*	*0.0*	*0.0*	0.0	*0.0*	0.0	*0.0*	*0.0*	*0.0*	*0.0*	0.0	*0.1*	*0.0*	*0.1*	*0.1*
Handling food	*0.0*	0.0	*0.0*	*0.0*	*0.0*	*0.0*	*0.1*	*0.0*	*0.0*	0.0	*0.0*	*0.0*	*0.1*	0.0	0.0	*0.1*	*0.1*	0.0
Handling medication	0.2	0.0	*0.0*	*0.0*	0.3	0.1	0.1	0.1	0.1	0.2	0.1	0.4^	*0.1*	*0.0*	*0.2*	*0.1*	0.4	*0.0*
Cleaning	0.5	0.4	0.4	0.3	0.3	0.3	0.8	0.4	0.4	0.4	0.3	0.7	0.5	0.5	0.4	0.5	0.9	0.8
Additional indirect activities	1.5	1.7	1.2	1.6	1.2	1.5	1.0	1.6	1.3	1.9	1.3	1.7	0.2	0.8	0.8	1.5	1.2	1.0
Total frequency indirect care	4.0	3.9	3.4	4.5	3.8	5.1	5.5	4.9	4.6	5.3	4.2	5.9	3.2	4.6	4.8	6.2	6.1	4.9

Som = Somatic residents; PG = Psycho-geriatric residents
^ Significant change in comparison to T1 *Values in italic*: value not significant at alpha = 5% (two-sided test)
* This activity took place at two levels (for an individual resident and for the entire ward). The frequency has been measured at both levels and thus represents an aggregated value.

Table 5. Average duration per LPN per day (in minutes per LPN)

Type of care	Traditional care		Transitional care		Integrated care	
	Som	PG	Som	PG	Som	PG
1. Direct resident care						
T1	126	112	133	124	87	17
T2	145	108	125	114	86	64
T3	181	159	89^	148	102	72
Average T1-T3	*151*	*126*	*116*	*129*	*92*	*51*
2. Indirect care						
T1	139	171	105	121	87	92
T2	126	139	108	127	90	95
T3	111	156	91	145	100	133
Average T1-T3	*125*	*155*	*101*	*131*	*93*	*107*

T1, T2, T3 = First, second, third measurement point, respectively.
^ Significant change in comparison to T1.
Som = Somatic residents; PG = Psycho-geriatric residents.

Then, the duration of all separate direct and indirect activities were added up in order to determine the average duration of direct care and indirect care (in minutes) per LPN per day, respectively.

Finally, per measurement point and per type of resident, we compared the type of activities and the average frequency and duration per care type. In nursing home B, which delivered transitional care, we also compared the activities at T1 (before the introduction of integrated care) with the activities at T2 and T3 (after the introduction of integrated care).

Results

Type of Activities

Table 3 shows the type of activities conducted by LPNs and the degree of involvement in each activity.

The table shows that, to some extent and with respect to several activities, the degree of involvement differed between traditional, transitional and integrated care. The LPN in integrated care, for instance, was less involved in morning care and additional indirect activities and more involved in consultation and administration compared to traditional care and transitional care. Furthermore, LPNs in transitional care and integrated care were more involved in indirect care (on the whole) compared to traditional care. With respect to transitional care, table 3 also shows that, after the introduction of integrated care, the LPN became more involved in indirect care and less involved in direct care. For instance, while 81.5 per cent of all performed activities at T1 were related to direct care, this percentage decreased to 73.3 per cent at T3. This was mainly caused by a decrease in the degree of involvement in medication and toileting. At the same time, involvement increased for all indirect care activities (except for schooling and handling food).

Despite these differences, the LPN did not perform a completely different role with respect to the type of activities. In all care types, more than 72 per cent of the activities were related to direct care. The remaining part was related to indirect care. Additionally, in all care types, the LPN was involved in 22 activities of which 14 were related to direct care and eight to indirect care. In the three care types, the LPN was also more involved in medication, toileting, meal activities, consultations and additional indirect activities and less involved in general activities, club activities, schooling, handling supplies, handling food and handling medication.

Frequency

Table 4 shows the average frequency per LPN per day for traditional, transitional and integrated care. The frequency shows how many times, on average per day, LPNs conducted certain activities for somatic and psycho-geriatric residents. A frequency of 2 for instance indicates that the LPN on average performed this activity twice a day. A frequency of 0.5 indicates that the LPN on average performed this activity once in two days.

The table shows that, to a limited extent, there were differences between the three care types. For instance, at T2, the total frequency of direct care activities was lower in integrated care compared to traditional care and transitional care. Furthermore, at most measurement points, the total frequency of indirect activities was higher in transitional care and integrated care than in traditional care. With respect to transitional care, table 4 also shows that the frequency of activities performed by the LPN changed after the introduction of integrated care. For instance, the total frequency of direct and indirect care for somatic residents became lower.

Nevertheless, there were also similarities with respect to the frequency of the activities performed by the LPN. In all care types, for instance, medication and toileting were activities which were frequently performed for somatic residents. In traditional and transitional care, morning care, evening care, transfer/transport and additional indirect activities were also frequently conducted. In transitional and integrated care, this was also the case for meal activities. Additionally, in all care types, activities with a low frequency included general activities, club activities, schooling, handling supplies and handling food.

Duration

Table 5 shows the average total duration per LPN per day. Duration indicates the average time per day (in minutes) it takes an average LPN to deliver direct care or indirect care to somatic or psycho-geriatric residents.

The table shows that, to a limited extent, there were differences between the three care types. The average duration of direct care and indirect care (both calculated as the average of the durations at T1, T2 and T3) was lower in integrated care compared to traditional and transitional care (see italics in Table 5). The introduction of integrated care in the latter type of care also reduced the average duration of activities for somatic residents (e.g. from 133 minutes at T1 to 89 minutes per day at T3 for direct care) and increased the duration for psycho-geriatric residents (the average duration of direct and indirect care both increased with 24 minutes per day at T3, compared to T1).

In all care types (except for transitional care at T3), however, the duration of direct care for somatic residents was always higher compared to care for psycho-geriatric residents. Additionally, the duration of indirect care was always higher for psycho-geriatric residents.

Furthermore, in all care types, the average duration of indirect care (calculated as the average of the durations at T1-T3) for psycho-geriatric residents outweighed the duration of direct care for these residents (see italics in Table 5).

Conclusions and Discussion

With the aim of finding out if LPNs perform different roles in different types of care, we compared the role of the LPN in traditional, transitional and integrated nursing home care in the Netherlands. Our study showed that the LPN was involved in 22 activities with similar high and low-frequent activities in all types. Comparable patterns in the duration of activities for somatic residents proportionally to psycho-geriatric residents were also found. However, there were also differences between LPNs delivering integrated care and those providing traditional care. The more nursing home care became integrated, the more (frequently) the LPN became involved in indirect care activities (and less in direct activities) and in activities for psycho-geriatric residents. The duration of these activities either decreased (in integrated care and transitional care for somatic residents) or increased (in transitional care for psycho-geriatric residents). It can therefore be concluded that, to a limited extent, LPNs performed different roles in different types of care.

Our findings indicate that the LPN remained a generalist in all types of nursing home care. There are two possible explanations. First, the routine nature of many care activities may explain the low potential for change in these activities [Becker 2004, Van Raak *et al.* 2008b]. Secondly, integrated care requires that a lot of activities have to be geared to one another. Coordination among different providers and activities, however, is more difficult for specialists than for generalists [Paulus *et al.* 2006]. This may explain why the LPN remained a generalist even after the introduction of integrated care. The fact that many parts of the role of the LPN remained unaffected by the type of care is in line with findings from several other studies on care for older people in the Netherlands. These studies show that the impact of emerging care types (such as integrated care) on the work of caregivers in nursing homes is generally limited [Berkhout *et al.* 2004, Finnema *et al.* 2005, Boumans *et al.* 2008]. Not unlike the Netherlands, LPNs in countries such as the United States and the United Kingdom are also involved in direct care and indirect care activities Although this provides some potential for generalization of part of our results, certified/skilled nursing assistants, enrolled nurses or other roles may also perform comparable activities in these countries [Manthey 1989, Deutschendorf 2003, Perry *et al.* 2003, Iley 2004, Kelsey 2006].Our study is limited in the sense that we did not compare the differences or similarities between these roles in- or outside the Netherlands. A comparative study is therefore strongly recommended.

Our findings also indicate that, to a certain extent and for certain residents, the introduction of integrated care seems to affect the frequency and duration of the activities traditionally performed by the LPN as well as the degree of involvement in these activities. Our study is limited by the fact that we did not ask LPNs about their experiences with these changes. We also did not investigate whether emerging care types changed the relation of the LPN with other roles. Several studies demonstrate that the quality of care and resident outcomes are related to a proper mixture of roles [Bostick *et al.* 2006]. Future research on these topics is therefore also recommended.

Despite these limitations, our findings indicate that the future role of the LPN in nursing home care is not expected to become less important in emerging care types. Because of the match between the features of the LPN and the attributes of integrated care (i.e. coordination of activities among all care providers), the role of the LPN as the main generalist may even become a crucial one in the process of successfully delivering integrated care to older people.

Acknowledgments

The authors would like to thank Femke Keijzer for her contribution to the data-collection. Furthermore we are grateful for the financial sources of support that we obtained from the Dutch Ministry of Health; the Province of Limburg; VGZ Insurers; the Boncura Foundation/Care Group 'Noord-Limburg'; the Foundation Stimulating Scientific Research on Nursing Home Care. We also thank Suus Koene for her convenient support.

References

Barber, J., Bland, C., Langdon, M.B., and Michael, S. (2000). LPN role advancement: from blueprints to ribbon cutting. *Journal of Nursing Staff Development*, 16 (3), 112-17.

Becker, M.C. (2004). Organizational routines: A review of the literature. *Industrial and Corporate Change*, 13 (4), 643-78.

Berkhout, A.J.M.B., Boumans, N.P.G., van Breukelen, G.P.J., Huijer Abu-Saad, H., and Nijhuis, F.J.N. (2004). Resident-oriented care in nursing homes: effects on nurses. *Journal of Advanced Nursing*, 45 (6), 621-32.

Bostick, J.E., Rantz, M.J., Flesner, M.K., and Riggs, C.J. (2006). Systematic review of studies of staffing and quality in nursing homes. *Journal of the American Medical Directors Association*, 7 (6), 366-76.

Boumans, N.P.G., Berkhout, A.J.M.B., Vijgen, S.M.C., Nijhuis, F.J.N., and Vasse, R.M. (2008). The effects of integrated care on quality of work in nursing homes: A quasi-experiment. *International Journal of Nursing Studies*, 45 (8), 1122-36.

Coile, R.C. (1995). Integration, capitation and managed care: Transformation of nursing for the 21st century health care. *Advanced Practice Nursing*, 1 (2), 77-84.

Deutschendorff, A. L. (2003). From past paradigms to future frontiers. Unique care delivery models to facilitate nursing work and quality outcomes. *Journal of Nursing Administration*, 33 (1), 52-9.

Faithfull, S., and Hunt, G. (2005). Exploring nursing values in the development of a nurse-led Service. *Nursing Ethics*, 12 (5), 440-52.

Finnema, E., Dröes, R-M, Ettema, T., Ooms, M., Adèr H., Ribbe, M., and van Tilburg, W. (2005). The effect of integrated emotion-oriented care versus usual care on elderly persons with dementia in the nursing home and on nursing assistants: a randomized clinical trial. *International Journal of Geriatric Psychiatry*, 20 (4), 330-43.

Hay, C.L. (2004). Leading towards the future: Implementing nursing leadership. *Canadian Journal of Nursing Leadership*, 17 (2), 69-81.

Iley, K. (2004). Occupational changes in nursing: the situation of enrolled nurses. *Journal of Advanced Nursing*, 45 (4), 360-70.

Jooste, K. (2004). Leadership: A new perspective. *Journal of Nursing Management*, 12 (3), 217-23.

Kelsey, L.R. (2006). Use 'em or lose 'em: The licensed practical nurse. *Gastroenterology Nursing*, 29 (1), 37-41.

Kümpers, S. (2005). *Steering Integrated Care in England and the Netherlands: The Case of Dementia Care.* Printpartners Ipskamp, Enschede. Manthey, M. 1989. The role of the LPN or…the problem of two levels. *Nursing Management*, 20 (2), 26-8.

Paulus, A, Boumans, N., Keijzer, F., Vijgen, S., and Mur, I. (2003). Geïntegreerde vraaggestuurde verpleeghuiszorg. Een longitudinaal en transversaal onderzoek naar de effecten, kosten en het proces van verandering van aanbod- naar geïntegreerde vraaggestuurde vormen van verpleeghuiszorg (Integrated demand-oriented nursing home care. A longitudinal and transversal research of the effects, costs and process of changing from supply-oriented towards integrated demand-oriented types of nursing home care). Maastricht: University of Maastricht.

Paulus, A., van Raak, A., and Keijzer, F. (2005). Informal and formal caregivers' involvement in nursing home care activities: impact of integrated care. *Journal of Advanced Nursing*, 49 (4), 354-66.

Paulus, A., van Raak, A., and Keijzer, F. (2006). Nursing home care: whodunit? *Journal of Clinical Nursing*, 15 (11), 1426-39.

Paulus, A., and van Raak, A. (2008). The impact of integrated care on direct nursing home care. *Health Policy*, 85 (1), 45-59.

Paulus, A., van Raak, A., and Maarse, H. (2008). Is integrated nursing home care cheaper than traditional care? A cost comparison. *International Journal of Nursing Studies*, 45 (12), 1764-77.

Perla, L. (2002). The future role of nurses. *Journal for Nurses in Staff Development.* 18 (4), 194-97.

Perry, M., Carpenter I., Challis, D., and Hope, K. (2003). Understanding the roles of registered general nurses and care assistants in UK nursing homes. *Journal of Advanced Nursing*, 42 (5), 497-505.

Porter-O'Grady, T. (2003a). A different age for leadership, part 1: New context, new content. *Journal of Nursing Administration*, 33 (2), 105-10.

Porter-O'Grady, T. (2003b). A different age for leadership, part 2: New rules, new roles. *Journal of Nursing Administration*, 33 (3), 173-78.

Reeves, D.L. (1997). A licensed practical nurse/licensed vocational nurse's (LPN/LVN) guide to the changing health care system. *Gastroenterology Nursing*, 20 (20), 54-6.

Richardson, A., and Cunliffe, L. (2003). New horizons: the motives, diversity and future of 'nurse led' care. *Journal of Nursing Management*, 11 (2), 80-4.

SGNA, (2006). Role delineation of the Licensed Practical/Vocational Nurse in Gastroenterology. *Society of Gastroenterology Nurses and Associates (SGNA)*, 29 (1), 60-1.

Sherman, A., Bohlander, G., and Snell, S. (1998). *Managing Human Resources.* South Western College Publishing (11th edition), Cincinnati.

Valanis, B. (2000). Professional nursing practice in an HMO: the future is now. *The Journal of Nursing Education*, 39 (10), 13-20.

Van der Windt, W., Arnold, E., and F. Keulen (2007), Regiomarge 2007. De arbeidsmarkt van verpleegkundigen, verzorgenden en sociaal-agogen 2007-2011 (The labour market for nurses and social workers 2007-2001). Utrecht: Stichting Prismant.

Van Raak, A., Mur-Veeman, I., Hardy, B., Steenbergen, M., and Paulus, A. (eds) (2003) *Integrated Care in Europe. Description and Comparison of Integrated Care Delivery and its Context in Six EU Countries*. Reed Business Information, Maarssen.

Van Raak, A., Paulus, A., and Groothuis, S. (2008a), Integrated care delivery: process redesign and the role of rules, routines and transaction costs. In: Klein, L.A. and Neumann E.L. (eds), *Integrated Health Care Delivery*, Nova Science Publishers, Inc., Hauppage NY, 115-35.

Van Raak, A., Paulus, A., Cuijpers, R., and Te Velde, C. (2008b), Problems of integrated palliative care: A Dutch case study of routines and cooperation in the region of Arnhem, *Health and Place*, 14 (4), 768-778.

Williams, A., McGee, P., and Bates, L. (2001). An examination of senior nursing roles: challenges for the NHS. *Journal of Clinical Nursing*, 10 (2), 195-203.

In: Palliative and Nursing Home Care
Editor: Samuel E. Plunkett

ISBN 978-1-61122-417-7

Chapter 6

Special Considerations for Providing Care for Obese Nursing Home Residents

Holly C. Felix[1], Christine Bradway[2], Irene Fleshner[3], Amy Heivly[3] and Lawrence S. Powell[4]

[1]Fay W. Boozman College of Public Health
University of Arkansas for Medical Sciences
Little Rock, AR, USA
[2]School of Nursing, University of Pennsylvania
Urology Health Specialists, Philadelphia, PA, USA
[3]Genesis HealthCare Corporation, Kennett Square, PA, USA
[4]College of Business, University of Arkansas at Little Rock
Little Rock, AR, USA

Abstract

The demographics and care needs of nursing home residents in the United States (US) are changing. Nursing homes are now seeing increasing numbers of obese (body mass index [BMI] $\geq$ 30) persons seeking long-term care. Current estimates indicate approximately 25% of nursing home residents are obese, and this percentage is likely to increase as rates of obesity among the US pre-elderly (55-64 years of age) and elderly ($\geq$65 years of age) population increases. The experience of providing care for obese patients in hospital settings reveals that obese patients often have complex medical profiles with multiple co-morbidities, unique care needs, and greater health care resource utilization. Emerging research reveals that the differences in the process of care between obese and non-obese patients experienced in hospital settings persists into nursing home settings and presents unique care challenges for the long-term care system, such as the need for bariatric medical supplies and equipment, increased staffing levels, and greater personal care assistance. This chapter will review this emerging research on the long-term care needs of obese persons in the US, present several case studies to highlight specific care needs of obese residents around continence care and bathing, review best practices and OSHA worker safety recommendations for patient handling, and conclude with the description of a model program to provide quality care for obese nursing home residents (developed and implemented at Genesis Healthcare Corporation).

Introduction

More than 1.5 million persons currently reside in nursing homes in the US. The average nursing home resident is at least 75 years old, white, female, and resides in the facility for 835 days. About 20% of persons enter nursing homes for short periods of time (less than 90 days) for recuperation or rehabilitation. More than half of residents require extensive assistance with the five basic activities of daily living – bathing, dressing, toileting, transferring, and eating.[1] In the last quarter of the 20th Century, reductions in rates of disability among older Americans have been observed, resulting in lower rates of long-term care usage. However, current forecasts suggest that a reversal of that trend will occur, leading to higher rates of long-term care usage in the future.[2] Certainly, the aging of those in the Baby Boom Generation will increase demand for home and community-based and institutional long-term care services in the immediate future;[2] however, one of the key factors that will also drive this forecasted demand trend is obesity.[3] Although obesity impacts the delivery of home and community-based long-term care services, the purpose of this chapter is to discuss the issues and challenges of providing long-term care services to obese persons residing in nursing homes.

Obesity Epidemic in the US

The proportion of Americans who are considered obese has been steadily increasing over the last 40 years. Obesity and other weight categories are defined by ranges of the BMI, which is a standardize measure of weight categories based on the ratio of weight and height. It is calculated by dividing weight (in kilograms) by height (in measures) squared.[4] See Table 1. Results of the first National Health and Nutrition Examination Survey conducted between 1960 and 1961 indicated about 13.7% of adults in the US were obese.[5] By 2008, one-third (33.8%) of adults in the US were obese and another third (34.2%) were overweight.

Table 1. Weight Categories and Corresponding Body Mass Index (BMI) Ranges

Weight Category	BMI Range
Underweight	<18.5
Normal Weight	18.5–24.9
Overweight	25.0–29.9
Obesity I	30.0–34.9
Obesity II	35.0–39.9
Obesity III	>40.0

Source: NHLBI. [4].

This US obesity epidemic has been well covered in the popular media. Since 2000, the number of newspaper articles published on obesity has increased significantly.[6] It has also been extensively covered the scientific literature.[7] However, most media and scientific coverage of obesity is focused on its prevalence and impact among children and younger adults; yet, the obesity epidemic also affects older adults. In 1960-61, 18.0% of persons 60-69 years of age and 15.7% of persons 70-79 years of age were obese.[5] By 2007-08, 33.6% of persons ≥ 60 years of age were obese.[8] Researchers have projected that the prevalence of obesity among persons ≥ 60 years of age will be as high as 40% by the end of 2010.[9]

The great concern with the obesity epidemic is the burden it presents to individuals and society alike. A well established body of literature has identified a wide range of chronic conditions and diseases associated with obesity, and is not fully reviewed here.[4, 10] However, in general, research has identified type 2 diabetes, cardiovascular disease, hypertension, stroke, osteoarthritis and some cancers to be associated with obesity. For example, using data from the third National Health and Nutrition Examination Survey, Must and colleagues found that the prevalence ratios of type 2 diabetes, high blood pressure, gallbladder disease, and osteoarthritis increase as overweight or obesity increases in both men and women.[11] Similarly, analysis of Behavior Risk Factor Surveillance Survey System data found extremely obese (BMI ≥ 40) individuals had substantially higher odds of having diabetes (OR=7.4), high blood pressure (OR=6.4), asthma (OR=2.7), high cholesterol (OR=1.9), arthritis (OR=4.4) and fair to poor health status (OR=4.2) in comparison to their normal weight peers after controlling for age, education, smoking status, gender, and race/ethnicity.[12] Among older individuals aged 50-76 years, there were significant, positive associations between increasing levels of obesity and a high number and wide range of health conditions for men and women.[13]

Many are aware of the before mentioned associations between obesity and many chronic health conditions. Fewer are aware of the association between obesity and functional limitations; yet, research shows that obesity is also related to declines in cognitive and physical functioning. Goropse and Dave conducted a systemic review of eight longitudinal population-based studies published between 1995 and 2005 that examined the connection between obesity and dementia. They concluded that increased BMI independently increases the risk of dementia as supported by the findings of the studies they reviewed.[14] An association has also been detected between obesity and Alzheimer's disease (AD). A study by Whitmer et al examined the risk of both AD and vascular dementia later in life among persons who were obese at midlife compared to persons who were normal weight at midlife (study n=10,136). After controlling for age, education, race, gender, marital status, smoking, hyperlipidemia, hypertension, diabetes, ischemic heart disease and stroke, persons obese at midlife were 3.1 times more likely to have AD and five times more likely to have vascular dementia than persons of normal weight at midlife [15].

Obesity is also associated with functional decline. Using data from the Asset and Health Dynamics Among the Oldest Old (AHEAD) survey, Jenkins found that obesity was independently associated with strength loss, lower body mobility impairment, and the inability to perform activities of daily living (ADL) (e.g. grooming and dressing, and transferring) and instrumental activities of daily living (IADL) (e.g. using the telephone and preparing meals) among older (≥70 years) adults living in the community.[16] In addition, Strum et al determined that the probability of having ADL limitations increases 50% for moderately obese men and 100% for severely obese women; and the probability of IADL limitations increases 200% for severely obese men and 400% for severely obese women.[3] The high rate of obesity and the association between obesity and cognitive and functional decline should be of particular concern for the long-term care system as cognitive and functional limitations are primary reasons for nursing home placement, and for society as nursing home care is primarily paid for with public funds. In fact, research has now shown an association between obesity and nursing home placement. Elkins et al used data from nearly 9,000 members of a medical care insurance plan to identify characteristics at midlife that were associated with nursing home admission later in life. They found that obesity in midlife independently predicted admission to a nursing home some 25 years later, even after controlling for co-morbid conditions, with the odds of later life nursing home admission being 30% higher among individuals obese at midlife compared to those of normal weight at midlife.[17]

Current Estimates of Obesity in Nursing Homes

Weight-related characteristics of nursing home residents are not regularly reported, resulting in limited information on the proportion of current nursing home residents who are obese. However, two studies provide some evidence, both of which used the Minimum Data Set (MDS). The MDS contains federally required assessments of all US nursing home residents and enables the federal Centers for Medicare and Medicaid Services to monitor socio-demographic and health related characteristics, including height and weight which can be used to calculate BMI, as well as physical and cognitive changes of residents and quality indicators of nursing homes.[18] Lapane and Resnik assessed obesity rates among residents in nursing homes in five states (Kansas, Maine, Mississippi, New York, and South Dakota). They found that 15% of residents were obese in 1992; however, the prevalence of obesity among nursing home residents increased to 25% by 2002.[19] Felix examined obesity rates among elderly nursing home residents newly admitted to nursing homes in Arkansas and documented the prevalence rate of obesity to be 15%.[20] The single state examination may be responsible for the lower prevalence rate. Felix also documented that newly admitted obese elders were significantly younger (~4 years) than newly admitted non-obese elders and have significantly more need for assistance from two or more persons to perform ten ADLs than non-obese persons.[20]

Nursing Home Care for Obese Residents

Little is known about caring for obese nursing home residents; however, the experience of caring for obese persons in hospital settings provides evidence of special considerations that may be required for care of obese nursing home residents. In two separate studies, hospital-based nurses have reported significant challenges in providing care for obese patients, which include increased staff time and more staff numbers for basic care.[21] For example, in a field study conducted at a large hospital affiliated with an academic medical center, Rose et al observed nursing staff providing bathing and walking assistance to obese (n=30) and non-obese (n=30) patients. They found that significantly ($p<0.01$) more total staff time was required for the bathing of obese patients compared to the bathing of non-obese patients (63.8 minutes vs 45.1 minutes) and to assist obese patients in walking compared to non-obese patients (99.6 minutes vs 20.6 minutes).[22] However, another study of hospital nurses reported that algorithms used to set staffing levels in hospitals do not account for the prevalence of obesity among the patient population and inadequate staffing levels produce safety issues for both obese patients and the nursing staff.[21] Other studies have shown that increased body weight and differences in metabolism can affect the therapeutic benefit of certain medications and can require individualized medication dosage adjustments to ensure therapeutic benefit while avoiding drug toxicity for the obese patient.[23, 24] Likewise, there are issues related to proper nutrition. Finally, poor vascularization in adipose tissue, fungal infections in skin folds, and improperly sized hospital beds can increase the risk for pressure ulcers among obese patients and special precautions are necessary to care for the skin of obese patients.[24-26] These issues – staffing requirements, medication management and pressure ulcer risk – among others, are likely to be issues that are encountered in nursing home settings as well.

Hospital settings also provide some evidence of structural factors which can affect the care of obese patients. In a survey of nurses across inpatient, outpatient and community practice settings (n=109), 33% of all nurses and 36% of hospital-based nurses reported the lack of specialized bariatric equipment was a significant barrier to providing quality care to obese patients. A third of hospital-based nurses also reported that attitudes of nurses were a significant barrier for quality care for obese patients.[27] Although nurses' attitudes were not specifically defined in that study by Drake et al, it is most likely prejudicial or negative attitudes toward obese patients, as negative attitudes have been documented among nurses in other studies. [28] An emerging body of research is providing some indication of the experience of providing care for obese persons residing in nursing homes. Using nursing home resident assessment data, Felix found that newly admitted obese nursing home residents were significantly more likely than their non-obese peers to require two or more persons to assist with bed mobility, transfer, walking in their room, walking in halls, locomotion on unit, locomotion off unit, dressing, toileting, personal hygiene and bathing, after controlling for age, gender, race, admission year, and other health conditions (ps >0.01).[20] Bradway et al conducted the first known study to explore and describe the care practices employed by nursing home staff for the continence care needs of obese residents. They identified three themes as it relates to providing continence care to obese nursing home residents: "obese and incontinent day to day", "fitting in the environment, and "it's rough…but we want to do it.". The "day to day" theme related primarily to resident experiences including social isolation, preferences related to catheterization, bathing, and skin challenges. The "fitting in" theme related to the limited physical space in resident rooms to attend to obese residents using necessary equipment and products, and higher numbers of staff. Finally, the third theme related to the time and physical demand required of staff to manage urinary and fecal incontinence issues of obese residents. [29] The following two case studies illustrate some of the challenges nursing home staff may encounter when providing regular personal care for obese nursing home residents:

Case Study One -- Incontinence Care

Bradway and colleagues conducted a mixed methods study to explore current continence related care practices for obese nursing home residents.[29] The study collected observational and experiential data which is used here to describe the experience of one obese nursing home resident in receiving care for bladder and bowel incontinence. In this case, the resident is a 75 year old female with a BMI of 53.4. This resident reported that she is transferred out of bed to a geriatric chair each day by certified nursing aides (CNAs) who use a Hoyer lift because the resident cannot weight bear or transfer. This process requires two to three staff members. The resident had previously had an indwelling catheter but now wears an adult absorbent brief because she cannot use the toilet or a bedside commode. Because the brief is too small given her size, it is not properly fastened and the sharp plastic closure tabs lie against her skin and scratch and stick her. The resident reported a history of constipation and loose bowels which was problematic for her because it was so difficult to transfer her for a bowel movement and harder to clean her after a bowel movement. The resident also described having to sit in a soiled brief for extended periods of time before staff were available to transfer her back to bed to change her brief and had experienced some skin problems as a result. In fact, the resident also noted that she was often being faced with the decision of staying out of bed for an extended period of time (from 11:00am to 7:00pm) and risk sitting in a soiled brief versus staying out of bed for a shorter period of time (11:00am to 4:00pm) and thereby decreasing her risk of having an episode of urinary or fecal incontinence or if she did experience incontinence, having the soiled brief remain in place for a shorter period of time.

Case Study Two – Bathing

The study examining the incontinence care of obese nursing home residents conducted by Bradway et al[29] recorded the experience of nursing home staff in showering a morbidly obese nursing home resident. In this case, a 72 year male with a BMI of 50.2 was provided a shower that required two CNAs a combined total of 105 minutes of staff time. Specifically, the showering process entailed one CNA administering a modified bed bath and readying the obese resident for transfer to a shower stretcher using a Hoyer lift. The room was also rearranged to allow space for the Hoyer lift and the shower stretcher. A second CNA was called to assist the first CNA in transferring the obese resident to the shower stretcher and transport the obese resident to the shower room. After completing the shower, the first CNA called for the second CNA to assist in transporting the obese resident back to his room. Because the Hoyer lift pad remained under the obese resident during the showering process, the two CNAs had to mop a significant amount of water from the room floor after completing the transfer. The first CNA applied anti-fungal power in the groin folds and deodorant, and dressed the resident.[30, 31]

Special Considerations for Caring for Obese Nursing Home Residents

A review of the scientific literature published between 1990 and 2007 conducted by Bradway and colleagues found little evidence to guide optimal care for obese nursing home residents.[32] However, the two case studies, emerging literature (published since 2007) on challenges in providing care to obese nursing home residents as well as the literature on providing care for obese hospital patients highlight care challenges and provide some guidance for nursing homes. The following discussion highlights some of the critical areas in which nursing homes may need to make special considerations in order to meet the needs of current and potential residents who are obese:

Admission Assessments

Nursing homes must be able to meet the individual care needs of all their residents. Most nursing homes use a pre-placement assessment to determine admission appropriateness. In this process, admissions personnel consider the specific needs of the potential resident as well as the nursing home's current capabilities to meet those needs.[33, 34] The pre-placement assessment process should include components that assess the specialized needs of potential residents who are obese to determine if the nursing home is equipped and staffed to meet their bariatric-specific care needs. Some nursing homes, including those operated by Genesis Healthcare Corporation (GHC), one of the largest providers of nursing home care in the US, have developed an addendum to their standard pre-admission assessment which determines potential residents' specific bariatric-related care needs. If the pre-admission assessment identifies a bariatric-related need for which the GHC nursing home cannot respond, the potential resident who is obese is referred to another nursing home within the GHC system that can meet her/his individual care needs.[35] However, some obese individuals seeking admission may find themselves without access to needed long-term care if nursing homes cannot meet their needs or find an alternative facility that can.[34]

Staffing

Previous research showing an association between staffing levels and quality of care prompted the federal government (under the Omnibus Budget Reconciliation Act of 1987) and states to pass regulations imposing minimum staffing levels for nursing homes.[36, 37] These staffing regulations do not take into account the case mix of the nursing home or the prevalence of obesity among nursing home residents. Yet, the day to day care of an obese resident may require higher staff levels than required by state and/or federal regulations given the extensive assistance obese residents require to perform basic ADLs compared to non-obese residents.[20, 35] For example, as illustrated in Case Study Two, up to 105 minutes of total staff time may be required to bathe one obese nursing home resident. With facilities having an average of 96 residents,[38] extensive time to care for one resident may reduce the time available for caring for other residents. Nursing homes administrators may need to develop and use special staffing algorithms which consider the case mix of their nursing home as well the prevalence of obesity among residents in order to ensure there are adequate numbers of staff to meet the needs of all residents.

Some doctors, nurses and other health care workers have been found to hold prejudicial or negative attitudes toward obese patients and such attitudes negatively affected the care they provided.[28, 39, 40] A survey of hospital-based nurses found that one-third thought attitudes of nurses were a significant barrier for quality care for obese patients.[27] Given this experience in other care settings, it is probable that some nursing home staff may also have negative opinions of obesity which could affect resident outcomes; however, no known study has made such an assessment. Nevertheless, nursing homes should consider developing a bariatric sensitivity training program and require staff who provide direct care to obese nursing home residents to complete the training. Vacek provides guidance for positive interactions between nursing staff and obese patients -- such as being thoughtful with comments so they cannot be misinterpreted as obesity-related insults and record weights in private and without comment -- which could be incorporated into sensitivity training programs to be offered to nursing home staff.[41]

Environmental Modifications, Equipment and Supplies

State and federal regulations govern the size of nursing home resident rooms.[42] These regulations do not specify space requirements for resident rooms for obese persons. However, additional space as well as bariatric furniture and fixtures in common areas and in at least some resident rooms within nursing homes are necessary to accommodate obese residents. Some hospitals are allotting three[43] to five feet[44] on both sides of hospital beds to provide adequate space for lift equipment and extra nursing staff that may be needed to provide care for obese patients. In the absence of specific requirements for room space for obese nursing home residents, these hospital space allowances may serve as a guideline for nursing homes. In some cases, this may require the conversion of a standard double occupancy resident room to a single occupancy bariatric resident room. In addition, doorways and hallways need to be sufficiently wide to accommodate bariatric wheelchairs and stretchers.

In addition to room space, furnishings and fixtures in resident rooms (e.g. bed, bedside chair), bathrooms (e.g. wall mounted commode, wall railings) and common areas (e.g. dining table and chairs, lounge furniture) should also accommodate obese residents. Standard furniture and medical equipment typically has a maximum weight limit of 250 to 300 pounds. However, this weight maximum may be insufficient to accommodate a morbidly obese person seeking admission to a nursing home. The Joint Commission for the Accreditation of Healthcare Facilities has recommended that at least 10% of all hospital furniture accommodate bariatric patients.[45] Nursing homes could adopt this recommendation in furnishing the facility to ensure the needs of obese residents are met.

Medical equipment and supplies, such as blood pressure cuffs, wheelchairs, bedside commodes, stretchers, continence care products, and gowns and clothing, appropriate for use with obese residents should also be available.

Lift Policies

Health care workers, including nursing home staff, are at high risk for workplace injury and illness.[46] Although at least one study investigating the rates of injuries among nursing home aides did not find obesity to be a risk factor for shoulder and/or back injury,[47] the increasing rates of obesity within nursing homes[19] and the extensive assistance obese residents require to perform ADLs[20] should raise concern for nursing home administrators about potentially increasing rates of work-related injuries associated with caring for obese residents.

Specific evidence-based guidelines for handling obese nursing home residents are not known. However, the Occupational Health and Safety Administration recommends that nursing homes minimize the lifting of all residents – which would include obese residents -- whenever possible.[48] Minimal lift / no-lift policies require the availability of mechanical lift equipment. Such equipment should have weight allowances sufficient to accommodate obese residents. Furthermore, best practices for the safe handling of obese patients in hospital settings as well as the experience of some nursing homes can provide guidance to other nursing homes in this area.

The safe handling recommendations developed by the National Association of Bariatric Nurses include common elements such as staff training in safe lifting practices and use of lift equipment with bariatric patients, establishing lift protocols, and using proper assistive and lift equipment. However, they also recommend a multidisciplinary approach as "no one person or group has all the answers" and insist on effective communication among staff to ensure all staff are knowledgeable and aware of resident needs and available lift assistance equipment (including weight limits on such equipment).[49] A significant amount of work has been conducted by staff of the US Department of Veterans Affairs in the development of a Bariatric Patient Safe Handling Toolkit, which is available online.[50] Although developed for a hospital setting, many aspects of the toolkit, including handling algorithms, the equipment checklist, and a policy template may be applicable to the nursing home setting.

Skin Care

Obese nursing home residents, especially those with limited mobility, present specific skin care challenges for nursing home staff. Poor vascularization in adipose tissue, moisture in skin folds, and pressure or rubbing from medical appliances (e.g. catheter tubes and bed railings) elevate risks for pressure ulcers in obese persons.[25] For example, a federal report investigating nursing home quality reported that an obese person newly admitted to a nursing home with no pressure ulcers had four stage II ulcers and three stage I ulcers within 7 days due to the nursing home staff's inability to turn the obese resident due to the inappropriately sized bed and mattress that did not facilitate turning.[51]

To address this risk, nursing homes should develop special skin care protocols specific for obese residents. The National Association of Bariatric Nurses developed evidence-based skin care guidelines for morbidly obese persons based on a review of the published literature on the subject.[52] Nursing homes should consider reviewing and adapting these guidelines for use in nursing homes. Nursing home staff should also be given specific training on the skin care for obese residents.

Development of Model Obese Nursing Home Resident Care Program

In response to the specialized care needs of obese hospital patients, an interdisciplinary team in a large trauma center developed a comprehensive protocol which listed specific care needs of obese patients and provided guidance for hospital staff in managing their care. They published a template based on their protocol for other hospitals to adapt for their own use.[53] Although the protocol was designed for hospitalized patients, it covers many topics (e.g. skin care, respiratory care, and mobility) of likely interest to nursing homes and may provide a template for adaption for such facilities.

GHC has developed a six component model to address the care needs of obese nursing home residents. The model includes a specialized pre-admission assessment (see above), a staff injury reduction program, a bariatric education protocol, bariatric equipment inventory standards, environmental modifications, and higher staffing ratios. Although GHC has experienced some positive outcomes (e.g. reductions in worker' compensations costs associated with resident handling), there is a need to fully evaluate the model.[35] Nevertheless, it serves as a guide for other nursing homes interested in developing a bariatric care program.

Public Policy Considerations

Given the myriad special considerations we suggest are necessary in caring for obese nursing home residents, there are clearly substantial increases in cost associated with such care. These increased costs present significant challenges for nursing homes now and in the future as the US population grows older and larger. This problem is exacerbated in an economic context because, unlike costs, daily reimbursement rates do not vary systematically with size of the resident. This presents a classic example of increasing demand (obesity) with unchanging supply (reimbursement). Without question, such a scenario left unchecked will lead to unnatural scarcity in the supply of care for obese nursing home residents.

If a facility earns greater profits by declining to admit obese residents, and prospective residents are able to assess quality before entering a facility, the best facilities will not be available to obese residents. While private markets have built in mechanisms to mitigate scarcity problems, the large role of public funding in long-term care leaves all consumers vulnerable to obesity as a negative externality. In this setting, we could expect a substantial difference in available long-term care resources by levels of income and wealth. In addition, this difference could manifest across levels of obesity, where potential residents are matched to scarce nursing home beds by a sorting process of weight. In the latter scenario, obese residents would receive inferior care as lighter members of their cohort select the highest quality facilities.

More research is needed in this area to measure the cost of care for obese nursing home residents and to develop and test policy and programmatic interventions that could mitigate problems associated with obesity in the delivery of long-term care.

Conclusion

The US long-term care system is seeing increasing numbers of persons seeking care who are obese and it is likely that this trend will continue and may accelerate as the proportion of elderly in the US population increases. The experience of providing health care to obese patients in hospital settings and emerging research on providing long-term care to obese nursing home residents reveals that obese persons have unique care needs that often present significant challenges to their care environments. These unique care needs also raise questions about access to long-term care, quality of long-term care, and the cost of long-term care for obese persons needing such care.

This discussion highlighted some of the critical areas in which nursing homes may need to make special considerations in order to provide optimal care for obese residents. Other areas of caregiving consideration include nutrition, medication management, best practice guidelines for continence care, access to socialization and recreation activities, and behavioral and mental health issues. Although additional research is needed in this area to develop and test specific care protocols for obese nursing home residents as well as research into the cost of providing such care, some of the protocols and guidelines developed for the care of obese persons in hospital settings and reviewed here may provide some assistance to nursing homes in this area.

References

[1] Jones A, Dwyer L, Bercovitz A, Strahan G. The National Nursing Home Survey: 2004 overview. *Vital Health Statistics* 2009; 13.

[2] Lakdawalla D, Goldman DP, Bhattacharya JM, Hurd MD, Joyce GF, Panis CWA. Forecasting the nursing home population. *Medical Care* 2003; 41:8-20.

[3] Strum R, Ringel J, Andreyeva T. Increasing obesity rates and disability trends. *Health Affairs* 2004; 23:199-205.

[4] NHLBI Obesity Education Initiative Expert Panel on the Identification, Evaluation and Treatment of Overweight and Obesity in Adults. *Clinical guidelines on the identification, evaluation and treatment of overweight and obesity in adults: The evidence report*. Washington DC: National Institutes of Health, 1998.

[5] Flegal K, Carroll M, Kuczmarski R, Johnson C. Overweight and obesity in the United States: prevalence and trends, 1960-1994. *International Journal of Obesity* 1998; 22:39-47.

[6] Sullivan K, McDivitt J, Melcher C, Brunner S. Getting the skinny on obesity: A content analysis of newspaper coverage of obesity from 2000 to 2006 (APHA Abstract #160469). American Public Health Association Annual Meeting. Washington, DC, 2007.

[7] Vioque J, Ramos J, Navarrete-Muñoz E, García-de-la-Hera M. A bibliometric study of scientific literature on obesity research in PubMed (1988-2007). *Obesity Research* 2010; 11:603-11.

[8] Flegal K, Carroll M, Ogden C, Curtin L. Prevalence and trends in obesity among US adults, 1999-2008. *Journal of the American Medical Association* 2010; 303:235-41.

[9] Arterburn D, Crane P, Sullivan S. The coming epidemic of obesity in elderly Americans. *Journal of the American Geriatrics Society* 2004; 52:1907-12.

[10] Villareal D, Apovian C, Kushner R, Klein S. Obesity in older adults: technical review and position statement of the American Society for Nutrition and NAASO, The Obesity Society. *American Journal of Clinical Research* 2005; 82:923-34.

[11] Must A, Spadano J, Coakley E, Field A, Colditz G, Dietz W. The disease burden associated with overweight and obesity. *Journal of the American Medical Association* 1999; 282:1523-9.

[12] Mokdad A, Ford E, Bowman B, al e. Prevalence of obesity, diabetes and obesity related health risk factors, 2001. *Journal of the American Medical Association* 2003; 289:76-9.

[13] Patterson R, Frank L, Kristal A, White E. A comprehensive examination of health conditions associated with obesity in older adults. *American Journal of Preventive Medicine* 2004; 27:385-90.

[14] Gorospe E, Dave J. The risk of dementia with increased body mass. *Age and Ageing* 2007; 36:23-9.

[15] Whitmer R, Gunderson E, Quesenberry C, Zhou J, Yaffe K. Body mass index in midlife and risk of Alzheimer disease and vascular dementia. *Current Alzheimer Research* 2007; 4:103-9.

[16] Jenkins K. Obesity's effects on the onset of functional impairment among older adults. *The Gerontologist* 2004; 44:206-16.

[17] Elkins J, Whitmer R, Sidney S, Sorel M, Yaffe K, Johnston S. Midlife obesity and long-term risk of nursing home admission. *Obesity* 2006; 14:1472-8.

[18] Wunderlich G, Kohler P. *Improving the Quality of Long-term Care*. Washington, DC: National Academy Press, 2001.

[19] Lapane K, Resnick L. Obesity in nursing homes: An escalating problem. *Journal of the American Geriatrics Society* 2005; 53:1386-91.

[20] Felix H. Personal care assistance needs of obese elders entering nursing homes. *Journal of the American Medical Directors Association* 2008; 9:319-26.

[21] Drake D, Dutton K, Engelke M, McAuliffe M, Rose M. Challenges that nurses face in caring for morbidly obese patients in the acute care setting. *Surgery for Obesity and Related Diseases* 2005; 1:462-6.

[22] Rose M, Baker G, Drake D, Engelke M, McAuliffe M, Pokorny M, Pozzuto S, Swanson M, Waters W, Watkins F. A comparison of nurse staffing requirements for the care of morbidly obese and non-obese patients in the acute care setting. *Bariatric Nursing and Surgical Patient Care* 2007; 2:53-6.

[23] Lee J, Winstead P, Cook A. Pharmacokinetic alterations in obesity. *Orthopedics*, 2006.

[24] Markoff B, Amesterdam A. Impact of obesity on hospitalized patients. *Mount Sinai Journal of Medicine* 2008; 75:454-9.

[25] Mathison C. Skin and wound care challenges in the hospitalized morbidly obese patient. *Wound Care* 2003; 30:78-83.

[26] Gallegher S, Langlois C, Spacht D, Blackett A, Henns T. Preplanning with protocols for skin and wound care in obese patients. *Advances in Skin and Wound Care* 2004; 7:436-43.

[27] Drake D, Baker G, Engekle M, McAuliffe M, Pokorny M, Swanson M, Waters W. Challenges in caring for the morbidly obese: differences by practice setting. *Southern Online Journal of Nursing Research*, 2008:1-12.

[28] Brown I. Nurses' attitudes toward adult patients who are obese: literature review. *Journal of Advanced Nursing* 2006; 53:221-32.

[29] Bradway C, Miller E, Heivly A, Fleshner I. Continence care for obese nursing home residents. *Urologic Nursing* 2010; 30:121-9.

[30] Powell L, Felix H, Bradway C, Miller M, Heivly A, Fleshner I. Additional research on the cost of caring for obese nursing home residents is critical to maintaining adequate resources in the long-term care industry. *Journal of the American Medical Directors Association* 2010; 11:222.

[31] Felix H, Bradway C, Miller E, Heivly A, Fleshner I, Powell L. Obese nursing home residents: A call to research action. *Journal of the American Geriatrics Society*. 58(6):1197-97.

[32] Bradway B, DiResta J, Fleshner I, Polomano R. Obesity in nursing homes: A critical review. *Journal of the American Geriatrics Society* 2008; 56:1528-35.

[33] Allen J. *Nursing Home Administration*. New York: Springer Publishing Company, 2008.

[34] Rotkoff N. Care of the morbidly obese patient in a long-term care facility. *Geriatric Nursing* 1999; 20:309-13.

[35] Bradway C, DiResta J, Miller E, Edmiston M, Fleshner I, Polomano R. Caring for obese individuals in the long-term care setting. *Annals of Long-Term Care* 2009; 17:17-21.

[36] Zhang N, Unruh L, Liu R, Wan T. Minimum nurse staffing ratios for nursing homes. *Nursing Economics* 2006; 24:78-85.

[37] Harrington C. Nursing staffing in nursing homes in the United States. *Journal of Gerontological Nursing* 2005; 32:18-23.

[38] CDC. *National Nursing Home Survey, 2004*. Washington, DC: USDHHS, 2006.

[39] Hebl M, Xu J. Weighing the care: physicians' reactions to the size of a patient. *International Journal of Obesity* 2001; 25:1246-52.

[40] Puhl R, Brownell KD. Bias, discrimination and obesity. *Obesity Research* 2001; 9:788-805.

[41] Vacek L. Sensitivity training for nurses caring for morbidly obese patients. *Bariatric Nursing and Surgical Patient Care* 2007; 2:251-3.

[42] Evashwick C. *The Continuum of Long-term Care*. Clifton Park, NY: Thomson Delmar, 2005.

[43] Muir M, Heese G. Safe patient handling of the bariatric patient: Sharing of experiences and practical tips when using bariatric algorithms. *Bariatric Nursing and Surgical Patient Care* 2008; 3:147-58.

[44] Wignall D. Design as a critical tool in bariatric patient care. *Journal of Diabetes Science and Technology* 2008; 2.

[45] Williams D. Design with dignity: The design and manufacutring of appropraite furniture for the bariatric patient population. *Bariatric Nursing and Surgical Patient Care* 2008; 3:39-40.

[46] BLS. *Workplace injursing and illness -- 2008*. Washington, DC: Bureau of Labor Statistics, 2009.

[47] Myers D, Silverstein B, Nelson N. Predictors of shoulder and back injuries in nursing home workers: A prospective study. *Am. J. Industrial Medicine* 2002; 41:466-76.

[48] OSHA. *Guidelines for Nursing Homes: Ergonomics for the Prevention of Musculoskeletal Disorders*. Washington, DC: US Department of Labor, 2009.

[49] McGinley L, Bunke K. Best practices for safe handling of the morbidly obese patient. *Bariatric Nursing and Surgical Patient Care* 2008; 3:255-60.

[50] VISN 8 Patient Safety Center of Inquiry. *Safe Bariatric Patient Handling Toolkit.* Washington DC: USVA, n.d.

[51] GAO. Nursing home quality: Prevalence of serious problems, while declining, reinforces importance of enhanced oversight. Washington, DC: General Accounting Office, 2003:1-97.

[52] Rose M, Dreosti A. Best practice for skin care of the morbidly obese. *Bariatric Nursing and Surgical Patient Care* 2008; 3:129-34.

[53] Arzouman J, Lacovara J, Blackett A, McDonald P, Traver G, Bartholomeaux F. Developing a comprehensive bariatric protocol: a template for improving patient care. Medsurg nursing: *Official Journal of the Academy of Medical-Surgical Nurses* 2006; 15:21-6.

In: Palliative and Nursing Home Care
Editor: Samuel E. Plunkett

ISBN 978-1-61122-417-7

Chapter 7

Palliative Care and Dementia: Is a Good Death Possible at Home?

Barbara Anderson
Royal District Nursing Service of SA Inc, South Australia

Abstract

Introduction: The suggestion has been made that modern medicine has diverted attention from preparing for death and helping people to die a good death. The branch of medicine which has addressed the care of the dying, palliative medicine, has seemed to give the impression that dying can be dignified through the management of terminal pain. However, many patients dying from cancer and non-cancer diagnoses have a range of symptoms which are less easily managed in old age. The principles of a good death have been outlined and are used to answer the question "Can people with end-stage dementia have a good death at home?"

Conclusion: there are complex issues associated with the care of people with end-stage dementia at home, including the difficulties in prognostication. However, with committed informal carers, supported by appropriately funded home care organisations, and the use of advance care plans to minimise hospital admissions and unnecessarily invasive interventions, the desire of people with end-stage dementia to die a good death at home can be fulfilled.

Introduction

In an editorial in the BMJ addressing the need to help people die a good death, Smith (2000) has suggested that

> modern medicine may even have had the hubris to suggest implicitly, if not explicitly, that it could defeat death. If death is seen as a failure rather than as an important part of life then individuals are diverted from preparing for it and medicine does not give the attention that it should to helping people die a good death. (p 129)

One branch of medicine which has considered dying as an important part of life is palliative medicine. Yet, it has been suggested that the hospice movement has given the impression that dying can always be dignified due to the successful management of terminal pain. Nevertheless, many patients dying from cancer as well as those dying from the end-result of multiple co-morbidities have a range of other symptoms, such as delirium, urinary and faecal incontinence, sores and discharges, which are less easily managed when the body is failing in old age (Kafetz, 2002).

What Are the Principles of a Good Death?

The principles of a good death have been set out as follows:

- To know when death is coming and to understand what can be expected
- To be able to retain control of what happens
- To be afforded dignity and privacy
- To have control over pain relief and other symptom control
- To have choice and control over where death occurs (at home or elsewhere)
- To have access to information and expertise of whatever kind is necessary
- To have access to hospice care in any location, not only in hospital
- To have control over who is present and who shares the end
- To be able to issue advance directives which ensure wishes are respected
- To have time to say goodbye, and control over other aspects of timing
- To be able to leave when it is time to go, and not to have life prolonged pointlessly (Smith, 2000).

However, this view of a good death is not universally accepted. While Jones and Willis (2003) agree that access to good palliative care is important for all, they disagree with this construction of a good death. They acknowledge that if this is the kind of death a patient has specified in an advance directive, this is appropriate, but they question whether everyone wants such a death. They suggest that there should be resources and skills available to facilitate the type of death requested by individual patients (Jones and Willis, 2003).

Can People with End-Stage Dementia Have a Good Death at Home?

To answer this question, a number of the principles of a good death will be examined.

- To know when death is coming and to understand what can be expected

There are no reliable prognostic markers to predict life expectancy of less than 6 months with dementia. Prognosis models that attempt to estimate survival greater than 6 months in non-cancer patients have generally poor discrimination, reflecting the unpredictable nature of most non-malignant disease (Coventry, Grande, Richards and Todd, 2005). Indeed, Lee and Chodosh (2009) observe that in spite of an abundance of data, there is no unifying guideline for dementia prognostication. They highlight the need to create a risk score for dementia which could be helpful for patients and families in reassessing goals of care and possible enrolment in services, such as hospice or palliative care (p 466). Godwin and Waters (2009) observe that end of life dementia care may be delivered over a protracted period during which the patient's terminal status may not be acknowledged and addressed.

Further complicating the difficulty of prognostication in dementia is the lack of recognition that dementia is a terminal illness. For example, dementia is a leading cause of death in the United States (US), but is under-recognised as a terminal illness (Mitchell, Teno, Kiely, Shaffer, Jones, Prigerson, Volicer, Givens and Hamel, 2009). The survival of elderly people afflicted with Alzheimer's disease (AD) is known to be shortened compared with the life expectancy of the US population. In the US, a longitudinal study in 1966 monitored 327 patients diagnosed with probably AD. The rate of death for AD patients was more than double the rate in the general elderly population, when adjusted for age and gender (Wolf-Klein, Pekmezaris, Chin and Weiner, 2007).

Shega and colleagues reported the results of a study, which found that although 70 per cent of families interviewed knew that the patient was dying, prior to their death, more than two thirds of these family members thought that the patient was dying of another cause, rather than dementia (Shega, Levin, Hougham, Cox-Hayley, Luchins, Hanrahan, Stocking and Sachs, 2003).

Although reliable prognostication is difficult, nutritional status has been identified as being an indicator of survival (Schonwetter, Han, Small, Martin, Tope and Haley William E, 2003, p111). They report the findings of a longitudinal study, including 666 patients with AD, in which weight loss is a predictor of mortality, in particular, weight loss of 5 per cent in any year was a significant predictor of mortality. In another study, severe cachexia and severe cognitive impairment were associated with significantly higher mortality. Pneumonia, febrile episodes and eating problems are frequent complications in patients with advanced dementia, which are associated with high 6-month mortality rates (Mitchell *et al.*, 2009).

- To be able to retain control over what happens

The ability to retain control over what happens at end of life is closely related to 2 other aspects of a good death, namely the ability to make advance directives and the time to say goodbye.

The trajectory of the dementia patient is a gradual decline in health status, interspersed by declines caused by acute illness (Sachs, Shega and Cox-Hayley, 2004). Acute illnesses often result in the hospitalisation of people with end-stage dementia. Although negative experiences have been reported when such people had been hospitalised (Treloar, Crugel and Adamis, 2009), it is not necessary the case in all situations.

Case study 1, drawn from a broader study (Anderson, Kralik, March and Briffa, 2010) highlights the importance of appropriate support for people with dementia on admission to hospital, and the need for appropriate legal delegations to be in place such that inappropriate medical interventions can be avoided.

Case Study 1. "A Father's Journey": as related by Carer 4

Dad was diagnosed with Alzheimer's ten and a half years ago. His journey has been very slow. April 12 months ago, he was sitting eating his soup, and he froze. He had the spoon in his hand, but there was no response to me. I waited for quite a considerable period of time, hoping that something would change, then rang my brother and said, 'Dad's not responding; I don't know what's going on.' His wife is a nurse, and so she rang a few places to see what we should do, and I eventually rang my nephew who's a paramedic, and he said, 'Well, why don't you call the ambulance people and they can tell you we should take him to hospital.'

To put him in hospital was really, really hard, because even though he doesn't know who I am, he knows I'm really important. When he was in hospital, he got very, very distressed, very disorientated, very agitated, and didn't sleep and it's just cruel leaving him. However, he was in a special ward where they observe the patients. They have volunteers during the day, and at night time, he was banded so that if he did go out the door, alarms would go off.

The care was very good, and the volunteer section was just brilliant, just very, very caring. There are actually two volunteers in his bay from 8 o'clock in the morning to 8 o'clock at night, who will chat to them, help them eat, and if they start to get up, call a nurse. They have reduced their falls by about 97%, I think.

In March this year, a carer came in and found dad, in his chair, not breathing. An ambulance was called. He'd had a respiratory arrest; his pulse was only 40. Although he has a Palliative Care order, they gave him oxygen and adrenaline and took him off to a different hospital, to which he was admitted. I stayed with him, because they only had a private room and no staff to keep an eye on him. We didn't want a broken leg at that point in time! He did not sleep at all. He ripped out his drip. He was so agitated - he tried to crawl out the doors, the windows, and in the end, spent two hours crawling around the floor, fixing and fiddling with the bed and doing all sorts of things.

One of the doctors in Accident and Emergency had said 'Oh, we might have to put a pacemaker in'. To which I replied, 'Well no, you won't be doing that, we have an Enduring Power of Attorney and Guardianship and he is end-stage dementia'.

In the same study, several carers reported experiencing pressure from hospital personnel about the placement of their husbands in aged care facilities (Anderson *et al.*, 2010). In one situation, hospital personnel made the decision to place the person with dementia in such a facility, without ascertaining the wishes of the carer or the person with dementia, when able to do so:

> ...he had a fall in the bedroom, yet another fall ...[w]e went to the hospital. Now he wasn't hurt physically, but they discovered a urinary tract infection... that plays merry hell with dementia people and he became very aggressive ... it was another 2 or 3 weeks before they attempted to have him assessed. So he was assessed as needing high care, dementia, secure nursing. So it was taken out of my hands. ...[t]hey didn't really ask me [about him coming home], they just said 'this is how it should be'. (Carer 6)

A similar attempt was made to place another person with dementia in an aged care facility, however, their carer resisted the pressure from hospital staff to do so.

> ... there was a big conference at the hospital, trying to persuade me to put him into permanent care … [a]nd I said, 'we're going home'. And once he was home, he kind of came back to better than when he was in hospital. (Carer 9)

While the need for a diagnosis for dementia to allow advance care planning to occur has been highlighted by a number of researchers, including Leifer, 2003, Downs, Clibbens, Rae, Cook and Woods, 2002, the difficulties in addressing this sensitive issue cannot be underestimated. For example, Anderson *et al.*, (2010) report that for most of the carers interviewed, it was not a subject that had been able to be discussed mainly due to the lack of acceptance of the person with dementia of their condition and the all-consuming nature of day-to-day care.

> … [i]n terms of her recognizing her own illness - in the early days she refused to accept it was happening, and would become angry if it was mentioned. So no specifics were ever gone into once the problem arose. (Carer 1)
>
> [advance care planning discussions] there was nothing wrong with him! 'No, No, No', he said 'just a bit of a memory lapse now and then…there's nothing wrong with me'. (Carer 11)
>
> I don't think I was even contemplating that [advance care planning] at that stage… it was more of 'what can I do now?' not 'what will we have to do in the future?' (Carer 18)

The difficulties associated with the lack of advance care plans were reported by Anderson *et al.*, (2010).

> … I find it hard to make decisions for someone else…maybe because … we weren't together that long before this started… he's got 5 children, but they're useless… they don't want to know… so we don't see much of them… back in 2000, I had my first heart attack, so we tried to get a Will made up for [partner], but couldn't do so because he couldn't remember his children's names… there's nothing written down or anything… power of attorney's been passed on to son [name] who is the oldest son … mainly because he used to see most of [name], but in recent years, it's come down to once very 14 months maybe… so I just go ahead…sign the pieces of paper and all that sort of thing and nobody complains…I don't know whether that's good or bad. (Carer 17)

- To have control over pain relief and other symptoms, closely aligned with access to hospice care in any location, not only in hospital.

McCarty and Vollicer (2009) indicate that barriers to utilisation of hospice services was lack of recognition that advanced dementia is a terminal condition.

In the UK, a number of organisations are recorded as caring for patients with advanced cancer. In 1948, the Marie Curie Memorial Foundation opened terminal care homes. Prior to this, in 1911, the Cancer Relief Macmillan Fund was founded by Douglas Macmillan, who had watched his father die of cancer (Gamlin, 2001). Chatterjee (2008) acknowledges that as the philosophy and practice of palliative care has been based in the care of cancer patients, those dying of non-malignant diseases receive less of this type of care (p 29).

Australian data relating to patients admitted for palliative care in 1999-00 reveals that 69 per cent of palliative care separations had a principle diagnosis of cancer (Australian Institute of Health and Welfare (AIHW), 2003). Also, a number of US studies indicate palliative care is regularly provided to people with cancers, but not to people with end-stage dementia. For example, a survey of 796 hospice organizations revealed that 46.3 per cent of deaths were from cancers, 42.4 per cent were from other chronic conditions, and 11.3 per cent were from dementia. However they note that dementia is a leading cause of death in the USA (Mitchell, Kiely, Miller, Connor, Spence and Teno, 2007). Similarly in the UK, there is growing evidence that people with diseases other than cancer, have difficulty accessing specialist palliative care services (Birch and Draper, 2008).

People with end-stage dementia have been identified as having died with a high level of suffering (Aminoff and Adunsky, 2006). Although the principles of palliative care should be applicable to the care of people dying from dementia, many do not receive the same attention to symptom control and discussions about end-of-life care (Armitage and Evans, 2005). Unlike most people dying from cancers, those with end-stage dementia cannot relate their symptoms, which impacts on the assessment and management of their physical and psychological symptoms (Shega and Tozer, 2009).

In the acute setting, older people with a documented diagnosis of dementia, who died in hospital wards were identified as receiving significantly fewer palliative medications or referrals to palliative care teams prior to death (Sampson, Gould, Leed and Blanchard, 2006). Indeed, the care of the person with end-stage dementia is not generally considered to be within the bounds of the majority palliative care units (Lloyd-Williams, 1996).

There appears to be a difference of opinion in the literature about attention paid to palliative care in end-stage dementia. MacPhee and Bickel (2007) suggest that palliative care for dementia has received little attention, but the available literature is said to show its usefulness. They refer to a number of studies which have demonstrated that palliative care for dementia decreases cost, decreases use of inappropriate interventions and increases patient comfort, increases patient and family satisfaction, results in better symptom management and is preferred by patients and families.

However, Hughes, Jolley, Jordan and Sampson (2007) suggest that while the literature relating to palliative care in dementia is growing substantially, there is no generally agreed way in which services should be provided. They cite a review carried out by Sampson, Ritchie, Lai, Raven and Blanchard, (2005) which concluded that evidence of efficacy of palliative care was equivocal. Methodology of studies varied in rigour, however the study with the best methodology (Ahronheim, Morrison, Morris, Baskin and Meier, 2000) did not demonstrate any influence of the palliative care approach on care of patients with dementia in an acute hospital (Hughes *et al.*, 2007).

Roger (2006), who carried out a literature review of palliative care, end-of-life and dementia found that the primary themes were person-centred care, grief, agitation, aggression, pain management, care provision, training and education, decision-making, primary settings of care and spirituality and dignity. On the basis of her review, a number of recommendations were made, including:

- to develop a better understanding of the trajectory and experiences of people with dementia as they progress towards end-of-life
- to support the development of palliative care programs and hospices, with units that focus on the specific issues of those dying with dementia (Roger, 2006, p300).

A review of challenges of delivering effective palliative care to older people with dementia revealed four main themes:

- difficulties associated with diagnosing the terminal phase of the illness
- issues relating to communication
- medical interventions
- the appropriateness of palliative care intervention (Birch and Draper, 2008).

Case study 2. "Palliative care experience in late-stage dementia"
In this case study, a number of issues are highlighted, including:

- inadequate pain relief
- verbal abuse from hospital staff in relation to pain management
- no consultation with family members about care
- protracted, uncertain 'dying' period
- inadequate care provided in hospital
- value of supportive service organizations to allow quality in-home care
- no funding for palliative care services due to uncertain prognosis
- no palliative care services for people with late-stage dementia
- To have choice and control over where death occurs (at home or elsewhere)

While dying at home is the preferred location for many people, how many people with dementia actually there?

In the US, a number of studies have highlighted that the majority of dementia-related deaths occur in nursing homes. For example, one study revealed that the majority of dementia-related deaths (66.9%) occurred in nursing homes whereas the majority of older persons with cancer died at home (37.8%) or in a hospital (35.4%) (Mitchell, Teno, Miller and Mor, 2005).

In Australia, guidelines for the care of patients with dementia in general practice have been produced (NSW Department of Health, 2003). With respect to leaving home, these guidelines suggest that "institutionalisation offers the best duration of survival for people with dementia, survival in this context meaning time until death rather than quality of life" (NSW Department of Health, 2003, p25). They also acknowledge that often the patient and carer prefer a formal care package while remaining at home. Indeed, while care has traditionally occurred in the nursing home setting, over recent years with the growth of community support services, more people remain at home through this end-stage (Merl, 2006).

In the UK, research has found that the option to remain at home appears to be almost unachievable. In some cases, sufficient resources can be provided to fulfil a person's wish to stay at home, but the determination of the carer and support received from local services is critical in allowing this to happen (Hughes *et al.*, 2007). An Australian study has identified similar findings, with several general practitioners suggesting that there were inadequate resources available in the community to support people with anything more than mild dementia, and service organizations acknowledging the need for more resources to address the increasing care needs of people with dementia approaching death (Anderson *et al.*, 2010).

This study also revealed the determination of a number of carers to look after their relatives at home (Anderson *et al.*, 2010).

Case Study 2. "Palliative care experience in late-stage dementia": as related by Carer 4

My mother was in an awful lot of pain in hospital, both physical and emotional. The doctor said to her, 'You're in pain?' She said, 'Yes, my heart's broken.' Yet, at other times, they couldn't find it, but I'm sure there was something in the cerebellum, because she would fall unconscious and wake and scream in pain. I was called one night by my niece, who said, 'Rosie, please come, Nana is in so much pain.' They would not do anything because they'd given her all her quota of pain relief, and I said to them, 'Please give her some medication'. 'We're not here to do euthanasia' was the reply. Now, I was not asking for my mother to be euthanased. I was asking for my mother to have pain relief, so that she could be out of pain.

After this, we went to palliative care. The palliative care man said to me 'Well, if you're going to take her home, you're going to have to go and have some rest'. We were meant to have an assessment, but I don't know whether the assessment ever occurred. However, they actually sent an Aged Care Assessment through for mum to be put into a nursing home, without my permission.

By this point in time, my brothers and I had just about had enough of the way we were being treated. Mum was falling in and out of consciousness, so every night, my brother would sit with her until one o'clock in the morning, and then I'd be called in about two or three o'clock in the morning to say that she was Cheyne-Stoking, that you need to get there, we don't think she's going to last. I did that for about four and a half weeks. I was called at 6 am on a Saturday to be told 'You'd better get up here straight away, she's going to go within the hour.' We sat with her, she would stop breathing and you'd think, 'This is it,' and then she'd rally again.

We then decided to bring her home. In hospital, they had been doing hot bed sponges or blanket bath things and mum had become covered in rashes. I don't think anybody had seen a bowl of water and soap and had a good idea about scrubbing under her arms, breasts and between the groins, where she had developed thrush. Needless to say, we weren't really happy with the care. It sounds like I always complain, but I wrote a letter, again, being an advocate for people with dementia, who also need care. We had a meeting and the geriatric specialist said to me, 'Well, you know, you are going to have to look after her hygiene, when you take her home'. I'd actually been caring for my mother for three years. She did not have a rash when she went into hospital; she had not had a bed sore or anything. We brought her home; the ambulance people picked her up, and she was semi-comatose, and they said, 'Where are you taking her?' 'Oh, we're taking her home' said I. 'You're taking her *home*?' 'Yes, we're taking her home.' They said, 'How are we going to get her in the house?' And I said, 'The same way you got her out', because obviously they don't take many people home like that.

Anyway, we got her in the house and the home care organization provided me with Kylie sheets, with the nappies, or the incontinence sheets, some of those glycerin swabs, a slipper pan and a commode. I bought lambskins and we provided our own egg carton mattress. The organization provided two carers at breakfast, two carers at lunch, and two carers at tea, who would wash her, turn her, massage her. I did it again I got home from work and before she went to sleep. I often turned her once in the night, and then I did all this again before I went to work. Within a week, we got rid of every rash, using basic soap and water, lots of massaging, and lots of moisturiser, as she lay on the egg carton mattress in her bed, next to her husband.

She did not have a bed sore, when she left, which was due to the wonderful care given by the carers and the co-ordinator's support. She said, 'Rosie, tell us what you need.' My brother and his wife would come down every Sunday, which was shower day. We would get mum up, put her in the wheelchair, put her into the shower and we'd wash her. My sister-in-law would change the sheets, and then we would put her back into bed. We did that for the six weeks.

Both my brothers and their wives were away when mum died. This caring had been going on for three and a half years and you just don't know when someone's going to slip away. It could have gone on for a lot longer. We'd had many false alarms. Eighteen months beforehand, one of my brothers and his wife wondered whether they should go to Ireland. They ended up going to Ireland twice before mum died. My other brother wondered whether they should go on a cruise while mum was in hospital. We agreed that we have said our goodbyes, but also that 'She may last'. He went on his cruise, came back, and she did last. So, you just didn't know.

I worked through all of this, and to her last day, so I took the Tuesday off and she died Wednesday morning at 6am.

There was no funding for palliative care, to die in the home. The palliative care service could not provide mum with palliative care, because they didn't know how long she was going to take to die. Basically, you're allowed to have palliative care for the last two weeks of your life, but, she'd taken five weeks in hospital and hadn't done what they thought she should do, which was to die, so therefore, she wasn't entitled to any more. The care co-ordinator tried to get support from an organization providing palliative care, but at that point in time, you could only have it if you were dying of cancer or heart disease and mum wasn't dying of either of those. And so, there was no support and that's only nearly four years ago.

What resources are needed to assist carers to look after people with end-stage dementia who wish to die at home?

From interviews with carers who had been supported to look after people who died at home, (Treloar *et al.*, 2009) identified the following key themes:

- Professional expertise:
  - Carers accessed a wide range of professional expertise, including old age psychiatry, which was considered as 'indispensable'.

- Equipment needed:
  - continence pads and sheets, commode and wheelchair rated as 'indispensable'.
  - hospital beds, chair and pressure relieving cushions and electric hoists were rated 'very useful'.

- Feeding: in order to try and prevent weight loss, many techniques for maintaining the food intake were described, such as 'good nutritious food well laid out', 'Irish stews', 'thickened soups'.
- Support and services: need for a person who would visit regularly, advise and bring in other people, as necessary. Carers wanted a support of team, which understood the challenges of looking after a person with dementia.
- To be able to leave when it is time to go and not to have life prolonged pointlessly

McCarty and Vollicer (2009) have noted that when individuals with advanced dementia are transferred to hospital, treatment may often include invasive interventions, such as insertion of feeding tube, which are considered curative. A study has investigated the association of personal background factors with end-of-life decisions among Finnish doctors by presenting two scenarios involving a terminally ill cancer patient and a dementia patient. The findings indicate that their decisions are based not only on patients' preferences, but also their age, gender, marital status, attitudes, life values, life experiences and training.

> If the doctor is young, female single, internist and has not experiences of severe illness in her own family, then she is much more likely to make a decision in favour of active treatment for a terminal cancer patient then a doctor who is over 50, male, married, an oncologist and has experiences of severe illness in the family. If there exists an advance directive, there is very little variation in the decision-making. It the patient suffers from terminal dementia instead of terminal cancer, it is much more likely the treatment decision will be active (Hinkka, Kosunen, Lammi, Metsanoja, Puustelli and Kellokumpu-Lehtinen, 2002, p203)

Insertion of a feeding tube is one response to eating problems, which are a feature of end-stage dementia. Eating problems can be caused by:

- Oral dysphagia, manifesting as absent or continuous chewing with a tendency to pocket or spit food.
- Pharyngeal dysphagia, presenting with delayed swallowing initiation, multiple swallows and aspiration that often leads to pneumonia.

Some patients with advanced dementia lose the ability to perform the task of eating or to interpret the sensation of hunger while others, may simply refuse to eat (Mitchell, 2007).

With respect to the placement of a feeding tube, approximately one third of US nursing home residents with advanced dementia are tube fed. The most commonly cited reasons for tube feeding in advanced dementia include:

- prolonging life,
- improving nutrition,
- preventing aspiration and
- providing comfort (Mitchell, 2007).

However, a number of studies suggest that tube feeding:

- does not prolong survival in advanced dementia,
- does not improve nutritional status, or
- the clinical consequences of malnutrition, such as pressure ulcers.
- will not prevent aspiration of oral secretions or regurgitated gastric contents.
- is associated with a number of risks including:
  - gastro-intestinal adverse effects (ie vomiting, diarrhoea).
  - tube dislodgement, blockage and leakage

- agitated demented patients may require physical or chemical constraints to prevent tube dislodgement
- association with greater use of restraint.

Best available evidence fails to demonstrate any health benefits of tube feeding in advanced dementia (Mitchell, 2007).

Advance care planning plays a critical role in feeding decisions. The lack of advanced directives is a consistent risk factor associated with feeding tube insertion in dementia (Mitchell, 2007). Furthermore, clinicians should be knowledgeable about the potential risks and benefits of hand feeding vs tube feeding. However, although best available evidence does not demonstrate any health benefits of tube feeding in advance dementia, in a 2001 survey of 195 primary care physicians, the majority believed tube feeding in advanced dementia reduced aspiration pneumonia (76%), prolonged survival (61%) and improved nutrition (93.7%) (Mitchell, 2007). Hence, it is imperative that health professionals receive accurate information about procedures such as insertion of feeding tubes.

Conclusion

There are complex issues associated with the care of people with end-stage dementia, who wish to die at home, not the least of which are the difficulties in prognostication. However, with a committed informal carer, supported by adequately funded home care organizations and the use of advance care plans to minimise hospital admissions and unnecessarily invasive interventions, such as insertion of feeding tubes, the desire of people with end-stage dementia to die at home can be fulfilled.

References

Ahronheim J.C., Morrison R.S., Morris J., Baskin S. and Meier D.E. (2000) Palliative care in advanced dementia: a randomized controlled trial and descriptive analysis. *J. Palliat. Med.* 3 (3), 265-73.

Aminoff B.Z. and Adunsky A. (2006) Their last 6 months: suffering and survival of end-stage dementia patients. *Age and Ageing* 35, 597-601.

Anderson B.A., Kralik D., March G. and Briffa M. (2010) "Identification of the palliative care needs of home-based people with late-stage dementia and their carers" Project. Royal District Nursing Service SA Inc Research Unit, Adelaide.

Armitage D and Evans J. (2005) Improving end-stage dementia care: A practice development approach. *Geriaction* (Winter), 25-29.

Australian Institute of Health and Welfare (AIHW) (2003) Admitted patient palliative care in Australia 1999-00.edn. AIHW. Canberra. Accessed 16th February 2010, http://www.aihw.gov.au/publications/index.cfm/title/9045.

Birch D. and Draper J. (2008) A critical literature review exploring the challenges of delivering effective palliative care to older people with dementia. *Journal of Clinical Nursing* 17, 1144-1163.

Coventry P.A., Grande G.E., Richards D.A. and Todd C.J. (2005) Prediction of appropriate timing of palliative care for older adults with non-malignant life-threatening disease: a systematic review. *Age and Ageing* 34, 218-227.

Downs M., Clibbens R., Rae C., Cook A. and Woods R. (2002) What do general practitioners tell people with dementia and their families about the condition? *Dementia* 1 (1), 47-58.

Gamlin R. (2001) Palliative nursing: past, present and future Palliative Nursing: Bringing Comfort and Hope (S. Kinghorn and R. Gamlin, eds). Balliere Tindall, Edinburgh.

Godwin B. and Waters H. (2009) 'In solitary confinement': Planning end-of-life well-being with people with advanced dementia, their family and professional carers. *Mortality* 14 (3), 265-285.

Hinkka H., Kosunen E., Lammi U.-K., Metsanoja R., Puustelli A. and Kellokumpu-Lehtinen P. (2002) Decision making in terminal care: a survey of Finnish doctors' treatment decisions in end-of-life scenarios involving a terminal cancer and a terminal dementia patient. *Palliative Medicine* 16, 195-204.

Hughes J.C., Jolley D., Jordan A. and Sampson E.L. (2007) Palliative care in dementia: issues and evidence. *Advances in Psychiatric Treatment* 13, 251-260.

Jones J. and Willis D. (2003) What is a good death? *British Medical Journal* 327 (26 July), 224.

Kafetz K. (2002) What happens when elderly people die? *Journal of the Royal Society of Medicine* 95 (November), 536-538.

Lee M. and Chodosh J. (2009) Dementia and Life Expectancy: What Do We Know? *Journal of the American Medical Directors' Association* 10, 466-471.

Leifer B.P. (2003) Early Diagnosis of Alzheimer's Disease: Clinical and Economic Benefits. *Journal of the American Geriatrics Society* 51 (No 5, Supplement), S281-S288.

Lloyd-Williams M. (1996) An audit of palliative care in dementia. *European Journal of Cancer Care* 5 (1), 53-5.

MacPhee E. and Bickel K. (2007) Palliative Care for Patients with Dementia: From Diagnosis to Bereavement. *Annals of Long-Term Care* 15 (6), 41-47.

McCarty C.E. and Vollicer L. (2009) Hospice Access for Individuals With Dementia. *American Journal of Alzheimer's Disease and Other Dementias* 24 (6), 476-485.

Merl H. (2006) End-stage Dementia - a rocky journey or a tranquil passage. *ACCNS Journal for Community Nurses* 11 (1), 7-8.

Mitchell S.L. (2007) A 93-Year-Old Man With Advanced Dementia and Eating Problems. *Journal of the American Medical Association* 298 (21), 2527-2536.

Mitchell S.L., Kiely D.K., Miller S.C., Connor S.R., Spence C. and Teno J.M. (2007) Hospice Care for Patients with Dementia. *Journal of Pain and Symptom Management* 34, 7-16.

Mitchell S.L., Teno J.M., Kiely D.K., Shaffer M.L., Jones R.N., Prigerson H.G., Volicer L., Givens J.L. and Hamel M.B. (2009) The Clinical Course of Advanced Dementia. *The New England Journal of Medicine* 361 (16), 1529-38.

Mitchell S.L., Teno J.M., Miller S.C. and Mor V. (2005) A National Study of the Location of Death for Older Persons with Dementia. *Journal of the American Geriatrics Society* 53, 299-305.

NSW Department of Health (2003) Care of Patients with Dementia in General Practice. NSW Department of Health, North Sydney, Accessed 6 October 2009, http://www.health.nsw.gov.au.

Roger K.S. (2006) A literature review of palliative care, end of life, and dementia. *Palliative and Supportive Care* 4, 295-303.

Sachs G.A., Shega J.W. and Cox-Hayley D. (2004) Barriers to Excellent End-of-life Care for Patients with Dementia. *Journal of General Internal Medicine* 19, 1057.

Sampson E.L., Gould V., Leed D. and Blanchard M.R. (2006) Differences in care received by patients with and without dementia who died during acute hospital admission: a retrospective case note study. *Age and Ageing* 35, 187-189.

Sampson E.L., Ritchie C.W., Lai R., Raven P.W. and Blanchard M.R. (2005) A systemic review of the scientific evidence for the efficacy of a palliative care approach in advanced dementia. *International Psychogeriatrics* 17, 31-40.

Schonwetter R.S., Han B., Small B.J., Martin B., Tope K. and Haley William E (2003) Predictors of six-month survival among patients with dementia: An evaluation of hospice Medicare guidelines. *American Journal of Hospice and Palliative Care* 20 (2), 105-113.

Shega J. and Tozer C. (2009) Improving the care of people with dementia at the end of life. *Dementia* 8 (3), 377-389.

Shega J.W., Levin A., Hougham G.W., Cox-Hayley D., Luchins D., Hanrahan P., Stocking C. and Sachs G.A. (2003) Palliative Excellence in Alzheimer Care Efforts (PEACE): A Program Description. *Journal of Palliative Medicine* 6 (2), 315-320.

Smith R. (2000) A good death. *British Medical Journal* 320 (7728), 129-130.

Treloar A., Crugel M. and Adamis D. (2009) Palliative and end of life care of dementia at home is feasible and rewarding. *Dementia* 8 (3), 335-347.

Wolf-Klein G., Pekmezaris R., Chin L. and Weiner J. (2007) Conceptualizing Alzheimer's Disease as a Terminal Medical Illness. *American Journal of Hospice and Palliative Medicine* 24 (1), 77-82.

In: Palliative and Nursing Home Care
Editor: Samuel E. Plunkett
ISBN 978-1-61122-417-7

Chapter 8

Where and How Non Oncological Respiratory Patients Die: A Palliative Answer

Michele Vitacca*[*] *and Luca Barbano
Fondazione Salvatore Maugeri, IRCCS Institute of
Lumezzane (Brescia) Respiratory Unit and Weaning Center

Abstract

Death due to respiratory diseases is high, being chronic obstructive pulmonary disease (COPD) an important risk factor for death. The COPD dying trajectory is often unknown. Commonest cause of death after Intensive Care Unit (ICU) discharge is respiratory failure, while respiratory causes for death are often under-diagnosed. Among COPD patients, a lot of subjects may be defined under palliative and at risk of end of life conditions.

Three different situations emerge depending on the fact that patient is in hospital, at home or using mechanical ventilation. The hospital scenario often offers a high percentage of respiratory patients receiving end of life decisions by different professional figures involved in end of life (EOL) strategies. Major difficulties are represented by death prediction, particularly in those patients admitted in ICU, or by interaction with patient expressing different preferences for a life support or having a poor level of discussion among doctors and between doctors and patients. A second scenario is represented by chronic respiratory patients at home. More than 68% of all COPD admissions and 74% of all days in-hospital occurred in the 3.5 years before death, indicating longer stays closer to death. The last 6 months of life accounted for 22% and 28% of all COPD admissions and days, respectively. Poor symptom control remains an important cause of distress. The most frequent cause of death after discharge is heart disease. Lack of surveillance and inadequate services with absence of palliative care is a routinely experience. The more frequent request from COPD patients is education on diagnosis and disease process, treatments, prognosis for survival, quality of life and

[*] ☎ +39 30 8253168, 🖶 +39 30 8253188, ✉ michele.vitacca@fsm.it

advance care planning. They do not receive holistic care as patients with lung cancer. The last scenario is relative to patients with home mechanical ventilation. Despite these patients are usually pleased about their chose, they are well confident about the high burden imposed to their caregivers. Moreover, for these patients dyspnoea and secretion encumbrance remain the main unresolved symptoms. In comparison with mechanical invasively ventilated patients, non invasively ventilated patients are more aware of prognosis, use more respiratory drugs, change ventilation time more frequently and die less frequently when under mechanical ventilation.

Palliative home care programs and Hospice admissions for EOL care in respiratory patients are insufficient or absent. Individual approach to patients with non homogenous disease is often necessary. Hospital and home palliation protocols (milestones, skills and interventions) for non-oncological respiratory patients are urgently needed.

Introduction

It is well known that COPD is an important risk factor for death in particular in community-living frail elderly people with long-term care needs as demonstrated by Carey et al [1] and Sund-Levander et al [2]. Lindner et al [3] and Bordin et al [4] reviewing the complete clinical and autopsy records showed that vascular and respiratory diseases were the most common cause of death being the contribution of COPD to mortality often underestimated [5]. In USA, death from non oncological respiratory causes accounts for 8% of all deaths and 9.6% when patients have more than 65 years being chronic obstructive pulmonary disease (COPD) the 56 % of all respiratory causes [6]. COPD time course is characterized by a progressive worsening of dyspnoea, reduced effort tolerance, frequent exacerbations and hospitalizations. In COPD, oxygen therapy and mechanical ventilation (MV) are two fundamental instruments to improve survival and morbility in acute situation [7]. At home, oxygen therapy has been demonstrated useful to improve survival and quality of life (QOL). However, COPD time course is unknown and unpredictable as other chronic diseases [8]. In particular chronic illness at the end of life (EOL) generally follows 3 trajectories: (a) a short period of obvious decline at the end, which is typical of cancer; (b) long-term disability, with periodic exacerbations and unpredictable timing of death which characterize dying with chronic multiorgan failure; or (c) self-care deficits and a slowly dwindling course to death, which usually results from frailty or dementia. Effective and reliable care for persons coming to the EOL will require changes in the organization and financing of care, compassionate and skillful clinicians to match these different trajectories [8]. In a provocative paper, Curtis et al. proposed to identify/characterize, among our respiratory patients, who is an end of life [9]. He suggests that, after a serious analysis of the conditions and clinical status, we would define a patient needing palliative items when he shows poor reasonable chance of recovery, poor rehabilitation possibilities with a re-modulation of organizational complexity and instrumental needs [9].

Three areas may influence the quality of care for patients forthcoming into a palliative trajectory: 1) the role of anxiety and depression as common problems for patients with COPD, 2) the importance of advance care planning, and 3) the level of communication. Patients to be accompanied to their last days of life (with an estimatation of death within the next 7 days) may be defined as EOL patient. Caring for these patients should be defined as potentially "futile", i.e. disproportionate measures in terms of quality and quantity of care with poor expected quality of life (QOL). Table 1 shows a possible definition of a respiratory patient with palliative and EOL needs.

Table 1. Criteria to define a respiratory patient with palliative or end of life needs

A) Patient with palliative needs (Occurence of 1 major or three minor criteria)

Major criteria:

FEV1 <30% prd cachexia (BMI <18 or recent weight loss) COPD with unweanable tracheotomy previous surgery complications (within six months) *Minor criteria:* 2 hospitalizations in the last year (medical wards) 1 admission into a ICU in the last year disability above 75% with Barthel scale aged over 80 y

LTOT since 6 years

Dyspnoea at rest severe side effects under NMV or refusal of NMV during acute respiratory failure episode more than two comorbidities severe obesity (BMI> 40) senile dementia advanced bulbar symptoms diagnosis of advanced pulmonary fibrosis or Cystic fibrosis with decreased exercise tolerance, need for oxygen at rest and/or excluded from transplant list)

B) Patient with end of life needs (Occurrence of at least three of these conditions)

Reduction of free intervals of well-being (within the last week)

Repeated medical treatments care with risk of futility (need for repeated use of artificial ventilation, blood transfusions, cardiopulmonary resuscitation, use of inotropes and antibiotics in the same admission).

Difficulty taking oral therapy

Refusal of food and liquids

Refusal of medical and basic care

Not recoverable disability

Generalized asthenia

Disorientation and drowsiness

No therapeutic response to life-saving drugs

Poor response to pain therapy

Legend: *FEV1: forced expiratory volume; BMI: body mass index; COPD:* chronic obstructive pulmonary disease; *NMV: non invasive mechanical ventilation; LTOT: long term oxygen therapy; ICU: intensive care unit; ALS: amyotrophic lateral sclerosis .*

The first scenario we have to considered is the hospital. This is the condition in which end stage decisions are promptly requested being respiratory reason a common cause of death in hospital. Roberts at al. showed that significant differences in mortality may exist between hospital's types [10]: when respiratory patients were admitted in small hospitals with few doctors, few patients were treated under the care of a specialist physician and they may present an higher mortality rate [10]. Gordo et al. [11] demonstrated an high mortality rate of 19% (41/215 pts) for patients who were discharged from an intensive care unit (ICU) and died when they were admitted to general ward. A mean period of 9 days elapsed between discharge from the ICU and patient's death with 25% of patients dying within the first two days. The commonest cause of death was respiratory failure (37%). Three figures are involved in the EOL scenario: doctors, family and patients. All these figures present different perspectives and expectations. In a recent survey Nava et al [12] showed that, in European respiratory intermediate care units and high dependency units, an EOL decision is taken for 21.5% of the admitted patients. Withholding of treatment, do-not-intubate/do-not-resuscitate orders and noninvasive mechanical ventilation (NMV) as the ventilatory care ceiling are the most common procedures used and proposed [12]. This study agrees with the study of Ferrand et al. showing that about 21 % of chronic patients usually receive EOL decisions in hospital [13]. In the same survey Nava et al. [12] show that competent patients together with nurses are often involved in EOL decisions. European ICU physicians do not experience difficulties with EOL decisions in most cases [13]. However, Sprung et al. underline that EOL decisions change according to diagnosis, countries and doctors' religion [14]. Another important point is the well known difficulty to predict outcomes and death for COPD patients when admitted in ICU. Wildman and collegues investigated, in 92 ICU and three respiratory high dependency units in the United Kingdom [15], whether clinicians' prognoses in patients with severe acute exacerbations of COPD admitted to ICU matched the observed outcomes in terms of survival. Due to decisions on whether to admit patients with COPD or asthma to ICU for intubation depend on clinicians' prognoses, some patients who might otherwise survive may be probably denied to be admitted because of unwarranted prognostic pessimism [15]. Usually the need to prioritize care to the most unstable ICU patients lead to discriminate COPD patients which do not receive the proper attention by clinicians being usually undertreated [15]. Less than 15% of patients in ICU were competent, the majority of them lacking in written anticipated directives or in discussing on EOL preferences with their relatives [16]. Gerstel at al. explain that one of the main problems in ICU is the withdrawal of life support that is a complex process depending on patient and family's characteristics [17]. Intubation stuttering withdrawal is a frequent phenomenon that seems to be associated with family satisfaction, on the contrary extubation before death, if possible, should be encouraged by clinicians [17]. During hospitalization preferences for life support in COPD patients are similar to those of patients with oncological diseases, as explained by Claessens [18]. Hospitalized patients with lung cancer or COPD prefer comfort-focused care, yet dyspnoea and pain were problematic in both groups [18]. Patients with COPD are more often treated with life-sustaining interventions and short-term effectiveness is comparatively better than in patients with lung cancer [18]. In caring for severe COPD patients consideration should be given to implement palliative treatments in a more aggressive way, even while remaining open to provision of life-sustaining interventions [18]. Curtis and collegues [19] show that a fundamental problem related to EOL is the strategy of communication. Patients and caregivers suffer about the great difficulties to discuss with doctors due to the poor doctors's ability to speak with the family [19]. Among the clinical figures involved in the EOL decisions discrepancies between doctors and nurses have been demonstrated by Ferrand et al.[20]: fear of litigation was one of the main reason given by physicians for modifying information to competent patients, families, and nursing staff [20]. Perceptions by nursing staff may be a reliable indicator of the quality of medical decision-making processes and may serve as a simple and effective tool for evaluating everyday practice. Recommendations and legislation may help to build consensus and avoid conflicts among caregivers at each step of the decision-making process [20]. Strategies to improve family ratings may require interventions that have more direct contact with family members as explain by Curtis [21].

The second possible scenario takes into consideration the respiratory patients discharged from hospital or patients living at home for a long period. Andersson and collegues showed that more than 68% of all COPD admissions and 74% of all days in hospital occurred in the 3.5 years before death indicating a longer stay closer to death [22]. The last 6 months of life accounted for 22% and 28% of all COPD admissions and days, respectively [22]. Finally, COPD patients often have a number of concomitant diseases which may affect diagnosis and healthcare resource use [22]. Poor symptom control remains an important cause of distress in these patients and the importance of an individual approach to subjects with apparently homogenous disease is crucial. While the most frequent cause of in-hospital death is the respiratory disease, the main cause of death in COPD patients after discharge from hospital is heart disease, as described by Faustini [23]. However, the Torch study showed that, among patients with COPD, death can result in a number of disease categories), in part due to the strong association between COPD and exposure to cigarette smoke [24]. Indeed, in the Torch trial, 35% of deaths were due to pulmonary causes, 27% to cardiovascular disease, and 21% to cancer. Ten percent of deaths were attributed to other causes, whereas the primary cause of death could not be determined by the clinical end point committee in 7% of cases [24]. It is common experience a lack of surveillance, inadequate services and absence of palliative home care services for non oncological respiratory patients. Respiratory patients who are housebound with high levels of morbidity require high community health services: unfortunately respiratory nurse specialists are rarely involved in the home patients' care. Teno et al. examined differences in the pattern of functional decline among persons dying of cancer and other leading non cancer causes of death and explain that persons dying of cancer experienced sharp functional decline in the last months of life whereas other decedents' have a more gradual decline [25]. The more precipitous functional decline was associated with hospice involvement and dying at home [25]. In another study Curtis et al [26] subtitles that severe COPD patients approaching EOL time require, as main necessities, education on diagnosis and disease process, to know treatments, what they have to do and to expect, prognosis for survival and QOL. The patients with COPD, AIDS, and cancer demonstrated many similarities in their perspectives on important areas of physician skill in providing EOL care [26]. Physicians and educators should target patients with COPD for efforts to improve patient education about their disease and about end-of-life care [26]. Curtis et al [19] explain that only 32% of respiratory patients report discussing EOL care with physician because patients identified several barriers as "I would rather concentrate on staying alive than talk about death" or " I'm not sure which doctor will be taking care of me if I get very sick" [19]. Others barriers as "there is too little time to discuss everything we should" or "patient is not ready to talk about what kind of care he wants if he gets sick" have been also identified by physicians [19]. Thus, it is necessary to identify areas of communication that physicians do not address and areas that patients rate poorly, including talking about prognosis, dying and spirituality. These areas may provide targets for interventions to improve communication about EOL care for patients with COPD [19]. Gore et al suggest that patients with end stage COPD have significantly impaired QOL and emotional well being which may not be as well met as those of patients with lung cancer, nor do they receive holistic care appropriate to their needs [27]. Lynn et al [28] characterize the experience of dying from the perspective of surrogate decision makers, usually close to family members [28]. Pain and other symptoms were common place and troubling to patients [28]. Family members believed that patients preferred comfort, but life-sustaining treatments were often used [28].

The last scenario is relative to home patients with mechanical ventilation (MV). Marchese et al. [29] describe survival, predictors of long-term outcome and attitudes in patients treated at home by tracheostomy-intermittent positive-pressure ventilation (TIPPV) during a 10-year period.

Sixty -four out of 77 (83%) patients were pleased to have chosen MV with tracheostomy and 69 patients (90%) would choose it again [29]. Forty-two caregivers (55%) were pleased the patients had chosen home mechanical ventilation (HMV), but 29 (38%) reported major burdens [29]. TIPPV is well-received by patients, it is considered safe and provides survival for long periods of time [29]. In another study.

Fine Model

Singer et al [30] demonstrate that patients with long term respiratory failure require pain relief, avoiding prolongation of life, sense of control, relief of burden and strengthening relationship with beloved exactly as other chronic patients with AIDS or dyalisis. Vitacca et al describe the family's perception of care delivered to home mechanical ventilation (HMV) patients during the last 3 months of life [31].

Eleven Respiratory Units submitted a binary 35-item questionnaire with 6 domains (symptoms, awareness of disease, family burden, dying, medical troubles and technical problems) to close relatives of 168 deceased patients (41% COPD) [31]. The majority of patients complained respiratory symptoms and were aware of the severity and prognosis of the disease [31].

Family burden was high especially in relation to money need [31]. During hospitalisation, 74.4% of patients were admitted to ICU, 27% of patients received resuscitation manoeuvres. Hospitalisations and family economical burden were unrelated to diagnosis and MV. Families of the patients did not report major technical problems on the use of ventilators [31]. In comparison with mechanical invasively ventilated (MIV) patients, noninvasively ventilated (NIV) patients were more aware of prognosis, used more respiratory drugs, changed ventilation time more frequently and died less frequently when under MV [31].

Borgsteede et al explore aspects valued by both patients and general practitioners (GPs) in EOL care at home and conclude that future developments in the organization of primary care such as the restriction of time for home visits, more part-time jobs and GP cooperatives responsible for care after office hours, may threat valued aspects in EOL care [32]. Provision of interdisciplinary home-based palliative care at EOL can effectively increase the likelihood of dying at home for patients with chronic heart failure, COPD, and cancer while realizing significant cost savings [32]. Enguidanos et al explain how home care program is associated with significantly fewer hospital-based health care costs (with the exception of COPD) [33]. Steele et al describe how hospice care can offer expertize for palliation and may be used as a bridge between hospital and home [34].

Preliminary experiences on the use of telemedicine (TM) have beeen approached to care and assist patients during EOL decisions at home [35]. Scheduled phone calls, pulso-oxymetry recording, 24/24 H call centre, specialized nurse and doctor's second opinion were tested for 21 patients [35].

TM team was involved in counselling on hospital admission, on discussion for decisions, on all care options avoiding nihilistic position or aggressive and not proportional care chooses, GP or home nurse's consults, sedative or morphine prescription, solution of ventilators' troubles, oxygen saturimetric prescription, reinforcement speech about gravity of illness, coordination with home nurse service, psychological and spiritual help [35].

Indeed, a nurse centered TM program for terminal patients may improve communication between hospital staff and patients' relatives, optimize pain and respiratory symptoms management, improve health care assistance and rationalize hospitalizations and the health care necessities [35].

Communication with patients and families about EOL care is an important component of caring often neglected in the training of clinicians who provide this care. Vitacca et al. showed how to comunicate bad news to caregivers of patients with ALS [36]. Caregivers require major assistance in particular during the delicate time of discussing advanced care plans and directives or critical treatments decisions [36].

Different protocols have been presented in literature to improve the relationship between physicians and patients/caregivers on when and how to transmit *bad news* related to poor prognosis in particular for oncologic patients [37]. Interventions to improve this communication have been generally unsuccessful, suggesting that important barriers do exist [37]. The heterogeneity of barriers and facilitators between patients with progressive diseases and their clinicians suggest that interventions to improve communication about EOL care must be focused on individual needs and must involve counselling interventions and health system changes in addition to education as explained by Curtis [38]. Clinician barriers are more common and more strongly associated with the occurrence of EOL communication if compared with barriers relevant to patients/caregivers, suggesting that clinicians are an important target group for improving this type of communication [38]. Johnston concludes that much of the research relating to communication skills in EOL care has been developed in cancer care [39].

The Calgary–Cambridge model [37] for medical consultations and the SPIKES (Setting up, Perception, Invitation, Knowledge, Emotions, Strategy and Summary, [40] model for breaking *bad news* are examples of consultation guides that integrate the patient agenda with biomedical issues. Appendixes 1 and 2 show our talk protocol during and after bad communication speech.

An additional step in preparing for an EOL discussion is to plan where the discussion will take place and who will attend this discussion there. Ideally, the conversation should take place in a quiet and private room where there is some assurance that people, phones, or pagers will not interrupt the discussion as described by Vitacca [36]. It should be a room that is comfortable for all the participants, without a lot of medical machinery or other distractions such as medical diagrams.

All parties should be sitting around a table or chairs in a circle [36]. It would be better to avoid the clinician sitting behind a desk with the family in front of it. If the patient can participate to the discussion but is too ill to stay out of bed, efforts should be made to make the room comfortable for everyone present [36]. Communication of advance care planning, defined as an ongoing discussion among patients and family members may be a more effective mean to meet patients' wishes [36]. Such discussions require great sensitivity and some patients do not wish to discuss death issues [41,42].

The principle of medical futility need to be proposed in our meetings: the principle of medical futility states that a therapy is futile if there is no likelihood or a very low likelihood that the therapy will be successful [36].

According to literature and our personal experience, future care proposals for non oncological respiratory patients will focus desired outcomes, skills and interventions for doctors, nurses and respiratory therapists.

Appendices from 3 to 6 summarize our proposed, used outcomes and interventions for palliative care in non oncological respiratory patients.

In conclusion, in respiratory patients presenting EOL conditions we need to:

- Offer the best practice to cure the disease
- Think that medicine doesn't save anyone or doesn't win death
- Control physical (dyspnoea) and psychological symptoms
- Take care of our patient
- Allow a continuous presence of family, friends and religious assistance
- Give time and place to our patient to say everyone "good bye"
- Talk to our patients and relatives using their languages
- Listen because we have one mouth and two ears
- Consider patients' preferences (i.e. control the symptoms, use drugs and/or NMV, organize a home care program to relief their burden)
- Imagine together their future
- Take in advance the right decision about EOL
- Unduly prolong life and suffering
- Consider Hospice and "palliative care" as opportunities for our patients

Appendix 1.

Interview with caregiver (36)
Items of the talk:

1. Disease and its evolution
2. Prognosis
3. Treatments to be proposed
4. Side effects of treatments
5. Risk of sudden exacerbations
6. How it is possible to treat the symptoms
7. What might be the cause of death
8. Decisions on advanced planning (start treatment or discontinue treatment = futility)
9. Preferences at the end of life
10. How to talk/inform the patient
11. To seize family contrasts
12. To listen to family needs
13. Future perspective on place of care (home?, nursing home?, Hospice ?)
14. How the team may help family at home
15. Information on the hospital, on relatives' visits
16. Information on how to stay around the hospital, how to eat and drink
17. To invite the caregiver to take breaks

18. To ask if there are frail economic dynamics
19. To ask if there are frail job dynamics

Mode of talk

1. To find a comfortable place
2. To take adequate time (a minimum of 30 minutes)
3. To sit
4. To make all sit
5. To speak calmly with decision and authority
6. To explain with drawings if necessary
7. To look for partnerships (no conflicts or collusion)
8. To classify the type of caregiver (compliant or absent)

Final report after interview
Confirm a value from 0 to 10 (0 = minimum value; 10 = maximum value)

1. Has the caregiver understood the content?
2. Is the caregiver satisfied?
3. Is the caregiver confused?
4. Is the caregiver calm?
5. Can the caregiver help the patient?
6. Does the caregiver need a new interview?
7. Strategies for the interview:

- To upload the fear of death
- To avoid despair or sense of futility
- Do not mention abandonment of care
- To use neutrality
- To solicite the patient
- To target the audience
- To understand the specific objectives of the patient
- To clarify strategies
- To avoid details

Appendix 2.

Check list for individual and advanced written treatment plan (IATP) for all the team

Patient :_______________
Disease :_______________
Date :_________________

	YES	NO
To talk with the patient		
Interview with the relatives		
Prescription of non-invasive mechanical ventilation in acute situation		
Suspension for non-invasive mechanical ventilation when in use		
Prescription of high flow oxygen therapy		
Suspension oxygen therapy		
Cardio Pulmonary Resuscitation		
Endotracheal intubation		
Tracheotomy		
ICU Transfer		
Central vein if necessary		
Terminal sedation		
Gastrostomy		
To suspend feeding and hidratation		
To suspend drugs and avoid blood transfusion		

Appendix 3.

NON ONCOLOGICAL PALLIATION/END OF LIFE OUTCOMES FOR RESPIRATORY PATIENTS

Palliative time	End of life time
Stabilisation of quality of life Symptoms control (pain, dyspnoea, encumbrance, agitation, costipation) Listening and communication with patient/relatives To give hope about assistance Searching for an individual and advanced written treatment plan (MV, gastrostomy, CPR, access to ICU, terminal sedation) Psychological aid to caregiver To reduce disability To improve privacy To humanize the place of care Cough Assistance Communication among Hospital team for palliative stage (subdivision of the burden of decision making) To use residual resources (family and community) To learn strategies (behavioural, cognitive and spiritual)	Quality of a good death To give dignity To give policy To provide hope To provide spiritual support To give free access to relatives Terminal sedation Communications to the Hospital's team Home discharge if requested by the patient/relative Empathic listening To improve privacy To provide assistance to family's members after death

Legend: MV: mechanical ventilation; CPR: cardiopulmonary resuscitation; ICU: intensive care unit;

Appendix 4.

NON ONCOLOGICAL PALLIATION/END OF LIFE MEDICAL INTERVENTIONS FOR RESPIRATORY PATIENTS

Palliative time	End of life time
Interview with caregiver/family To check list for individual and advanced written treatment plan Counselling Request of occupational therapist for ADL Prescription aids (Walker, Wheelchair, PEG, tracheocannula, Communication) Educational Program Link with home care service Bronchial assistance Reshaping of blood tests and instrumental prescription Psychotherapy	Communication with patients/relatives about the end of life protocol and subsequent approval To begin prescription of drugs (pain controller, sedatives, symptomatic, neuroleptics, prokinetics, morphine, midazolam, lorazepam) To allow H 24 family's presence To deny access to people do not like to patient Psychological care for family Material aid to the family NMV if dyspnoea Oxygen therapy if the patient breathes spontaneously (to reduce dyspnea) Bronchial assistance only on demand To eliminate dry mucous To reset the MV Morphine IV (even if on SB) Sedation if under controlled ventilation Suspension of visual monitoring To prefer comfortable and minimally invasive medications Drugs Suspension Antibiotic suspension Oxygen suspension when under MV Blood chemistry Suspension Re-assessment of feed with possible suspension To reduce the hydration

Legend: ADL: activity daily life; PEG: percutaneous endoscopy gastrostomy; NIV: non invasive ventilation; MV: mechanical ventilation; IV: intravenous; SB: spontaneous breathing

Appendix 5.

NON ONCOLOGICAL PALLIATION/END OF LIFE PHYSIOTERAPIC INTERVENTIONS FOR RESPIRATORY PATIENTS

Palliative time	End of life time
Muscular rehabilitation in order to save ADL and the prevention of contractures and sores Passive and active mobilization Training in walking Adaptation to prostheses or aids (walker, wheelchairs, communicators) Prescription aids Bronchial assistance NMV as needed (if the presence of dyspnoea can not be corrected by other means and only if it can produce symptomatic benefit) Delivery home care assistance Caregivers education programs for MV home management and discharge	NMV as needed (if the presence of dyspnoea can not be corrected by other means and only if it can produce symptomatic benefit) Bronchial assistance on demand

Legend: ADL: activity daily life; NIMV: non invasive mechanical ventilation; PEG: percutaneous endoscopy gastrostomy; MV: mechanical ventilation

Appendix 6.

NON ONCOLOGICAL PALLIATION/END OF LIFE NURSING INTERVENTIONS FOR RESPIRATORY PATIENTS

Palliative time	End of life time
To design quiet environment with family Hygiene (control / help) Mobilization (control / help) Feed (control/help) Sores' prevention (aids) Control symptoms/response to therapy Caregiver educational training Management of tracheostomy /gastrostomy Management of aids Execution of blood chemistry/instrumental prescription Briefing with referents (medical, respiratory therapist, psychologist)	To design quiet environment with family Mouth Care General Hygiene Mobilization/positioning in bed Feed supply if required Sores' prevention (aids) Control symptoms / response to therapy Management of tracheostomy / gastrostomy Briefing with referents (medical, respiratory therapist, psychologist) To propose religious assistance, if desired

References

[1] Carey EC, Covinsky KE, Lui LY, Eng C, Sands LP, et al. (2008) Prediction of mortality in community-living frail elderly people with long-term care needs. *J. Am. Geriatr. Soc.* 56(1): 68-75.

[2] Sund-Levander M, Grodzinsky E, Wahren LK. (2007) Gender differences in predictors of survival in elderly nursing-home residents: A 3-year follow up. *Scand. J. Caring Sci.* 21(1): 18-24.

[3] Lindner JL, Omalu BI, Buhari AM, Shakir A, Rozin L, et al. (2007) Nursing home deaths which fall under the jurisdiction of the coroner: An 11-year retrospective study. *Am. J. Forensic Med. Pathol.* 28(4): 292-298.

[4] Bordin P, Da Col PG, Peruzzo P, Stanta G, Guralnik JM, et al. (1999) Causes of death and clinical diagnostic errors in extreme aged hospitalized people: A retrospective clinical-necropsy survey. *J. Gerontol. A Biol. Sci. Med. Sci.* 54(11): M554-9.

[5] Hansell AL, Walk JA, Soriano JB. (2003) What do chronic obstructive pulmonary disease patients die from? A multiple cause coding analysis. *Eur. Respir. J.* 22(5): 809-814.

[6] Lynn J. (2001) Perspectives on care at the close of life. serving patients who may die soon and their families: The role of hospice and other services. *JAMA* 285(7): 925-932.

[7] Curtis JR. (2008) Palliative and end-of-life care for patients with severe COPD. *Eur. Respir. J.* 32(3): 796-803.

[8] Roberts CM, Barnes S, Lowe D, Pearson MG, Clinical Effectiveness Evaluation Unit, Royal College of Physicians, et al. (2003) Evidence for a link between mortality in acute COPD and hospital type and resources. *Thorax* 58(11): 947-949.

[9] Gordo F, Nunez A, Calvo E, Algora A. (2003) Intrahospital mortality after discharge from the ICU (hidden mortality) in patients who required mechanical ventilation. *Med. Clin.* (Barc) 121(7): 241-244.

[10] Nava S, Sturani C, Hartl S, Magni G, Ciontu M, et al. (2007) End-of-life decision-making in respiratory intermediate care units: A european survey. *Eur. Respir. J.* 30(1): 156-164.

[11] Ferrand E, Robert R, Ingrand P, Lemaire F, French LATAREA Group. (2001) Withholding and withdrawal of life support in intensive-care units in france: A prospective survey. french LATAREA group. *Lancet* 357(9249): 9-14.

[12] Sprung CL, Woodcock T, Sjokvist P, Ricou B, Bulow HH, et al. (2008) Reasons, considerations, difficulties and documentation of end-of-life decisions in european intensive care units: The ETHICUS study. *Intensive Care Med.* 34(2): 271-277.

[13] Wildman MJ, Sanderson C, Groves J, Reeves BC, Ayres J, et al. (2007) Implications of prognostic pessimism in patients with chronic obstructive pulmonary disease (COPD) or asthma admitted to intensive care in the UK within the COPD and asthma outcome study (CAOS): Multicentre observational cohort study. *BMJ* 335(7630): 1132.

[14] Goodridge D, Duggleby W, Gjevre J, Rennie D. (2008) Caring for critically ill patients with advanced COPD at the end of life: A qualitative study. *Intensive Crit. Care Nurs* 24(3): 162-170.

[15] Gerstel E, Engelberg RA, Koepsell T, Curtis JR. (2008) Duration of withdrawal of life support in the intensive care unit and association with family satisfaction. *Am. J. Respir. Crit. Care Med.* 178(8): 798-804.

[16] Claessens MT, Lynn J, Zhong Z, Desbiens NA, Phillips RS, et al. (2000) Dying with lung cancer or chronic obstructive pulmonary disease: Insights from SUPPORT. study to understand prognoses and preferences for outcomes and risks of treatments. *J. Am. Geriatr. Soc.* 48(5 Suppl): S146-53.

[17] Curtis JR, Engelberg RA, Nielsen EL, Au DH, Patrick DL. (2004) Patient-physician communication about end-of-life care for patients with severe COPD. *Eur. Respir. J.* 24(2): 200-205.

[18] Andersson FL, Svensson K, Gerhardsson de Verdier M. (2006) Hospital use for COPD patients during the last few years of their life. *Respir. Med.* 100(8): 1436-1441.

[19] Faustini A, Marino C, D'Ippoliti D, Forastiere F, Belleudi V, et al. (2008) The impact on risk-factor analysis of different mortality outcomes in COPD patients. *Eur. Respir. J.* 32(3): 629-636.

[20] Rabe KF. (2007) Treating COPD--the TORCH trial, P values, and the dodo. *N. Engl. J. Med.* 356(8): 851-854.

[21] Teno JM, Weitzen S, Fennell ML, Mor V. (2001) Dying trajectory in the last year of life: Does cancer trajectory fit other diseases? *J. Palliat Med.* 4(4): 457-464.

[22] Curtis JR, Wenrich MD, Carline JD, Shannon SE, Ambrozy DM, et al. (2002) Patients' perspectives on physician skill in end-of-life care: Differences between patients with COPD, cancer, and AIDS. *Chest* 122(1): 356-362.

[23] Gore JM, Brophy CJ, Greenstone MA. (2000) How well do we care for patients with end stage chronic obstructive pulmonary disease (COPD)? A comparison of palliative care and quality of life in COPD and lung cancer. *Thorax* 55(12): 1000-1006.

[24] Lynn J, Teno JM, Phillips RS, Wu AW, Desbiens N, et al. (1997) Perceptions by family members of the dying experience of older and seriously ill patients. SUPPORT investigators. study to understand prognoses and preferences for outcomes and risks of treatments. *Ann. Intern. Med.* 126(2): 97-106.

[25] Marchese S, Lo Coco D, Lo Coco A. (2008) Outcome and attitudes toward home tracheostomy ventilation of consecutive patients: A 10-year experience. *Respir. Med.* 102(3): 430-436.

[26] Singer PA, Martin DK, Kelner M. (1999) Quality end-of-life care: Patients' perspectives. *JAMA* 281(2): 163-168.

[27] Vitacca M, Grassi M, Barbano L, Galavotti G, Sturani C, et al. (2010) Last 3 months of life in home-ventilated patients: The family perception. *Eur. Respir. J.* 35(5): 1064-1071.

[28] Borgsteede SD, Graafland-Riedstra C, Deliens L, Francke AL, van Eijk JT, et al. (2006) Good end-of-life care according to patients and their GPs. *Br. J. Gen. Pract.* 56(522): 20-26.

[29] Enguidanos SM, Cherin D, Brumley R. (2005) Home-based palliative care study: Site of death, and costs of medical care for patients with congestive heart failure, chronic obstructive pulmonary disease, and cancer. *J. Soc. Work End Life Palliat Care* 1(3): 37-56.

[30] Steele LL, Mills B, Hardin SR, Hussey LC. (2005) The quality of life of hospice patients: Patient and provider perceptions. *Am. J. Hosp. Palliat Care* 22(2): 95-110.

[31] Vitacca M, Assoni G, Gilè S, Fiorenza D, Bianchi L, Barbano L, Porta R, Bertella E, Scalvini E (2009) Telemedicine to support end of life in severe chronic respiratory failure patients at home. *J. Med. Person* 7:85-90.

[32] Vitacca M. (2010). How to communicate bad news to caregivers of patients with Amiotrophic Lateral Sclerosis. *Journal of medicine and Person* 8:19-24.

[33] Baile WF, Buckman R, Lenzi R, Glober G, Beale EA, Kudelka AP (2000) SPIKES-A six-step protocol for delivering bad news: application to the patient with cancer. *Oncologist* 5(4):302-311.

[34] Curtis JR, Patrick DL, Caldwell ES, Collier AC (2000) Why don't patients and physicians talk about end-of-life care? Barriers to communication for patients with acquired immunodeficiency syndrome and their primary care clinicians. *Arch. Intern. Med.* 160(11):1690-1696.

[35] Johnston M, Earll L, Mitchell E, Morrison V, Wright S (1996). Communicating the diagnosis of motor neuron disease. *Palliative Medicine* 10: 23–34.

[36] Silverman J, Kurtz S, Draper J (2005) Skills for communicating with patients. Abingdon, Radcliffe publishing ltd.

[37] National Health Service (2008) The preferred priorities for care (ppc) document: guidelines for health and/or social care staff. www.endoflifecareforadults.nhs.uk/eolc/files/f2111-ppc_staff_guidance_dec2007.pdf date last accessed: November 3 2008. Date last updated: December 2007.

[38] Connolly M, Duck A (2008) Communication skills in endstage respiratory disease: managing distressed patients and breaking bad news. *Breathe* 5(2):147-154.

In: Palliative and Nursing Home Care
Editor: Samuel E. Plunkett
ISBN 978-1-61122-417-7

Chapter 9

Can Data Envelopment Analysis Be Used to Study Performance Efficiency in Nursing Homes?

Daniel G. Shimshak
University of Massachusetts Boston, USA

Abstract

One area that has been the focus of growing attention has been the nursing home sector, which constitutes a large and increasingly costly segment of the health care industry. Nursing home administrators have come under great pressure to control costs while maintaining or increasing the quality and level of care. However, administrators in the industry have had difficulty in developing a useful measure of nursing home performance and strategies for improving nursing home care. Currently, large amounts of data are collected on numerous aspects of performance, including cost, utilization, case-mix severity, and quality. These data are typically compiled into summary reports that are prepared on a regular basis for individual nursing homes. Often values on these profile reports are benchmarked against normative values representing averages for other nursing homes in the state, region, or nation. It is anticipated that nursing homes will use the results of these benchmark reports to identify aspects of their performance that may need improvement.

There are some inherent problems with this technique for evaluating nursing home performance. First, it is cumbersome to inspect a long list of performance measures and their rankings compared to other homes. Second, without an objective means of prioritizing or combining the various measures, it is difficult to determine which nursing homes are performing well overall. Finally, this technique provides very little guidance on how nursing homes can change their operations to improve their performance.

Given the limitations on existing techniques, it is apparent that the nursing home industry needs better tools for converting the vast amounts of available data into information that is useful for managers. Here we will discuss the possibility of using Data Envelopment Analysis (DEA) for studying performance in nursing homes. DEA is a mathematical technique that converts multiple input and output measures into a single comprehensive measure of performance. Thus, DEA can calculate a single "performance rating" for each nursing home. Not only can DEA evaluate the utilization efficiency of a nursing home's resources, but it can construct performance targets for each home based on a comparison with a selected group of the best-performing nursing homes. In this way, DEA can help administrators of nursing homes to conduct a comprehensive evaluation of their performance and to devise strategies for improvement.

Introduction

One of the most costly components of the health care industry is the nursing home sector. The graying of the population of the United States in coming years suggests that this area will continue to grow. Expenditures for nursing home care amounted to $144.1 billion in 2009 and are projected to increase by over 70% over the next 10 years. The financial picture for the nursing home industry has resulted in greater pressure on nursing home administrators to control costs while maintaining or increasing the quality and level of care that is provided.

However, administrators of nursing homes have had difficulty in establishing a useful and equitable notion of efficiency in nursing home performance and in identifying specific improvement strategies. In manufacturing and financial businesses, for example, it is often possible to develop a single summary measure of performance, such as profit or market share. In nursing home settings, though, there must be multiple measures of performance because outcomes such as the quantity of services provided and the quality of care are all of vital consideration.

Currently, nursing home data is gathered through surveys or self reporting. Large amounts of data are gathered on numerous aspects of performance and are compiled into profile reports that are prepared on a regular basis for individual nursing homes. These profile reports include detailed information regarding a nursing home's costs, utilization, case-mix severity and quality. These indicators, many of which are in the form of ratios, are compared against performance averages for other nursing homes.

Profile reports are designed to generate a specific action if the performance indicators for a particular nursing home differ from the average by a certain amount. In this way, ratio-based indicators used in profile reports attempt to highlight nursing home performances that are exceptionally high or low. For example, a large expenditure on nursing aides per resident would stand out as an indication of inefficiency. However, because indicators are limited to one measure of input and/or one measure of output, they can't easily accommodate situations where multiple outputs are produced using multiple inputs, as is true for nursing homes.

To compensate for the one-dimensional nature of the indicators, a large set of ratios and normative values need to be calculated in the profile reports. Unfortunately, with multiple indicators, there is no objective way of identifying inefficient nursing homes. For example, a nursing home whose expenditure on nursing aides per resident is greater than the average value might be considered potentially inefficient. But it is not possible to determine how much larger than the average a nursing home must be to be considered inefficient or even if the average itself is efficient. Additionally, with multiple indicators, a nursing home may appear efficient for one group of measures but inefficient for another group. Without an objective means of prioritizing these indicators, identification of a truly efficient nursing home becomes difficult. Also, existing methods provide very little guidance on how nursing homes can change their operations to improve their performance.

Given the limitations on existing techniques, it is apparent that the nursing home industry needs better tools for converting the vast amounts of available data into information that is useful for administrators. This article proposes the use of one such tool, Data Envelopment Analysis (DEA). DEA can help administrators of nursing homes conduct a comprehensive evaluation of their performance and devise strategies for improvement.

Data Envelopment Analysis

In their seminal work, Charnes, Cooper and Rhodes [1] presented DEA as a mathematical programming approach that converts multiple input and output measures into a single comprehensive measure of performance (an "efficiency score") for each of a group of "decision-making units" (DMUs). One advantage of DEA is that the relative importance or weights of the input and output measures are not required to be known a priori. Also, each input and output variable can be measured independently in any useful unit, without being transformed into a single metric, provided the same variables are utilized for every DMU.

Each DMU (representing a nursing home in this article) is evaluated by comparing its performance with the hypothetical performance of composite DMUs that are constructed as weighted combinations of the other DMUs in their peer group. A DMU is deemed "efficient" when no other DMU, or hypothetical composite of two or more of them, can produce the same outputs with fewer inputs (the "input-oriented" model) or can produce more outputs with the same inputs (the "output-oriented" model). Otherwise, the DMU is deemed to be "inefficient." Efficient DMUs represent "best practice" and are given an efficiency score of 100%. Inefficient DMUs are given lower scores, based on how efficiently they use their inputs to generate outputs compared to the "best practice" ones.

The original model proposed by Charnes, Cooper and Rhodes [1] was referred to as a constant-returns-to-scale model (CRS) since it assumed that an increase in input values would result in a proportional increase of output levels. A second model was developed by Banker, Charnes and Cooper [2] which used variable-returns-to-scale (VRS) in that it assumed that an increase in inputs would result in a non-proportional increase in outputs. This occurs when the linear combination of inputs and outputs for the hypothetical composite DMU is constrained to be a convex combination (i.e., the sum of the weights is equal to 1). Both models could be either input-oriented (seeking reductions in inputs) or output-oriented (seeking increases in outputs).

The two DEA models are illustrated in Figure 1, which shows a graph of a single output and single input for six hypothetical nursing homes (labeled A through F). The input is total labor in full-time equivalents (FTEs) and the output is total number of residents. For the CRS model, the efficient frontier is the line AB and its extension; for the VRS model, it is the figure ABCD.

The major strength of DEA is that it identifies, for each inefficient DMU, a benchmark set (also known as a reference set) of efficient or "best practice" DMUs. The units in this peer group are used to set performance targets for the inefficient unit. If the DMU can reduce its inputs (or increase its outputs) as suggested, then it potentially can become as efficient as the "best practice" units. One way of realizing this potential is for the inefficient DMU to study and evaluate the practices and procedures of the units in its benchmark group. In effect, the

DMUs in the benchmark set can serve as role models for the less efficient unit. In Figure 1 the benchmark set for nursing home E is a composite of A, B and C.

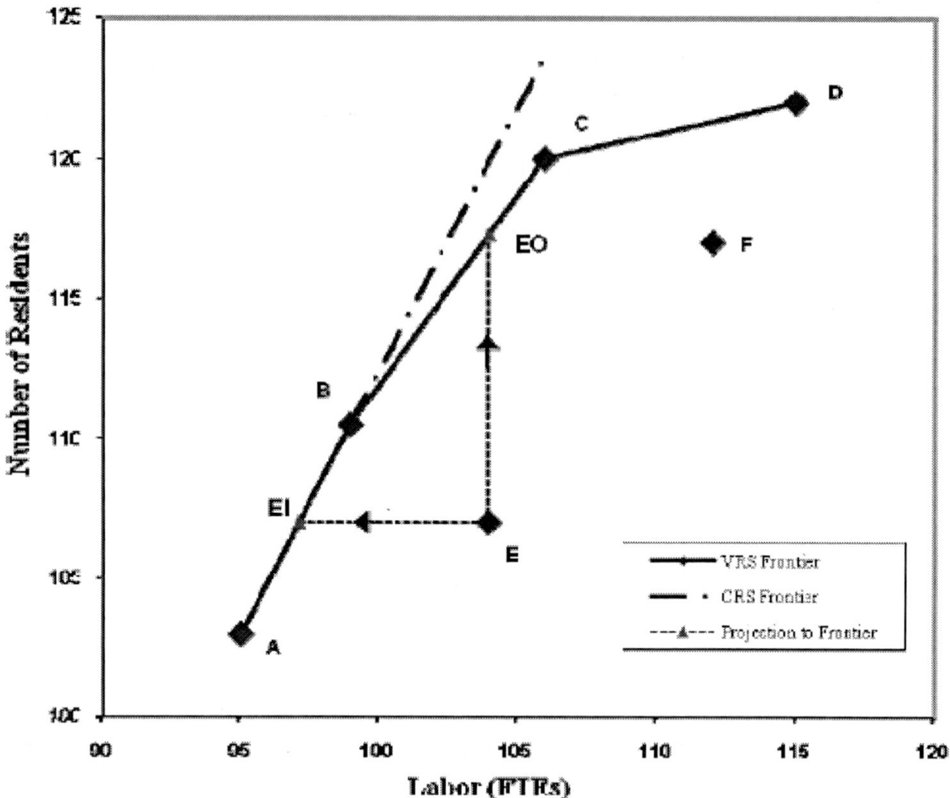

Figure 1. Efficient Frontier for DEA.

Many applications of DEA have been reported in a variety of managerial contexts [3]. A substantial amount of the DEA research has been done on applications in the health care sector. Most early studies concerned themselves with efficiency of hospital services and nursing services [4, 5]. DEA was extended to other types of health care institutions, including Veterans Administration medical centers [6], rural health programs [7], public health centers in Europe [8], organ procurement organizations [9] and health maintenance organizations [10]. More recently, the focus of DEA has turned to the study of the efficiency of physician practices [11-13].

In the area of nursing homes, DEA has been used more as a research tool than as a tool for performance improvement. Most studies have treated the DEA efficiency scores as the dependent variable in regression models in which characteristics of the nursing home or the market area were the independent variables [14-19]. The regression models attempted to explain which variables were related to nursing home efficiency. Some of the findings from these studies included: for-profit nursing homes were more efficient than not-for-profit homes; efficiency was positively related with chain membership, size, location in a big city and a wage index variable; and the existence of nurse trainees and patient turnover had a negative association with efficiency.

The study by Kleinsorge and Karney [20] took a somewhat different approach and demonstrated the usefulness of DEA for operational decision-making in nursing homes. It was a pilot study that experimented with several models of efficiency in nursing homes based on financial, economic, and quality measures. This study compared DEA with the results found using more traditional measures of performance, such as financial ratios. A more recent study applied DEA to benchmarking nursing home performance at the state level [21] while other research used nursing home applications to evaluate the problems that arise by incorporating quality measures into DEA models [22].

In this paper, we attempt to show how DEA can be used by administrators of nursing homes in a wide variety of settings to conduct a comprehensive evaluation of their performance and devise strategies for improvement. Taking advantage of the benchmarking features of DEA can prove to be an effective aid to operational decision-making in nursing homes.

DEA Applied to Nursing Homes

One widely used source of data on nursing homes is the Online Survey, Certification and Reporting (OSCAR) database. The OSCAR database, maintained by the Centers for Medicare and Medicaid Services (CMS), provides information on every nursing home in the United States that is certified by Medicare and/or Medicaid. OSCAR data are collected in two different ways. Self-reported data, including facility characteristics, resident characteristics and staffing levels are gathered annually for individual nursing homes. Next, states are required to conduct inspection surveys of each facility no less often than every 15 months. During the survey, data are gathered on facility deficiencies based on the evaluation of the processes and outcomes of care in the nursing homes.

When a nursing home fails to meet a standard, a deficiency is given to the facility for that individual standard. Deficiencies, which are limited to whether or not the facility meets each of the minimum standards, are also rated on the basis of severity. The deficiencies are given for problems which can result in negative impact on the health and safety of residents. Each OSCAR survey reports on nearly 190 nursing home deficiencies.

The data used in this paper came from OSCAR surveys. In order to apply DEA methodology to nursing homes, it is important to select relevant measures from the large amounts of available OSCAR performance data, and to divide these measures into inputs and outputs. Measures that are traditionally taken as inputs are resources consumed such as operating expenses or costs. Typically, this might include labor costs and capital expenditures. In the nursing home industry, salaries of health care personnel comprise the highest cost item. Some examples of other operating expenses would be housekeeping, laundry and food services. Capital expenditures, such as an investment to increase the bed size, should not be included as part of the inputs because they are highly regulated in this industry and are generally not subject to managerial control in the short term. With respect to inputs, using fewer of these resources could realize productivity gains. On the output side, organizations want to increase output measures in order to increase productivity. For service organizations, these outputs are typically measures representing both the quantity and quality of services provided. In the nursing home industry, outputs are represented by such categories of measures as number of residents, their case-mix severity and quality indicators.

This study considered nursing homes in the state of Massachusetts from a recent OSCAR database. There were a total of 399 nursing facilities in Massachusetts comprised of 40,649 nursing home residents in all 14 different state counties. The bed sizes in the facilities ranged from 16 to 366. Of the 399 facilities, 68% were for-profit, 30% not-for-profit and 2% were government run. Also, 55% of the facilities were part of a chain. As the basis for this study, we selected the 34 nursing homes that comprised the largest for-profit chain in Massachusetts. These facilities were located in 9 counties through the state of Massachusetts with bed sizes between 64 and 196.

The primary input category for our model of nursing home performance was labor. The OSCAR database provides many measure of staffing data. We aggregated these into six measures, namely the FTEs of registered nurses (RN), licensed practical nurses (LPN), nursing aides (AIDES), ancillary non-nursing professional staff (ANCPRO), ancillary non-nursing non-professional staff (ANCNON) and administrative staff (ADMIN).

On the output side, we selected measures of both quantity of services and quality of services provided. To represent the quantity of services provided, we used the total number of residents (TOTRES) in the nursing home along with the case-mix severity, as measured by the number of residents needing assistance with the five Activities of Daily Living (ADLs). Thus, the five measures of case-mix severity were the number of residents who are dependent on assistance with bathing (BATH_DEP), dressing (DRESS_DEP), transferring (TRANS_DEP), toileting (TOIL_DEP), and eating (EAT_DEP). The choice of these quantity output measures is supported by a number of previous studies that report a strong relationship among staffing levels and the number of nursing home residents and resident characteristics measured by case-mix severity [23-25].

With regard to quality measures, we chose three measures that focus on the prevalence of various conditions among the residents of a nursing home. These were selected from a list of quality measures that were generated and reported for all Medicare and Medicaid certified nursing homes by the CMS (fourteen long-term measures and five short-stay measures) and available on their Internet site [26]. The measures chosen were the number of residents with an indwelling catheter, residents who lose too much weight (5% or more in the last 30 days or 10% or more in the last 6 months), and residents with pressure sores. A high prevalence of any of these conditions is often taken as an indication of poor quality care by a nursing home. We used the OSCAR variables for the number of residents with catheters, who lose too much weight and with pressure sores, subtracted these variables from the total number of residents to get the following quality measures: the number of residents without a catheter (NOCATH), number of residents who don't lose too much weight (NOWTLOSS), and number of residents without pressure sores (NOSORE). In this way these quality measures satisfy the DEA assumption that efficiency scores increase when output measures increase.

The use of staffing levels as inputs and quality measures as outputs is an appropriate model for nursing homes. Studies in the literature have suggested that there is a positive relationship between staffing and quality in nursing homes. It has consistently been shown that higher staffing levels were associated with improved quality of care as measure through a number of outcome indicators [27-29]. In many of these studies, quality of care was determined on the basis of the prevalence of resident conditions including, but not limited to, the three that have been chosen in this paper.

Table 1 presents a summary of the input and output measures that were just described for the chain of 34 nursing homes considered in this paper. The table includes values of the mean, standard deviation, coefficient of variation, and minimum and maximum values for each of the input and output measures.

Interestingly, the input measure and the quantity output measure with the lowest mean value (ADMIN and EAT_DEP, respectively) also exhibited the highest coefficient of variation. The three quality output measures all show patterns that are relatively similar across all of the descriptive statistics.

Table 1. Summary of Input and Output Variables for 34 Nursing Homes

		Standard	Coefficient of		
Input Measures	Mean	Deviation	Variation	Minimum	Maximum
RN	7.63	3.58	47.0%	0.8	16.7
LPN	12.09	4.94	40.8%	4.0	25.5
AIDES	40.17	9.98	24.8%	23.2	67.5
ANCPRO	21.83	7.61	34.9%	9.5	48.3
ANCNON	14.44	4.02	27.8%	6.4	26.0
ADMIN	5.60	3.40	60.8%	2.0	14.4
Quantity		Standard	Coefficient of		
Output Measures	Mean	Deviation	Variation	Minimum	Maximum
RESIDENTS	101.79	25.91	25.4%	64	172
BATH_DEP	94.65	24.95	26.4%	57	160
DRES_DEP	92.79	25.11	27.1%	53	160
TRANS_DEP	74.21	23.86	32.1%	40	124
TOIL_DEP	79.88	23.20	29.0%	37	126
EAT_DEP	50.32	24.01	47.7%	19	117
Quality		Standard	Coefficient of		
Output Measures	Mean	Deviation	Variation	Minimum	Maximum
NOCATH	97.35	25.23	25.9%	56	165
NOWTLOSS	97.21	25.09	25.8%	58	163
NOSORE	95.44	26.28	27.5%	55	167

The input-oriented CRS model was used in this paper. We chose the input orientation because we believed that the categories of labor, representing the measures from the input side, were more directly under the control of management than the output measures. The CRS model represents constant return to scale among the nursing homes. This seemed appropriate because the nursing homes used in this paper were relatively homogeneous with respect to size and therefore we didn't expect to observe scale effects. Since DEA is an application of mathematical programming, modeling can be performed using the Solver add-in that comes with Microsoft Excel. Many other commercial DEA software products are available, including some that accompany books on DEA [3].

Results

The DEA model used for analysis included the following variables: six labor measures as inputs; and six quantity measures (total residents and five case-mix severity measures) and three quality measures as outputs. Table 2 shows the results of the DEA analysis in terms of efficiency scores. Of the 34 nursing homes in the for-profit chain, 23 were found to be fully efficient with 100% performance scores. The other 11 inefficient nursing homes had performance scores ranging from 80% up to 100%. The efficient nursing homes serve as a reference set for less efficient homes trying to improve their performance. With regard to facility size, nursing homes with either large or small numbers of beds did not consistently perform best. (The correlation of the bed size with efficiency score was +0.18). Similarly, the nursing homes with the largest or smallest number of total FTEs of labor did not have the highest efficiency scores (correlation of +0.11). It is impossible to generalize about nursing home performance with respect to measures such as facility size or amount of labor. Rather, efficiency is a much more difficult concept to study, one in which DEA modeling provides some useful insight. Table 3 provides an analysis of the efficient nursing homes by county in Massachusetts. The number of nursing homes belonging to this for-profit chain varies widely by county. It is also true that nursing home efficiency is not dominated by specific counties. (The correlation of number of homes by county and % of homes with 100% efficiency scores was -0.06). This dispels the notion that nursing homes belonging to this chain and clustered in

Table 2. Distribution of DEA Efficiency Scores

Efficiency Score (%)	Number of Homes
80-84.9	1
85-89.9	2
90-94.9	1
95-99.9	7
100	23
Total	34

Table 3. Distribution of Nursing Homes by County

County	Number of Homes	% Homes with 100% Efficiency Scores
Barnstable	1	100
Berkshire	2	50
Bristol	4	100
Essex	5	80
Middlesex	4	100
Norfolk	6	67
Plymouth	3	33
Suffolk	5	60
Worcester	4	25
Total	34	

a particular county are all either high or low performers. Thus, on the macro-level, efficiency in nursing homes is very unpredictable.

DEA has the capability of providing in-depth analysis of the nursing homes that have been found to be inefficient, including information for the purposes of performance improvement through benchmarking. Consider nursing home 10 which was found to be inefficient with a performance score of 95.0%. As seen in Table 4, the three homes that serve as its "best practice" reference set are nursing homes 9, 14 and 18. The target or benchmark values for the input and output measures are a composite found by using the weights shown in Table 4 to determine a weighted linear combination of the actual inputs and outputs for nursing homes 9, 14 and 18. For example, the ADMIN target value of 2.0 is the sum of the products of the ADMIN values for nursing homes 9, 14 and 18 and their respective weights (i.e., 2.0 = 2.1 X 0.384 + 2.3 X 0.366 + 14.4 X 0.025). These target values represent a composite nursing home that is more efficient than nursing home 10. The table also shows the differences between the target values and the actual values for nursing home 10 along with the percentage decrease in its inputs (and percentage increase in its outputs) necessary for nursing home 10 to reach the target. It can be seen in the table that the target for its inputs is a decrease of at least 5.0%, which caused its efficiency rating to be 100% minus 5.0%, or 95.0%.

Table 4. Detailed Performance Report for Nursing Home 10

	Reference Set[1]					Home 10[2]	
	Home 9	Home 14	Home 18	Target	Actual	To Reach Target	
Inputs						Decrease	% Decrease
RN	4.6	10.1	16.7	5.9	6.4	0.5	8.2%
LPN	10.8	10.9	5.3	8.3	9.1	0.8	9.2%
AIDES	39.3	47.0	46.0	33.4	35.2	1.8	5.0%
ANCPRO	12.0	19.9	26.0	12.5	13.2	0.7	5.0%
ANCNON	25.2	24.1	29.4	19.2	20.5	1.3	6.2%
ADMIN	2.1	2.3	14.4	2.0	2.5	0.5	19.8%
Quantity Outputs						Increase	% Increase
TOTRES	112	132	131	94.6	90	4.6	5.1%
BATH_DEP	102	132	119	90.4	86	4.4	5.1%
DRES_DEP	102	132	117	90.4	83	7.4	8.9%
TRANS_DEP	71	110	88	69.7	68	1.7	2.5%
TOIL_DEP	71	121	99	74.0	74	0.0	0.0%
EAT_DEP	65	109	39	65.8	65	0.8	1.3%
Quality Outputs						Increase	% Increase
NOCATH	106	130	127	91.4	87	4.4	5.1%
NOWTLOSS	112	128	126	93.0	89	4.0	4.4%
NOSORE	106	126	129	90.0	90	0.0	0.0%

[1]The weights for Homes 9, 14 and 18 are 38.4%, 36.6% and 2.5%, respectively.
[2]The efficiency score for Home 10 is 95.0%.

Generally, nursing home 10 has slightly lower numbers of residents needing assistance with the five ADLs and lower numbers of residents without a catheter, weight loss and pressure sores than in the composite nursing home that defines its benchmark set. However, nursing home 10 operates with higher levels of staff than the composite nursing home in every one of the six labor categories. Therefore, nursing home 10, with an efficiency score of 95.0%, must decrease its labor inputs by at least 5.0% in order to reach the target levels (while maintaining the same level of quality measures). Most noticeable is that nursing home 10 should attempt to lower the number of administrative staff (ADMIN) by 19.8%, licensed practical nurses (LPN) by 9.2% and registered nurses (RN) by 8.2 %. For each of these labor categories, the number of FTEs is considerable higher than the benchmark composite nursing home that defines the target levels.

The three nursing homes that comprise the reference set for nursing home 10 are worthy of further investigation. It would not be obvious to the management of nursing home 10 to select these three homes for benchmarking. The total residents in the benchmark homes vary considerably (range from 112 to 132 as compared to 90 total residents in nursing home 10).

The variation is also great across the three benchmark homes when considering staff levels, case-mix severity measures and the quality measures. DEA has the ability to identify those nursing homes that can best serve as the reference set for inefficient homes. Nursing homes 9 and 14 are particularly important for the purpose of benchmarking within this chain since they serve in the reference set for 90.9% and 81.8%, respectively, of all of the inefficient nursing homes. These two homes certainly deserve the attention of the administrators of the nursing home chain in addition to those at other facilities.

The administrators and decision-makers at the inefficient nursing homes, such as home 10, can use these results to improve the performance of their nursing home. Improving performance goes beyond just allowing a nursing home to compare itself to another home in the same geographic area or of the same bed size. The DEA results have shown that the reference set for nursing home 10 is comprised of three homes of varying size, two of which are located in different counties in the state. The nursing home chain could open their nursing homes to study and observation so that nursing home 10 could adopt the policies and procedures used by the reference set of nursing homes 9, 14 and 18. If they were successful in doing so, then nursing home 10 could potentially provide their residents with at least the same level of service quantity and level of service quality, but at a lower cost for labor.

Conclusion

Economic conditions have creating an environment in which developing a useful measure of nursing home performance and strategies for improving nursing home care is of growing importance. Existing methods that involve gathering large amounts of data on numerous aspects of performance and generating profile reports for individual nursing homes have several inherent problems. First, it is cumbersome to inspect a long list of performance measures and their rankings compared to other homes. Second, without an objective means of prioritizing or combining the various measures, it is difficult to determine which nursing homes are performing well overall. Finally, this technique provides very little guidance on how nursing homes can change their operations to improve their performance.

DEA is a mathematical technique that can overcome the aforementioned problems. DEA can be used to identify the most efficient nursing homes and to set performance benchmarks for less efficient homes. Administrators of a nursing home chain can use data from internal sources to evaluate the homes in their chain. Not only will they be able to identify good performers in their chain but they will also be able to provide guidance to the less successful facilities on how they could improve, thereby moving closer to their goal of providing better service at lower cost. Similarly, administrators in individual facilities could apply DEA to data from public sources to study comparable homes. Results could be used to evaluate their own performance compared to that of their peers.

The most powerful aspect of DEA is that it provides administrators with a multitude of options to improve performance. Efficiency is determined with a single measure and a small reference set of "best practice" nursing home performance patterns is identified. Hence, administrators may realize new approaches for controlling costs, increasing the quantity of services and improving quality levels. DEA is far superior to profiling methods of evaluating nursing home performance and allows individual facilities or entire nursing home chains to better oversee their operations.

We have illustrated DEA by studying the performance of nursing homes that are part of a for-profit chain. We had selected a particular set of input and output measures in this application. The input measures, represented by categories of labor, could be affected by the administrators' decisions in response to projected DEA targets. The output measures attempted to capture nursing home performance in terms of the quantity and quality of services delivered. Many other measures could have been chosen for study. Some researchers use profitability efficiency models or customer behavior models and include the selection of other types of input and output variables, such as customer satisfaction and a variety of other quality measures for inclusion in the models [30, 31]. Another model that could be considered would be a risk-adjusted model that ignored costs. Its inputs would be measures of case-mix and its outputs would be quality measures. Nursing home administrators have the flexibility to select the input and output variables that best fit their respective homes.

Another factor that influenced our choice of input and output measures were the data that comprise the OSCAR database. While OSCAR is a readily available source of nursing home data, there are other sources such as the minimum data-set (MDS) which is maintained by CMS. The MDS contains extensive and detailed data on individual residents reported by every Medicare and Medicaid certified nursing home. As a result of privacy concerns, the extent to which MDS data are available to the public is limited. CMS has been using MDS data to generate the set of quality measures for nursing homes which are reported on their Internet site [26]. This site could be used to select additional quality measures for DEA modeling of nursing homes. It is hoped that in the future, CMS will expand their lists of nursing home performance measures to be publicly shared.

Unfortunately, there is no cost data in the MDS. As a result, cost data would have to come from OSCAR or from some other data sources. One such source is from the individual states. In general, each state gathers and compiles data on their nursing homes. Some of these state data have been used by researchers in their study of nursing homes [14, 15]. However, since there is no national standard for the collection of financial data, the data and formats vary from state to state.

In the Commonwealth of Massachusetts, the Department of Medical Assistance uses the Management Minutes Questionnaire (MMQ), a survey instrument intended to reflect nursing care needs of individual residents (i.e., minutes of daily nursing care) to measure the case-mix of a nursing home's Medicaid residents. Also, the Massachusetts Division of Health Care Finance and Policy collects extensive financial data from nursing home cost reports. Many other states have systems for collecting nursing home data which could provide further input and output measures for DEA modeling. In addition to these public sources, administrators of nursing home chains will have available their own internal data that they could use in DEA.

The answer to the original question is yes. We have shown that DEA can be used to study performance efficiency in nursing homes. DEA affords the nursing home administrator the opportunity to select performance variables that are particularly relevant to the specific nursing home or chain of homes from an assortment of available data bases. Using readily available software, DEA generates results that allow nursing homes to develop multiple paths towards increasing efficiency and continuous performance improvement.

References

[1] Charnes, A., Cooper, W.W., and Rhodes, E. (1978). Measuring the Efficiency of Decision Making Units. *European Journal of Operational Research*, 2, 429-444.

[2] Banker, R.D., Charnes, A., and Cooper, W.W. (1984). Some Models for Estimating Technical and Scale Inefficiencies in Data Envelopment Analysis. *Management Science,* 30, 1078-1092.

[3] Cooper, W.W., Seiford, L.M., and Tone, K. (2000). *Data Envelopment Analysis: A Comprehensive Text with Models, Applications, References and DEA-Solver Software.* Boston, MA: Kluwer Academic.

[4] Sherman, H.D. (1984). Hospital Efficiency Measurement and Evaluation: Empirical Test of a New Technique. *Medical Care*, 22, 922-938.

[5] Nunamaker, T.R. (1983). Measuring Routine Nursing Service Efficiency: A Comparison of Cost Per Patient Day and Data Envelopment Analysis Models. *Health Services Research*, 18, 183-205.

[6] Sexton, T.R., Leiken, A.M., Nolan, A.H., Liss, S., Hogan, A., and Silkman, R.H. (1989). Evaluating Managerial Efficiency of Veterans Administration Medical Centers Using Data Envelopment Analysis. *Medical Care*, 27, 1175-1188.

[7] Huang, Y.L. and McLaughlin, C.P. (1989). Relative Efficiency in Rural Primary Health Care: An Application of Data Envelopment Analysis. *Health Services Research*, 24, 143-158.

[8] Pina, V. and Torres, L. (1992). Evaluating the Efficiency of Nonprofit Organizations: An Application of Data Envelopment Analysis to the Public Health Service. *Financial Accounting and Management*, 8, 213-224.

[9] Ozcan, Y.A., Begun, J.W., and McKinney, M.M. (1999). Benchmarking Organ Procurement Organizations: A National Study. *Health Services Research*, 34, 855-874.

[10] Draper, D.A., Solti, I., and Ozcan, Y.A. (2000). Characteristics of Health Maintenance Organizations and Their Influence on Efficiency. *Health Services Management Research*, 13, 40-56.

[11] Chilingerian, J.A. and Sherman, H.D. (1996). Benchmarking Physician Practice Patterns with DEA: A Multi-Stage Approach for Cost Containment. *Annals of Operations Research*, 67, 83-116.

[12] Ozcan, Y.A., Jiang, H.J., and Pai, C.W. (2000). Do Primary Care Physicians or Specialists Provide More Efficient Care? *Health Services Management Research*, 13, 90-96.

[13] Wagner, J.M., Shimshak, D.G., and Novak, M.A. (2003). Advances in Physician Profiling: The Use of DEA. *Socio-Economic Planning Sciences*, 37, 141-163.

[14] Nyman, J.A. and Bricker, D.L. (1989). Profit Incentives and Technical Efficiency in the Production of Nursing Home Care. *Review of Economics and Statistics*, 71, 586-594.

[15] Fizel, J.L. and Nunnikhoven, T.S. (1993). The Efficiency of Nursing Home Chains. *Applied Economics*, 25, 49-55.

[16] Chattopadhyay, S. and Heffley, D. (1994). Are For-Profit Nursing Homes More Efficient? Data Envelopment Analysis with a Case-Mix Constraint. *Eastern Economic Journal*, 20, 171-186.

[17] Kooreman, P. (1994). Nursing Home Care in the Netherlands: A Non-Parametric Efficiency Analysis. *Journal of Health Economics*, 13, 301-316.

[18] Rosko, M.D., Chilingerian, J.A., Zinn, J.S., and Aaronson, W.E. (1995). The Effects of Ownership, Operating Environment, and Strategic Choices on Nursing Home Efficiency. *Medical Care*, 33, 1001-1021.

[19] Ozcan, Y.A., Wogen, S.E., and Mau, L.W. (1998). Efficiency Evaluation of Skilled Nursing Facilities. *Journal of Medical Systems*, 22, 211-224.

[20] Kleinsorge, I.K. and Karney, D.F. (1992). Management of Nursing Homes Using Data Envelopment Analysis. *Socio-Economic Planning Sciences*, 26, 57-71.

[21] Lenard, M.L. and Shimshak, D.G. (2009). Benchmarking Nursing Home Performance at the State Level. *Health Services Management Research*, 22, 51-61.

[22] Shimshak, D.G., Lenard, M.L., and Klimberg, R.K. (2009). Incorporating Quality into Data Envelopment Analysis of Nursing Home Performance: A Case Study. *OMEGA*, 37, 672-685.

[23] Weissert, W.G., Scanlon, W.J., Wan, T.T.H., and Skinner, D.E. (1983). Care for the Chronically Ill: Nursing Home Incentive Payment Experiment. *Health Care Financing Review*, 5, 41-49.

[24] Arling, G., Nordquist, R.H., Brant, B.A., and Capitman, J.A. (1987). Nursing Home Case Mix: Patient Classification by Nursing Resource Use. *Medical Care*, 25, 9-19.

[25] Fries, B.E. (1990). Comparing Case-Mix Systems for Nursing Home Payment. *Health Care Financing Review*, 11, 103-120.

[26] U.S. Department of Health and Human Services, Centers for Medicare and Medicaid Services (2010). Nursing Home Quality Initiatives. (http://www.cms.gov/. NursingHomeQualityInits/10_NHQIQualityMeasures.asp).

[27] Munroe, D.J. (1990). The Influence of Registered Nurse Staffing on the Quality of Nursing Home Care. *Research in Nursing and Health*, 13, 263-270.

[28] Spector, W.D. and Takada, H.A. (1991). Characteristics of Nursing Homes that Affect Resident Outcomes. *Journal of Aging and Health*, 3, 427-454.

[29] Rudman, D., Slater, E.J., Richardson, T.J., and Mattson, D.E. (1993). The Occurrence of Pressure Ulcers in Three Nursing Homes. *Journal of General Internal Medicine*, 8, 653-658.

[30] Kamakura, W.A., Mittal, V., DeRosa, F., and Mazzon, J.A. (2002). Assessing the Service-Profit Chain. *Marketing Science*, 21, 294-317.

[31] Soteriou, A. and Zenios, S.A. (1999). Operations, Quality, and Profitability in the Provision of Banking Services. *Management Science*, 45, 1221-1238.

In: Palliative and Nursing Home Care
Editor: Samuel E. Plunkett ISBN 978-1-61122-417-7

Chapter 10

Quality of Life for Older Persons Living in Nursing Homes: A Cross-Sectional Study

Mimi Tse[1] and Vanessa Wan[2]
[1]Assistant Professor, School of Nursing,
The Hong Kong Polytechnic University, Kowloon, Hong Kong
[2]Registered Nurse, Princess Margaret Hospital, Hong Kong

Abstract

Background: Given the increasingly ageing population ad the impact of diseases and disabilities during the ageing process, the need of older persons for some form of alternative accommodation and residential care facilities is expected to rise. The Hong Kong Association of Gerontology (2004) estimates that 5.5% of people aged 65 or older need institutionalized care for their later life.

Aim: To explore quality of life among older persons living in nursing homes

Method: This was an exploratory cross-sectional study. Six nursing homes were approached and 365 older persons invited to join the study. A questionnaire was administered to them to collect information on their demographic data, bowel habits and pain situation. We also investigated their physical function (assessed using Barthel ADL Scores and Elderly Mobility Scores) and psychological condition, including life satisfaction, depression, happiness and loneliness (using the Life Satisfaction, Geriatric Depression, Happiness and UCLA Loneliness Scales).

Results: There were 365 older nursing home residents (248 female and 117 male, mean age 84.7 ± 6.73) in the study, of whom 249 (70%) suffered from pain, mean pain scores of 4.55 indicating medium pain intensity. The location of pain was mainly in the knee, back and shoulder, possibly affecting the older persons' physical function and psychological health. Those with mildly limited physical function had Barthel ADL Scores of 16.55 ± 4.75 (mostly those with difficulty bathing and climbing stairs) and Elderly Mobility Scores of 14.55 ± 5.69 (difficulty walking 6 meters and functional reaching). As for their psychological health, they scored low life satisfaction 8.81 ± 4.05, mild depression 6.92 ± 3.93, fair happiness 17.70 ± 6.09, and moderate loneliness 42.83 ± 12.34. In addition, the correlation between the demographic data and the psychological parameters was tested: there was a weak positive correlation between age and depression, and weak negative correlations between gender and happiness (male older residents felt happier) and pain and depression (elderly people with pain felt more depressed than the group with no pain).

Conclusions and relevance to clinical practice: Overall, older persons suffer from moderate to severe physical and psychological impairment in nursing homes. Nurses and other healthcare professionals should encourage them to engage in various interventions to minimize these problems and enhance their quality of life at the end of their life journey.

Introduction

Thanks to improvements in health technology and healthcare delivery that have contributed to the decline in mortality, there have been increases in life expectancy in the 20th century that are anticipated to continue in the future. The Hong Kong population has the second longest life expectancy in the world (Hong Kong Policy Research Institute Ltd., 2006). The life expectancy at birth in 2008 is 79.3 for males and 85.5 for females (Centre for Health Protection, 2008). In 2033, the aged population will reach 27% of the total Hong Kong population.

Given the increasingly ageing population and the impact of diseases and disabilities during the ageing process, the need of older persons for some form of alternative accommodation and residential care facilities is expected to rise. According to The Hong Kong Association of Gerontology (2004), approximately 5.5% of people aged 65 or older need institutionalized care for their later life. In this connection, the quality of life of older persons living in nursing homes needed to be examined.

There have been insufficient government-subsidized homes in Hong Kong, thus the numbers of private old age homes or nursing homes have been increasing rapidly to meet the demands of the ageing population. However, private nursing homes vary in quality: some poor quality ones are crowded, and their limited numbers of trained staff lead to poor quality of care for the older residents, which directly affects their health in later life (Leung et al., 2000; Sim and Leung 2000). Living in nursing homes has been regarded as causing loss of autonomy due to the necessity of following a routine in the institution, feelings of being abandoned by family members, and fears of deterioration of health and nearness of death (Tse, 2007).

In fact, most older people live in nursing homes due to the decrease in physical mobility that is common in the normal aging process and associated with chronic illness, which causes limitations in self-care daily activities, including bathing, hygiene, feeding and grooming. Yet the change of the family structure from typical Chinese extended families to the small nuclear families in today's society is resulting in many older people living alone or with their spouse only. This transformation in the family structure has undermined the social support network among the elderly in the community, since the child or children have difficulty caring for them when they are not living together. Therefore, nursing homes with daily living assistance are often a better choice for them if they are facing health deterioration or decreasing self-care ability.

Living in a nursing home may have a great psychological impact on Chinese older people due to the loss of freedom and the need to follow a routine in the institution; feelings of being abandoned by family members must also be very hurtful to them. Most older people in nursing homes have limited physical ability, suffer lower life satisfaction and depression due to their illness, and feel isolated from their family (Baum et al., 2003; Owen, 2008). Thus, the present study aimed at examining the quality of life among nursing home residents so as to formulate interventions to improve their physical and psychological wellness, and to restore or maintain their function longevity.

Methods

Design and Sample

This study used an exploratory, cross-sectional design. After gaining approval from the Ethics Committee of the University, six nursing homes were approached and invited to join the study. Written consent was obtained from all participants. The inclusion criteria included being 60 or older, able to communicate in Cantonese, and oriented to time and place. By contrast, those with a history of mental disorders or cognitive impairment were excluded from the study. A total of 365 older persons were recruited.

Participants were invited to attend an interview and answer questions related to their demographic data, physical mobility and psychological parameters.

Demographic data including gender, age, marital status, education level, previous occupation, duration of stay in nursing home, past health history, bowel habit and bowel medication were collected. Pain situations were measured by the Geriatric Pain Assessment, which included assessing pain intensity using a verbal rating scale (a 0 to 10-point scale), pattern and location of pain, and the use of analgesic drug and non-drug therapy, including its type and frequency. Physical parameters were collected by Barthel ADL and Elderly Mobility Scores, while psychological parameters were collected using the Life Satisfaction, Geriatric Depression, Subjective Happiness and Revised UCLA Loneliness Scales.

Measurements

Physical Parameters

Both physical and psychological parameters were measured in the nursing home residents. In the study, Barthel ADL and Elderly Mobility Scores were used to assess the older people's physical ability.

Barthel ADL Scores

The Barthel ADL Scores measure the self-care functional ability of nursing home residents, and the 10 testing items include presence or absence of fecal and urinary incontinence, and help needed with grooming, toileting, feeding, transfers, walking, dressing, climbing stairs and bathing. The scores can vary from item to item, with a minimum total score of 0 and a maximum total score of 20. The greater the score, the more functionally independent the older person (Mahoney and Barthel, 1965; Shyu et al., 2008).

Elderly Mobility Scale

The Elderly Mobility Scale consists of seven questions focusing on mobility independence related to position changes, such as from a supine to a sitting position or from sitting to standing; it also assesses independence in walking mobility. The score varies from item to item, and the maximum total score is 20: the higher the score, the greater the level of mobility (Smith, 1994; Proser et al., 1997; Ng et al, 2008).

Psychological Parameters

The psychological well-being of the older people included life satisfaction (assessed by the Life Satisfaction Index – A Form), geriatric depression (assessed by the Geriatric Depression Scale), happiness (assessed by the Subjective Happiness Scale) and loneliness (assessed by the Revised UCLA Loneliness Scale).

Life Satisfaction Index-A Form Scale

The Life Satisfaction Index-A Form Scale consists of 18 questions related to five different components: zest, resolution and fortitude, congruence between desired and achieved goals, positive self-concept and mood tone (Neugarten et al., 1961). There were 18 yes-no questions that scored 1 point for "Yes" and 0 for "No". Thus the range of scores was from a minimum of 0 to a maximum of 18, higher scores showing higher levels of life satisfaction. In this study, a Chinese version of the Life Satisfaction Index-A form was used, with the Cronbach's alpha 0.7 for reliability and split half value 0.62 for internal consistency (Chi and Boey, 1992).

Geriatric Depression Scale

The Geriatric Depression Scale is one of the most commonly used tools in screening older adults for depression (Yesavage et al., 1983). In the study, a short form GDS was used, consisting of 15 yes-no questions; scores could vary from a minimum of 0 to a maximum of 15. Scores of 0-4 are considered normal, depending on age, education, and complaints; 5-8 indicate mild depression; 9-11 indicate moderate depression; and 12-15 indicate severe depression. (Kurlowicz and Greenberg, 2007). Cronbach's alpha of internal consistency was 0.89, and the test-retest reliability was 0.85. A Chinese version of the Geriatric Depression Scale was used (Chan, 1996; Mui, 1996).

Subjective Happiness Scale

The Subjective Happiness Scale is an instrument that includes four items addressing the degree of the participant's happiness (Sonja and Heidi, 1999). Each item is rated on a seven-point scale, the range of the scale being from point 1 = "not at all" to 7 = "a great deal". Two items ask participants to characterize themselves using both absolute ratings and ratings relative to peers, while the other two items offer brief descriptions of happy and unhappy individuals and ask participants the extent to which each characterization describes them. The total range of the scores is 4-28, with higher scores reflecting greater happiness. The Cronbach's alpha was 0.79 to 0.94. (Lyubomirsky and Lepper, 1999). The test-retest reliability ranged from 0.55 to 0.90.

UCLA Loneliness Scale

The revised UCLA Loneliness Scale (version 3) is a scale for measuring loneliness (Russell, 1996). There are 20 items, including nine positively worded items and eleven negatively worded items. Each of the 20 items is rated on a scale of 1 (never), 2 (rarely), 3 (sometimes) and 4 (often).

After summing all the items, the range of possible scores was from a minimum of 20 to a maximum of 80, the higher scores representing greater loneliness. Scores from 30 to 40 are considered a normal experience of loneliness, while scores above 60 indicate that a person is experiencing severe loneliness. In the study, a Chinese version of the Revised UCLA Loneliness Scale was used, and the Cronbach's alpha of the Chinese UCLA Loneliness Scale was 0.90 (Chou et al., 2005).

Data Analysis

Several statistical methods were used in data analysis. Descriptive statistical analysis of the quantitative data was conducted using the Statistical Package for the Social Sciences version 15, 2006.

The demographic variables included gender, age, marital status, education level, previous occupation, health history, and duration of working in a nursing home were measured. Also, correlation of psychological health and demographic variables was carried out. A p-value of <0.05 was considered statistically significant.

Results

Demographic Data

The study recruited 365 older persons from six nursing homes. The demographic data is shown in Table 1. Most of the participants were female (248 females and 117 males). Their ages ranged from 60 to 101, with a mean age of 84.7 ± 6.73.

Most had been in nursing homes for 1-3 years and were widowed. Over half of the nursing home residents had not received formal education. Their major underlying medical problems included hypertension (64.9%), cataract (37%), old stroke (29.6%), heart disease (26.6%) and diabetes mellitus (22.7%).

Their other health-related issues, including pain history, bowel habits, constipation and use of oral bowel medications, are also investigated in Table 1. 68.2% (n=249) of participants reported having experienced pain and had a mean pain score of 4.55 ± 2.44 (on a 10-point scale) in the previous 3 months. The most frequently cited pain types were knee pain (55.4%), back pain (34.1%), shoulder pain (24.9%), and hip pain (17.3%), the remainder being ankle pain (11.2%). The majority of older residents neither used bowel medications nor suffered from constipation.

Table 1. Demographic data (N=365)

		N	*(%)*
Gender	Male	117	*(32.1)*
	Female	248	*(67.9)*
Age	60 - 70	18	*(5.0)*
Mean: 84.70, SD: 6.73	71 - 80	89	*(24.3)*
	81 - 90	213	*(58.3)*
	91 - 100	44	*(12.1)*
	Above 101	1	*(0.3)*
Marital Status	Single	38	*(10.4)*
	Married	82	*(22.5)*
	Divorced	7	*(1.9)*
	Widowed	238	*(65.2)*
Education Level	No formal education	186	*(51.0)*
	Primary education	137	*(37.5)*
	Secondary education	38	*(10.4)*
	Tertiary education	4	*(1.1)*
Previous occupation	Primary industry	48	*(13.2)*
	Second industry	96	*(26.3)*
	Tertiary Industry	116	*(31.8)*
	Housework	105	*(28.8)*
Year(s) in nursing home	1 – 3 years	173	*(47.4)*
	4 – 6 years	77	*(21.1)*
	7 – 9 years	48	*(13.1)*
	10 years or above	67	*(18.4)*
Past health history	Hypertension	237	*(64.9)*
	Cataract	135	*(37.0)*
	Stroke	108	*(29.6)*
	Heart disease	97	*(26.6)*
	Diabetes Mellitus	83	*(22.7)*
	Previous fracture	78	*(21.4)*
	Arthritis	68	*(18.6)*
	Respiratory disease	61	*(16.7)*
	Dementia	41	*(11.2)*
	Psychiatric disease	31	*(8.5)*
	Urinary tract infection	24	*(6.6)*
	Parkinsonism	16	*(4.4)*
	Glaucoma	12	*(3.3)*
	Impaired renal function	12	*(3.3)*
With chronic pain	Yes	249	*(68.2)*
	No	116	*(31.8)*
Bowel medication	Yes	125	*(34.2)*
	No	240	*(65.8)*
Constipation	No	352	*(96.4)*
	Yes	13	*(3.6)*
Bowel habit	Daily	206	*(56.4)*
	Every two days	87	*(23.8)*
	Every three days	59	*(16.2)*
	Every four days	13	*(3.6)*

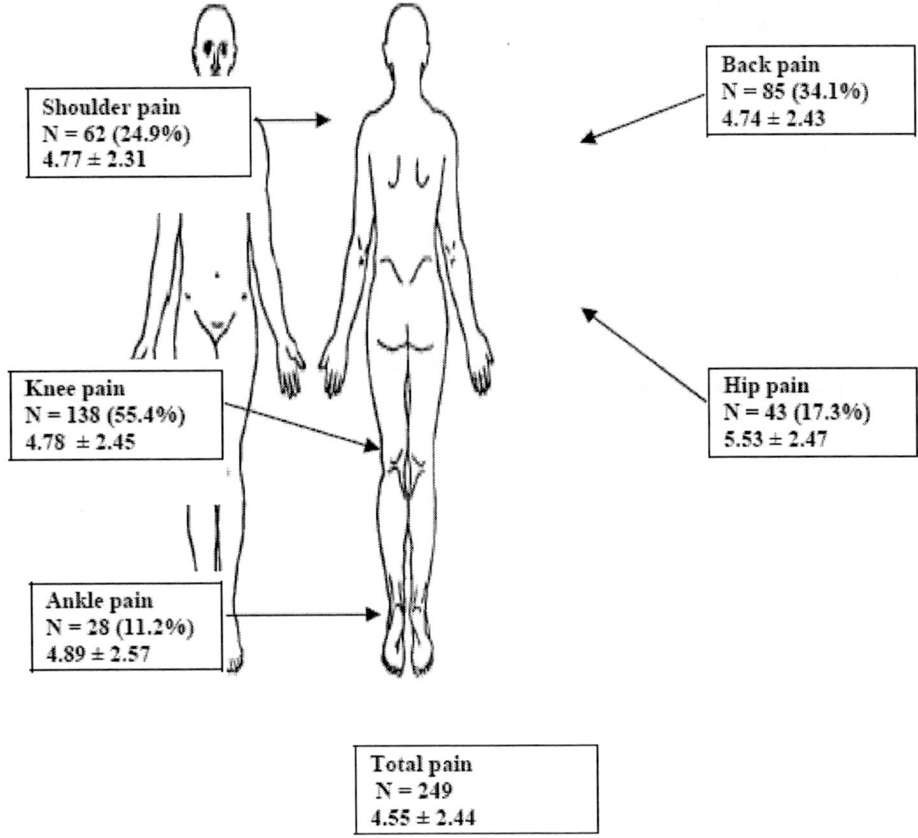

Figure 1. Pain intensity and site in pain group (N=249) Mean ± S.D.

Physical and Psychological Health

There were mild limitations in physical function among the nursing home residents surveyed: their Barthel ADL Score was 16.55 ± 4.75, most of them having difficulty in bathing (consisting of 0.6 out of a total score of 1) and climbing stairs (consisting of 1.24 out of a total score of 2); their Elderly Mobility Score was 14.55 ± 5.69, the weakest aspects being walking 6 meters and functional reaching, with around 60% of its full functioning.

Most nursing home residents have limitations in their physical ability, and such immobility and illness have some psychological consequences, such as lower life satisfaction, depression, loneliness, and decreased happiness.

In the study, the older people had lower life satisfaction at 8.81 ± 4.05 (18 yes-no questions); mild depression at 6.92 ± 3.93 (15 yes-no questions); fair happiness at 17.70 ± 6.09 (four questions on a 7-point scale); and moderate loneliness 42.83 ± 12.34 (20 questions on a 4-point scale).

Table 2. Physical condition (N=365)

Physical parameters	Total Mean ± S.D.	Range
Barthel ADL Scores		
Feeding	1.98 ± 0.20	0-2
Bathing	0.60 ± 0.49	0-1
Personal hygiene	0.96 ± 0.19	0-1
Dressing	1.78 ± 0.51	0-2
Bowel control	1.66 ± 0.71	0-2
Urinary control	1.75 ± 0.60	0-2
Toileting	1.68 ± 1.21	0-2
Moving from wheelchair to bed	2.51 ± 0.89	0-3
Walking	2.47 ± 1.02	0-3
Climbing stairs	1.24 ± 0.87	0-2
Total Score	16.55 ± 4.75	0-20
Elderly Mobility Scores		
From lying to sitting	1.82 ± 0.47	0-2
From sitting to lying	1.86 ± 0.45	0-2
From sitting to standing	2.35 ± 0.94	0-3
Standing	1.92 ± 1.14	0-3
Walking	2.28 ± 1.16	0-3
Walking 6 meters	1.88 ± 1.13	0-3
Functional reaching	2.51 ± 1.55	0-4
Total Score	14.55 ± 5.69	0-20

Table 3. Psychological condition (N=365)

Psychological parameters	Total Mean ± S.D.	Range
Life Satisfaction	8.81 ± 4.05	0-18
Depression	6.92 ± 3.93	0-15
Happiness	17.70 ± 6.09	4-28
UCLA Loneliness	42.83 ± 12.34	20-80

Demographic Data and Psychological Parameters

The relationship between the demographic data and the psychological parameters was measured and a weak positive correlation found between age and depression. This means that the old-old felt more depressed than the young-old. Two weak negative correlations were found, one between gender and happiness, which showed that males felt more happiness than female residents, and the other between pain and depression, the elderly with pain feeling more depressed than the group with no pain.

Table 4. Correlation: Psychological parameters and demographic variables

Spearman's Rho Correlations	Gender		Age		Marital status		Education level		Previous occupation		Duration in nursing home		Pain within 6 months	
	r	p-value	r	p-value	r	p-value	r	p-value	r	p-value	r	p-value	r	p-value
Life satisfaction	-0.068	0.193	-0.074	0.160	-0.041	0.440	0.023	0.660	0.021	0.686	0.004	0.936	0.092	0.078
Depression	0.094	0.073	0.134	0.010*	0.021	0.690	-0.005	0.920	-0.047	0.369	-0.025	0.637	-0.112	0.032*
Happiness	-0.129	0.014*	-0.099	0.059	-0.013	0.802	-0.035	0.500	-0.020	0.702	0.094	0.074	0.089	0.088
UCLA Loneliness	0.009	0.864	0.084	0.109	-0.071	0.179	0.099	0.060	-0.012	0.816	-0.041	0.432	-0.101	0.053

Note:
Spearman's Rho Correlations were used.
*$p \leq 0.05$ was considered statistically significant.

Table 5. Relationship between measurement scale and demographic variables

	N	Mean ± S.D.	Range
Total Happiness Score			
Gender			
Male	117	18.70 ± 6.21	1-28
Female	248	17.23 ± 5.99	4-28
Total Geriatric Depression Scores			
Age			
60-70	18	6.82 ± 3.61	2-13
71-80	89	5.88 ± 4.16	0-15
81-90	213	7.25 ± 3.89	0-15
91-100	44	7.39 ± 3.51	2-15
Above 101	1	-	10
Total Geriatric Depression Scores			
Pain within 6 months			
Yes	249	7.21 ± 3.97	0-15
No	116	6.28 ± 3.78	0-15

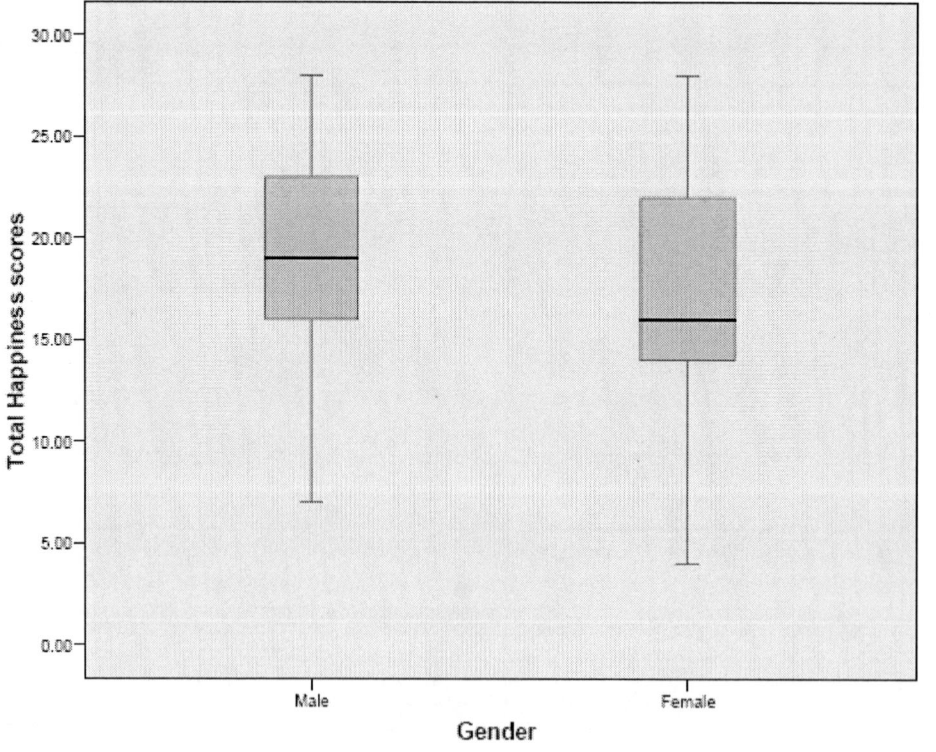

Figure 2. Relationship between Total Happiness Scores and Gender.

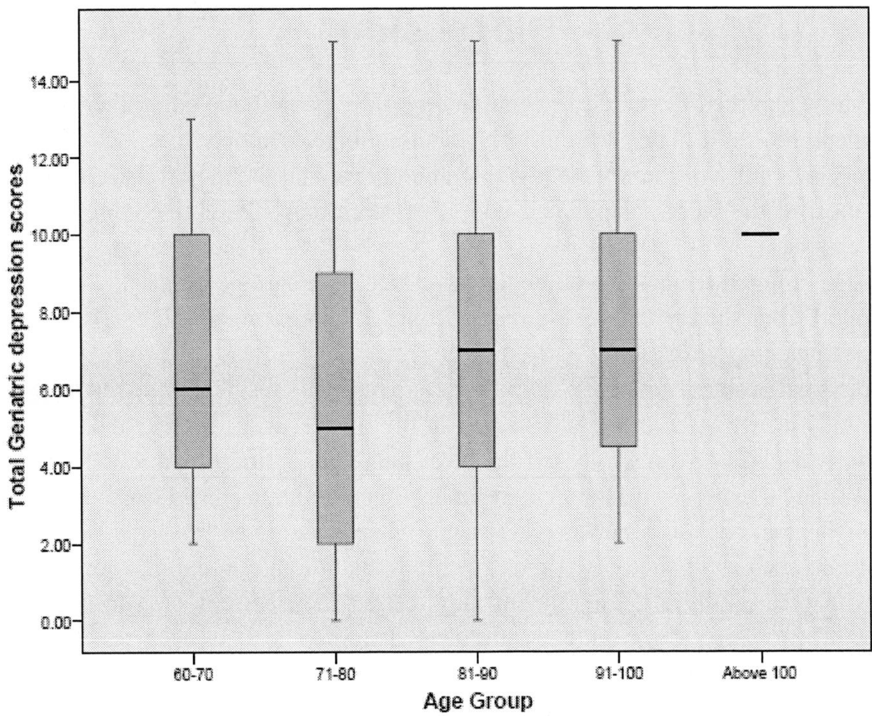

Figure 3. Relationship between Total Geriatric Depression scores and Age Group.

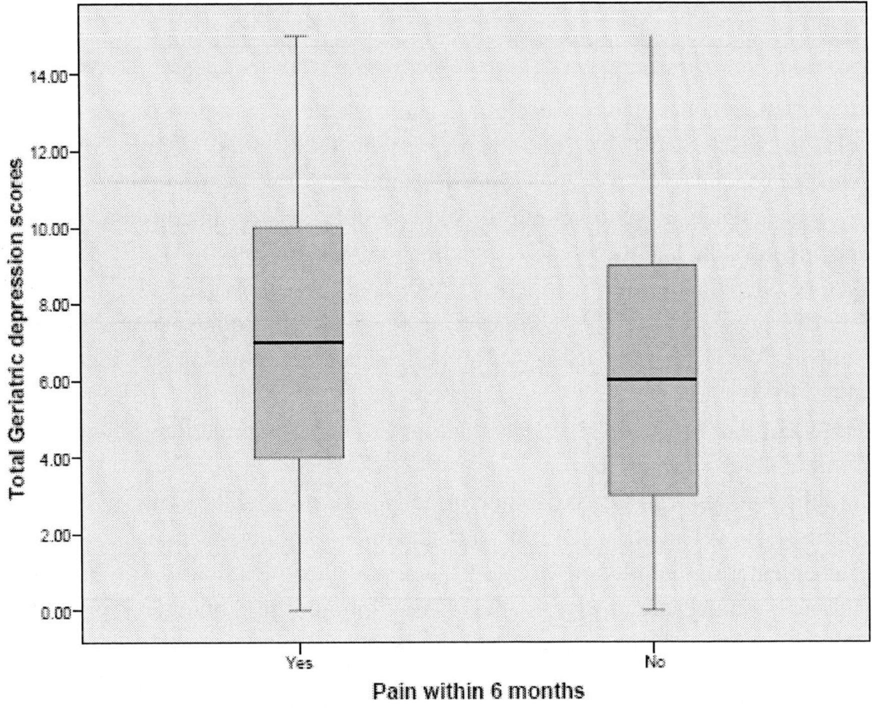

Figure 4. Relationship between Total Geriatric Depression scores and Pain within 6 months.

Discussion

This study explored the quality of life among older people, including their physical and psychological health in later life in the nursing home. Among the 365 older persons interviewed, over 60% of them were aged 81 and above, and the majority were widowed. In addition, most of the older persons had one or more chronic illness, including hypertension (64.9%), cataract (37.0%) and stroke (29.6%). Nearly 70% of them reported chronic pain. The decrease in functioning and well being associated with chronic disease, pain, and limited social support from society may cause older people to choose nursing homes as the place to spend their remaining years of life.

The physical problem among the surveyed nursing home residents was relatively serious: there was only nearly 80% of full functioning in the Barthel ADL Scores, and less than 75% in the Elderly Mobility Scores. Most of the older people had difficulty in climbing the stairs, bathing, walking 6 meters and functional reaching; such limitations may cause older people to depend on their nurses or healthcare assistants when needing to go a distance to another function room such as the activity room, TV room, bathroom and dining room. Some older persons with greater physical impairment may restrict their activity area in the absence of help from others, since they would be afraid to disturb others. In such cases, when older people limit their mobility, physical functioning may become worse and increase the risk of disability accompanied with inadequate coping factors such as poor health status, poor self-efficacy, depression, cognitive decline, negative appraisal and medication side-effects (Melding, 1997).

Chronic pain is a major problem among older persons, as documented in various articles (Mann and Carr, 2006; Clarke and Ryan, 2007). In earlier studies, 45 to 80% of older persons with more severe situation in long-term care settings had suffered from pain of moderate to severe intensity over the previous 3 months (Tse et al., 2005; Ferrell et al., 1990). However, many older persons believe that the chronic pain problem is a normal part of life when growing old. In our study, 68.2% (n=249) of participants reported having experienced pain, with a mean pain score of 4.55 ± 2.44 (on a 10-point scale) in the previous 3 months. There were many consequences of pain among the older people, such as impaired ambulation, sleep disturbance, depression and decreased socialization. According to Wells, Kaas and Feldt (1997), factors related to under-treatment of pain can be a knowledge deficit of the patient and healthcare provider for the analgesic used, and inadequate pain assessment and management in the long-term care setting. Besides pharmacological methods of pain management, healthcare workers can initiate simple activities for pain relief, such as physiotherapy, art therapy, deep breathing, and multisensory stimulation (Scudds and Scudds, 2005; Schofield, 2007; Tse, 2010).

In fact, older people can get assistance in daily activities while living in nursing homes. In the meantime, however, they need to face adjustment challenges and other mental health problems when entering the nursing home. In fact, poor life satisfaction, lower happiness and more loneliness among nursing residents were common psychological problems. Older people live with a loss of freedom and follow the routine and policy in the nursing home. Nursing home staff are busy in their own work and focus on the physical needs of older persons, and they may underestimate residents' emotional needs (Bagley et al, 2000). The cumulative unhappy psychological status may ultimately result in depression. According to various articles, depression is a significant mental health problem recognized in nursing homes (Hughes, 1997; Snowdon, 2007; Conn and Kaye, 2007). Appropriate pharmacological management of depression is effective for relieving the signs and symptoms of depression, and some group intervention programs can also be helpful in enabling residents to share their feelings and thoughts with their peers and nursing home staff.

According to Pearce (2006), therapeutic activities / programs can preserve physical well-being and encourage emotional self-expression and interaction with others when participating in the activities. It is recommended that therapeutic activities, including physiotherapy, art therapy, deep breathing and multi-sensory stimulation, be introduced in long-term care facilities.

There are various exercise programs, including group exercise programs and Tai Chi, that are recommended in nursing homes. These exercise programs are well documented as providing recreational and therapeutic effects among nursing home residents (Baum et al, 2003; Lee et al, 2009; Justine et al, 2010). Such primary health care can benefit the physical and psychological well-being of older persons, which can decrease crisis admission due to fall incidents in nursing homes as they improve in balance and their muscles strengthen. Other than the exercise program, deep breathing exercises and multi-sensory stimulation are well known for their effectiveness in relaxation and pain management (Tse, 2010).

Nowadays, end-of-life care among older people has become more challenging in long-term care facilities due to the expansion of the ageing population. The quality of life of older persons in nursing homes is not the responsibility of the nursing home staff alone; it is the responsibility of all of us. Better support for older persons in long-term care facilities can benefit to the health and social care system as a whole.

Conclusion

In recent years, the demand for nursing care homes and other forms of accommodation for older adults has been increasing due to the growth of the aging population. However, older persons suffer from moderate to severe physical and psychological impairment in nursing homes. There are activities such as physiotherapy, art therapy, deep breathing and multisensory stimulation that can help older people improve and maintain their physical impairment. Thus, older people can establish helpful neighborhood relationships with others during these activities, and meanwhile improve their psychological status. Therefore, nurses and other healthcare professionals should encourage older persons to engage in various therapeutic interventions and enhance the quality of life in nursing homes, which are likely to be their final stop on their journey of life.

Acknowledgments

The authors would like to thank all the study participants. Thanks also go to Professors Robert Kane, Rosaline Kane and Kerry Lam for their tremendous input in the study. Special thanks to CADENZA: A Jockey Club Initiative for Seniors, The Hong Kong Jockey Club Charities Trust, for providing financial support for this study.

References

Bagley, H., Cordingley, L., Burns, A., Mozley, C.G., Sutcliffe, C., Challis, D. and Huxley, P. (2000). Recognition of depression by staff in nursing and residential homes. *Journal of Clinical Nursing* 2000; 9: 445-450.

Baum E.E., Jarjoura, D., Polen, A.E., Faur D. and Rutecki G. (2003). Effectiveness of a group exercise program in a long-term care facility: A randomized pilot trial. *Journal of American Medical Directors Association 2003*, 4, 74-80.

Centre for Health Protection (2008). *Major health indicators in 2008 and 2009*. (on line) Available at: http://www.chp.gov.hk/ (accessed 23 May 2010).

Chan, A.C.M. (1996). Clinical validation of the geriatric depression scale (GDS). *Journal of Aging and Health (8)*, 238-253.

Chi, I. and Boey, K.W. (1992). *Validation of measuring instruments of mental health status of the elderly in Hong Kong*. Department of Social Work and Social Administration, University of Hong Kong.

Chou K.L., Jun L.W. and Chi I. (2005). Assessing Chinese older adults' suicidal ideation: Chinese version of the geriatric suicide ideation scale. *Aging and Mental Health* 9 (Suppl.2), 167-171.

Clarke, A. and Ryan, T. (2007). Creaking joints, a bit of arthritis, and aches and pains: older people's experiences and perceptions of pain. In P. Schofield (Ed.), *The management of pain in older people* (pp49-63). England: John Wiley and Sons.

Conn, D.K. and Kaye, A. (2007). Mood and anxiety disorders. In D.K. Conn, N. Herrmann, A. Kaye, D. Rewilak and B. Schogt (Eds.), *Practical psychiatry in the long-term care home: A handbook for staff* (pp79-101).Cambridge: Hogrefe and Huber.

Ferrell, B. A., Ferrell, B. R., Osterweil, D. (1990). Pain in the nursing home. *Journal of American Geriatric Society, 38,* 409-414.

Hong Kong Policy Research Institute Ltd (2006). *Health care for an ageing population – The challenge ahead for Hong Kong*. (on line) Available at: http://www.hkpri.org.hk/ (accessed 2 May 2006).

Hughes, C. (1997). Depression and mania in later life. In I.J. Norman and S.J. Redfern (Eds.), *Mental health care for elderly people* (pp141-161). New York: Churchill Livingstone.

Justine, M., Hamid, T.A., Kamalden, T.F.T. and Ahmad, Z. (2010). A multicomponent exercise program's effects on health-related quality of life of institutionalized elderly. *Topics in Geriatric Rehabilitation*, 26 (1), 70-79.

Kurlowicz, L. and Greenberg, S. A. (2007). *The Geriatric Depression Scale (GDS)*. (on line) Available at: http://consultgerirn.org/uploads/File/trythis/issue04.pdf (accessed 12 May 2010).

Lee, L.Y.K., Lee, D.T.F. and Woo, J. (2009). Tai Chi and health-related quality of life in nursing home residents. *Journal of Nursing Scholarship* 2009; 41:1, 35-43.

Leung J.Y.Y., Yu T.K.K, Cheung Y.L., Ma L.C., Cheung S.P. and Wong C.P. (2000). Private nursing home residents in Hong Kong – how frail are they and their need for hospital services? *Journal of Hong Kong Geriatric Society*, 10, 65-69.

Lyubomirsky S, Lepper H. (1999). A measure of subjective happiness: preliminary reliability and construct validation. *Social Indicators Research* 46, 137-155.

Mahoney F.I. and Barthel D.W. (1965). Functional evaluation: the Barthel Index. *Maryland State Medical Journal* 1965; 14: 56-61.

Mann, E. and Carr, E. (2006). *Pain management.* Oxford: Blackwell Publishing.

Melding, P.S. (1997). Coping with pain in old age. In D.I. Mostofsky and J. Lomranz (Eds.), *Handbook of pain and aging* (pp167-184). New York: Plenum Press.

Mui, A.C. (1996). Geriatric depression scale as a community screening instrument for elderly Chinese immigrants. *International Psychogeriatrics (8)*, 445-458.

Neugarten, B.L., Havighurst, R.J., Tobin, S.S. (1961). The measurement of life satisfaction. *Journal of Gerontology (16)*, 134-143.

Ng, M.F.W., Tong, R.K.Y. and Li, L.S.W. (2008). A pilot study of a randomized clinical controlled trial of gait training in subacute stroke patients with partial body-weight support electromechanical gait trainer and functional electrical stimulation: Six-month follow-up. *Stroke* 2008, 39, 154-160.

Owen, T. (2008). Healthcare in care homes: a vision for improvement. *Journal of Community Nursing* 2008, 22(5), 10-14.

Pearce, B.W. (2006). Therapeutic activity programs for assisted living facilities. In C.M. Brody and V.G. Semel (Eds.), *Strategies for therapy with the elderly: Living with hope and meaning* (2nd Ed.) (pp141-167). New York: Springer Publishing Company.

Proser L. et al. (1997). Further validation of EMS for measurement of mobility of hospitalised elderly people. *Clinical Rehabilitation* 11, 4, 338-343.

Russell, D.W. (1996). UCLA Loneliness Scale (Version 3): Reliability, validity and factor structure. *Journal of Personality Assessment* 66 (Suppl. 1), 20-40.

Schofield, P. (2007). Care homes and other settings. In P. Schofield (Ed.), *The management of pain in older people* (pp129-148). England: John Wiley and Sons.

Scudds, R.J. and Scudds, R.A. (2005). Physical therapy approaches to management of pain in older adults. In S.J. Gibson and D.K. Weiner (Eds.), *Pain in older persons* (pp223-237). Seattle: International Association for the Study of Pain.

Shyu, Y.I.L., Liang, J., Wu, C.C., Su, J.Y., Cheng, H.S., Chou, S.W., Chen, M.C. and Yang, C.T. (2008). Interdisciplinary intervention for hip fracture in older Taiwanese: Benefits last for 1 year. *Journal of Gerontology*, 63 (1), 92-97.

Sim T.C. and Leung E.M.F. (2000). Geriatric care for residents of private nursing homes. *Journal of Hong Kong Geriatric Society*, 10, 84-89.

Smith, R. (1994). Validation and Reliability of the Elderly Mobility Scale. *Physiotherapy* 80, 744-747.

Snowdon, J. (2007). Psychogeriatric services in the community and in long-term care facilities: needs and developments. *Current Opinion in Psychiatry* 2007, 20: 533-538.

Sonja, L., and Heidi, S.L. (1999). A measure of subjective happiness: preliminary reliability and construct validation. *Social Indicators Research, 46*, 137-155.

Tse, M. (2010). Multisensory environments and their effect on pain. *CyberTherapy and Rehabilitation*, 3 (1), 28-29.

Tse, M.Y. (2007). Nursing home placement: perspectives of community-dwelling older persons. *Journal of Clinical Nursing*, 16, 911-917.

Tse, M.M.Y., Pun, S.P.Y., and Benzie, I.F.F. (2005). Pain relief strategies used by older people with chronic pain: an exploratory survey for planning patient- centred intervention. *Journal of Clinical Nursing, 14*, 315-320.

Wells, N., Kaas, M. and Feldt, K. (1997). Managing pain in the institutionalized elderly. In D.I. Mostofsky and J. Lomranz (Eds.), *Handbook of pain and aging* (pp129-151). New York: Plenum Press.

Yesavage, J.A., Brink, T.L., Rose, T.L., Lum, O., Huang, V., Adey, M.B., Leirer, V.O. (1983). *Development and validation of a geriatric depression screening scale: A preliminary report. Journal of Psychiatric Research (17)*, 37-49.

In: Palliative and Nursing Home Care
Editor: Samuel E. Plunkett

ISBN 978-1-61122-417-7

Chapter 11

Neonatal Palliative Care: New Practice, New Challenges

***Pierre Bétrémieux*[1] *and Umberto Simeoni*[2]**
[1]Centre Hospitalier Universitaire, Hôpital Anne de Bretagne
16 boulevard de Bulgarie, F 35203 Rennes Cedex, France
[2]Université de la Méditerranée, hôpital de la Conception,
F13385 Marseille, France

Abstract

The delineation of Palliative Care (PC) in newborns recently opened a new practice. In the past and for years, neonatologists did not consider Palliative Care at the beginning of life. Nevertheless end of life procedures did exist but referred to either withholding or withdrawing active treatments, or even to active ending of life in desperate circumstances (what we now would call neonatal euthanasia). Four main domains can be recognized in the field of neonatology: 1) Babies born between 22 and 25 weeks: palliative care is the good alternative to life support therapy in some cases where the medical context and the parents' wishes are not in favour of such choice; 2) Babies born to a mother who knows that an intractable malformation affects the baby and wants to continue her pregnancy and meet her living baby, so that she does not ask for Termination of Pregnancy (TOP). This approach is quite new in France, for example, and concerns 3 to 5 % of mothers who could legally ask for TOP. Midwives, obstetrician and neonatologists give comfort care to the baby and sometimes help the family to bring the baby back home (most of prolonged PC occurs in severe hypoplastic left heart syndrome); 3) PC may also find its place in the neonatal intensive care unit when a baby who has been resuscitated at birth finally shows a dramatic neurologic outcome at a time when he/she is still dependent on intensive techniques such as mechanical ventilation or hemodynamic support. Withdrawing mechanical ventilation may sometimes lead to death but sometimes not and PC is the response to these situations.4) Finally PC may also be considered in an emergency context in any of the three previous situations occurring suddenly. Paediatricians must then decide in a while what would be the best choice for the baby. Each context modifies the way PC is provided, although in all cases basic compassionate and comfort care is delivered. Special attention is needed to ensure that parents and sometimes extended family may really meet their newborn baby, have their religious wills completed and are accompanied by a multiprofessional team attentive to their physical and psychological needs. This is conducted in the place the baby lives in, either delivery room, neonatal ward or even home if possible.

Introduction

Juxtaposition of both words "newborn" and "palliative care" is challenging. For years obstetricians, midwives and pediatricians have been concerned with neonatal death, nevertheless, palliative care spontaneously refers to end-of-life images in adults or elderly people.

Palliative care is defined as active care delivered in a global approach of a person affected by a life-threatening, evolutive or terminal illness. They aim at alleviating physical pain, uncomfort and at taking into account psychological, social and spiritual suffering. They consist in interdisciplinary care; they consider the patient as still living and death as a natural process. Palliative care-givers try to avoid obstinacy. They contribute to preserve the best quality of life for the patient as far as possible until death and provide support to the family before and after death.

In the Neonatal Domain, Four Main Situations Have Been Recognized as Possibly Opening the Field of Palliative Care

1. Situations Occurring in Intensive Care Units

They relate to newborns for whom intensive care was initiated at birth. Over times, these treatments may seem disproportionate to the actual condition of the baby when serious and irreversible injury leading to bleak prognosis has been diagnosed. As in numerous countries, the French law [1, 2] specifies that any treatment can be limited, suspended (withdrawn) or not be undertaken (withhold) in case of unreasonable obstinacy. The therapeutics that could be withdrawn in neonatalogy are for instance mechanical ventilation, haemodynamic support, peritoneal dialysis and total parenteral nutrition through a catheter.[3-6]]

Recognition and acceptance that the situation constitutes unreasonable obstinacy is the first step of the reflection leading to think of implementing a palliative care procedure. Recognizing unreasonable obstinacy is not so manifest in neonatal medicine and the procedure must be based on documented notes and expert advice [7, 8]. The second step is therapeutic renunciation i.e. rather than trying to save the patient's life at any price, it is collectively decided that the boundaries of curative care have been met and that the team and the parents have to turn to palliative care. The third step is the implementation of palliative care focusing on patient's comfort and family support. The care will not seek to hasten death but do not try to prevent or slow its spontaneous occurrence . The doctor will decide the limitation of intensive care and the implementation of palliative care after consulting the parents. It is certain that the weight of parental advisory is important in the decision, however, the French law clearly states that the physician, not the parents, is the decision maker and therefore responsible for the therapeutic limitations.

The clinical situations most covered with palliative care in neonatal intensive care units are currently severe neurological damage such as massive cerebral haemorrhage or extended bilateral cystic periventricular leukomalacia. Brain anoxia and ischemia as well as severely altered basal ganglia may also give rise to establishment of palliative care.

In most services the parents are now present during the withdrawal of respiratory device until death (although death is not the only possible outcome in this case); sometimes close relatives are welcomed. In most teams sedation and analgesia are maintained until death; for others, medications are first stopped and then adjusted to clinical findings if needed. The support of parents throughout the phase of death is important. The onset of dyspnea or terminal gasps often makes caregivers prescribe morphine although the painful component of these events is not well known so that this is an ethical more than a medical decision. Withdrawing the respirator is often accompanied by withdrawal of all other techniques including enteral nutrition. Withdrawing artificial nutrition in other context often raises ethical dilemmas in services where tube feeding is considered basic care and largely widespread [9].

2.Situations Related to Extreme Prematurity

They are also likely to put the child in a situation of unreasonable obstinacy. [10-13]

At 26 weeks gestation and over, ressuscitation techniques now allow a good chance of survival with little or no sequelae so that intensive care is started if needed without real ethical dilemmas.

Between 22 and 25 weeks gestation (roughly during the fifth month of gestation) it is somewhat different:

At 22 and 23 weeks prognosis is invariably dark and no team will now set off for ressuscitation or intensive treatment at this term. These children, if born alive, however, have the right to die with dignity and without suffering. Their death must no longer be hidden nor stolen to the parents. Palliative care is indicated. Recognizing their status as children (and not the status of the fetus) is a prerequisite for support in palliative care.

At 24 and 25 weeks, the prognosis is very uncertain: it is a gray area where mortality remains high but the risk of major sequelae gradually decreases and is certainly less than 100%. At the same time the risk of severe cognitive sequelae (reading, writing and arithmetic) is important even in the absence of motor impairment.

Arguments for prognosis can be drawn from clinical settings: female gender, black race, single fetal pregnancy, absence of maternal infection and premature rupture of membranes, a childbirth achieved in a "Level 3 centre", preceded by fetal lung maturation, are factors that positively influence the prognosis while the male gender, white race, multiple pregnancy, maternal infection, rupture of membranes, lack of antenatal steroids, birth in level 1 or 2 centre are factors that make the prognosis of a birth at 24 or 25 weeks more uncertain.

In these situations, parental investment will be key to cope with the needs of the child (prolonged hospitalization, sometimes repeatedly, necessity for physical therapy, psychomotility, orthophonist, schooling accompaniment...); the future of the child changes the future of Family and siblings. The views of parents therefore logically and significantly determine the behavior of paediatricians at birth [14-16].

An interview, even limited in time, shall take place with them: the obstetrician has to explain the inability or the medical hardship to prolong pregnancy, the paediatrician has to present the major risks of intensive care and the midwife has to accompany the course of birth including the elements discussed with them.

If parents do not want resuscitation to be started up, what we have seen may be permissible in some cases, teams need to implement supportive and palliative care for these children to be received the most humane way possible during their short lives.

This kind of accompaniment and support adapted to extreme prematurity are also now developing before the threshold of 22 weeks.

Indeed fetuses can be born alive before 22SA following a late miscarriage or medical termination of pregnancy (TOP) without feticide.

These children alive while not viable are not entitled to a declaration of birth and death, so that an act of lifeless child is written at the request of parents. This gives right to funerals and registration on "civil register" and in the family book. Those lives have long been denied, saying the children "stillborn" in a desire to "protect" parents, but we were told by parents that they are able to take decisions for the future of their child. Following clear and fair information, it is for them to say what they want for their child and what role they wish to take in this accompaniment.

What Care for These "Too-Small" and What Matters to Their Parents?

Over the past ten years the maternity teams have developed practices in perinatal bereavement support including the presentation of stillbirths and psychological support to parents.

To implement these new approaches caregivers need structure and guidance.

Information, listening and discussion with parents are essential to help them in their way. Even in a very short time, caregivers can describe what they provide to the newborn:

- Welcoming the baby without aggression, soft dry
- Wrap in a hot swaddle,
- install in a cocoon.

Speaking of the child with respect as a full human being, delivering care in the same room as parents (remember that the mother can not move right just after giving birth and the child will live maybe a few minutes only) allows them to imagine what they could not envisage before, a place and a role to play in assisting their child.

The agony, the gasps, color changes will be anticipated and explained simply. Parents often choose to take the baby in their arms, in the shadow of the delivery room, continuously or not. They sometimes want the presence of other people around them and this will be promoted. If they do not feel capacity to support their own child they know they can entrust it to the team.

These "too-small" are frequently soothed by skin to skin; they rarely show signs of discomfort which would be supported by curative dose of morphine through umbilical catheter (easy quick and painless to indwell). Parents should not have counted time with their child even after death with the discreet but containing presence of caregivers.

A psychological support, medical, administrative and social assistance will be offered in the maternity ward.

3.Situations Resulting from Prenatal Diagnosis

They represent a new approach of severe malformations of the fetus. From 1975 to 2005 or so, most women (or couples) who have been announced a severe malformation of the fetus demanded an abortion [17]. Now we see women and couples wishing to continue the pregnancy to its end in view to meeting the child alive despite severe malformations and diminished life expectancy [18-20]. Associations claim the right to such support for parents who choose this way (see the web site “SPAMA” created by a mom who chose this option). This possibility is now more often proposed at the announcement when the abnormality is probably lethal. This would represent around 2000 cases each year in France.

During the antenatal period Paediatricians must meet with parents together with the Obstetricians to describe what they know about the natural history of the pathology in question and to recall that, once the child is born, its status changes radically and it is forbidden to use euthanasia. At birth, it will be possible to implement palliative care. Recall that the duration of the life is unknown. We can also reassure parents about the management of possible pain, which will always be optimal, even if the use of painkillers can sometimes shorten the time of their child's life (the principle of "double effect" of the drugs is authorised by the French law : if the drug used to alleviate pain has the effect to shorten life, this is not considered euthanasia as far as the intention is to support pain, not to promote death).

The prenatal meetings are trying to identify parental expectations. If most couples agree that the child is neither resuscitated nor intubated, further support may become more complicated when life extends beyond the first hours:

- For example is it ethical to artificially feed the child if no suction exists?
- After time spent in the delivery room, does the baby go with mom to maternity ward or to neonatology ward?

Paediatricians believe that respect for the mother-child bond is critical but it is also true that the presence of a child at imminent risk of death in maternity ward raises questions. These new demands will lead to additional questions in obstetrics: the risk of fetal death is increased in such pregnancies, so that in case of fetal distress occurring during labour the question of the indication of a caesarean section may arise even though we know that the child is suffering from a lethal disease.

The obstetric teams meet on a case by case basis to these issues and it is not possible to generalize a consensus in this area. Decisions made antenatally necessitate several interviews with the parents (obstetrician, paediatrician, midwife, palliative team or palliative care network). These decisions should absolutely be included in the mother’s notes to ensure consistency with the actual conduct rulings, this consistency should be sought in particular by the on-call team, which has not always met the couple in advance. At birth, the immediate capabilities of the newborn will be assessed, and ensure that there is no need for additional post natal examinations that would be useful to the obstetrical future of the couple (ie, storage of DNA or checking a karyotype). Either the child has a very short life expectancy and clinical management will be the same as "too-small" newborns, or it exceeds the time spent in the delivery room (few hours) and other care will be provided. One of the situations where parents frequently demand for palliative care is hypoplastic left ventricle in its severe form; due to the permeability of the ductus arteriosus, the child can live a few days or few months before showing severe disorders. This is found in other situations that are not immediately lethal. After the time spent in the delivery room, a transfer to the maternity ward or to the neonatal unit or even at home may be considered, still promoting the non-separation of the child and his parents. These possibilities should be discussed prenatally with the couple. These interviews aim at determining with parents, continuity in the care of their child. It is important to determine what makes sense for them: for example the inclusion of this child in the family history, collection of memories, religious wishes, meeting with their child, presence of siblings and grandparents ...

From this collection of informations a project of life adapted to the child and the family will be drawn up in partnership with the various actors involved [20].

When the baby is taken in charge in a neonatal care unit, it is essential to have pre-determined, with parents and care-takers which care and support will be provided. Technical assistance implemented will be discussed: heart rate monitoring, glucose monitoring, umbilical catheterization, weighing, who gets visitation rights, presence of the father 24/ 24, preparation of a possible analgesic protocol ....

The project of life will be constantly evaluated based on the evolution of the clinical status of the child, the parental wishes and the difficulties encountered by the team. Some families state their desire to return home with their child if the clinical condition allows. The feasibility of this return home early is subject to local health workers. Home care for newborns is rarely implemented at the moment; it should be accompanied and coordinated by the paediatrician and the palliative care network. In the case of children with hypoplastic left ventricle, home support does not require any special care technique. Indeed, when the child begins to show deterioration in his/her clinical condition (signs of respiratory distress), it is readmitted to benefit from the administration of analgesics. In the future, it is possible that more parents wish for total accompaniment at home including last moments and death, as it is done for older children with terminal condition.

4.The Situations of Emergency

When the situations described above occur unexpectedly, teams may be helpless against the decisions and conduct to follow. Often it is EMS who is called and the teams involved in the transport of newborns must know the new practices of palliative care. Note first that, in France, there is no obligation to resuscitate in the delivery room an extremely premature infant when the term is certain, which would be in a state of apparent death at birth. The law of 22 April 2005 already cited above, is clear on this point: apparently useless acts can not be undertaken. Time must still be taken to discuss with parents to gather their opinions. Whether extreme premies "too small" to be managed actively or seriously malformed child, the conduct of palliative care will grow the same way, setting out the practical issues described above.

Current Developments

The development of these new approaches is encouraging: most of the situations of ethical dilemma are supported so soothed, under the law, which is extremely comfortable for the teams compared to past practices that were not based on clear legal conditions. Stopping resuscitation and implementing palliative care leads to death in respect of the patient with optimal management of pain.

But other dilemmas arise and we will mention some that have been encountered by the medical staff:

- The law providing that, if disproportionate, any treatment can be stopped, most teams recognize that it is possible, after collegial meeting and discussion, to stop parenteral nutrition on central catheter, but nobody knows if it is legal to suspend enteral feeding in Newborns. The placement of a nasogastric tube is actually a daily activity in neonatal units but it is an aggressive and potentially painful procedure and a technical act. If the child keeps some food self-sufficiency by breast or bottle feeding, it is perhaps possible to stop parenteral nutrition, but if he does not, what should we do? How provide hydration without feeding? Many teams consider the case of stopping tube feeding as difficult to accept in neonatology [9].

When mechanical ventilation is withdrawn in view to implement palliative care and the child becomes to breathe on its own, some teams have observed very prolonged survival in very altered condition, although, at the time of the decision to stop intensive care, nobody had considered this possibility. Parents therefore feel in great distress and teams do not know what to do: some of them consider that this is medical malpractice to sustain life, others consider that life, even extremely reduced, is intangible.

It is clear to all that the law represented an important progress and also that no legislation can anticipate all the situations encountered in clinical services. So is there currently a consensus of societies of obstetrics and neonatology to conduct these situations of end of life in the context of the 2005 Act and not to seek to amend this law.

Suggestions for Future

From these findings, the teams that focus actively on these issues feel the urgent need to disseminate palliative culture in maternity and neonatal units, where it was not widespread until now. The basic principles of palliative care just need to be exposed through both didactic sessions and during times of clinical situations reviewing. Meetings, round tables are increasingly being offered at a local and regional level. Establishing networks of perinatal care may be important in disseminating such knowledge. Similarly, mobile teams of palliative care and palliative care networks could be integrated early in clinical team discussions so that palliative support can be done smoothly from place of birth to home. We must also develop clinical research based on ground realities: how are assumed the "too small" or severely malformed children in maternity wards and how can we improve their treatment? What are the fears, misgivings, apprehensions of caregivers in these situations? What are the demands and parental expectations? These are questions we must begin to resolve [21-26].

Conclusion

Neonatal palliative care is a new approach in Western Old Continent. It applies to a series of situations which are finally not so exceptionnal in neonatal daily practice. Obstetricians, midwives, nurses and pediatricians have to appropriate basic concepts of palliative care. First of all it is necessary to recognize the status of the newborn at any term, who receives, by birth, all human rights. Thereafter the caregivers must stick to ethical principles : do no harm, do not hasten the death and do not slow its natural occurrence; avoid obstinacy. The important thing is that the knowledge gathered here, the culture of palliative care as applied to newborns, will bring good to these children, those who are most severely affected for several hours or for a long period. The palliative approach is a step towards a tolerant and caring society; sufficiently enlightened not to demonize the disability, the disease, the difference, but to fight with humanity and empathy, as well as by medical decision.

References

[1] Act No. 2005-370 of 22 April 2005 on patients' rights and end of life. *Official Journal of the French Republic* April 23, 2005 p7089.

[2] Dageville C, Rameix S, Andrini P et al (2007) End of life in neonatal medicine in the light of the law. *Arch. Pediatr.*; 14:1219-30.

[3] Cuttini M, Nadai M, Kaminski M et al. (2000) End-of-life decisions in neonatal intensive care : physicians'self reported practices in seven European countries. *Lancet* 355: 2112-2118

[4] Orfali K, Gordon EG (2004) Autonomy gone awry: a cross-cultural study of parents' experiences in neonatal intensive care units. *Theor. Med. Bioeth.* 25(4): 329-65.

[5] Catlin A, Carter B (2002) Creation of a neonatal end-of-life palliative care protocol. *J. Perinatol.* 22:184-195.

[6] Byrne S, Goldsmith JP (2006) Non initiation and discontinuation of resuscitation. *Clin. Perinatol.* 33:197-218.

[7] McHaffie HE, Lyon AJ, Fowlie PW (2001) Lingering death after treatment withdrawal in the neonatal intensive care unit. *Arch. Dis. Child Fetal Neonatal* Ed ;85(1):F8-F12.

[8] Dyregrov A, Matthiesen SB. (1991) Parental grief following the death of an infant--a follow-up over one year. *Scand. J. Psychol.* 32(3):193-207.

[9] Carter BS, Leuthner SR. (2003) The ethics of withholding/withdrawing nutrition in the newborn. *Semin. Perinatol.* 27(6):480-7.

[10] Tyson JE, Parikh NA, Langer J, et al. (2008) Intensive care for extreme prematurity--moving beyond gestational age. *N. Engl. J. Med.* 358 :1672-1681.

[11] Larroque B, Bréart G, Kaminski M, et al. (2004) Survival of very preterm infants : Epipage, a population based cohort study. *Arch. Dis. Child Fetal Neonatal Ed* 89: F139-144 .

[12] Marlow N, Wolke D, Bracewell M, et al. (2005) Neurologic and developmental disability at six years of age after extremely preterm birth. *N. Engl. J. Med.* 352 :9-19.

[13] PI Macfarlane, S Wood, J Bennet. (2003) Non-viable delivery at 20-23 weeks gestation: observations and signs of life after birth. *Arch. Dis. child fetal Neonatal*; 88:F199-F202.

[14] Saigal S (2000) Perception of health status and quality of life of extremely low-birth weight survivors. The consumer, the provider, and the child. *Clin. Perinatol.* Jun;27(2):403-19.

[15] Saigal S, Stoskopf B, Pinelli J, et al (2006) Self-perceived health-related quality of life of former extremely low birth weight infants at young adulthood. *Pediatrics*; 118(3):1140-8.

[16] Saigal S, Rosenbaum PL, Feeny D, et al (2000) Parental perspectives of the health status and health-related quality of life of teen-aged children who were extremely low birth weight and term controls. *Pediatrics*; 105:569-74.

[17] Garel M, Etienne E, Blondel B, Dommergues M (2007) French midwives'practice of termination of pregnancy for fetal abnormality. At what psychological and ethical cost ? *Prenat Diagn* 27: 622-628.

[18] Leuthner S (2004) Fetal palliative care. *Clin. Perinatol.* 31:649-665.

[19] Munson D, Leuthner SR (2007) Palliative care for the family carrying a fetus with a life-limiting diagnosis. *Pediatr. Clin. N. Am.* 54 :787-798.

[20] Leuthner SR (2004) Palliative care of the infant with lethal anomalies. *Pediatr Clin. N. Am.* 51:747-759.

[21] Crabtree BF, Miller WL (1991) A qualitative approach to primary care research: the long interview. *Fam. Med.* 23(2): 145-51.

[22] Hynson JL, Aroni R, Bauld C, Sawyer SM (2006) Research with bereaved parents : a question of how not why. *Palliat. Med.* 20(8): 805-11.

[23] Dyregrov K (2004) Bereaved parents' experience of research participation. *Soc. Sci. Med.* 58: 391–400.

[24] Toce SS, Andresen EM. (2002) The roles of data collection, evaluation, and research in pediatric palliative care. *Support Voice* 8:11-13.

[25] Greenhalgh T, Taylor R (1997) Papers that go beyond numbers (qualitative research). *BMJ* 315: 740-743.

[26] Pope C, Mays N. (1995) Reaching the parts other methods cannot reach: an introduction to qualitative methods in health and health services research. *BMJ* 1;311(6996): 42-5.

In: Palliative and Nursing Home Care
Editor: Samuel E. Plunkett

ISBN 978-1-61122-417-7

Chapter 12

Depression and Mood Distress Among Female Patients with Gynecological Cancer in a Program of Palliative Cancer Care

L. Slovacek
Department of Clinical Oncology and Radiotherapy of
Charles University Hospital and Faculty of Medicine,
Hradec Králové, Czech Republic

Introduction

Cancer can be characterized as an uncontrolled growth of cells, which is of autonomous means. This cell proliferation is connected with a defect of control mechanisms and an alteration of cell differentiation. Uncontrolled growth of cells leads to the expanding of affected tissue which can press the surrounding organs, or to a gradual invasion to surrounding structures and to metastasis [1-4].

Thanks to the growing average lifetime, the occurrence of carcinoma is rising. The number of people who survive the carcinoma is rising, too. Yet it is perceived as a death sentence for many people which consider it as chronic, or even incurable, disease. In every case, it is a shock for a patient to hear such a diagnosis . Patients must tie with a sense of uncertainty of their future life, with undesirable side effects of anti-tumoros therapy, with a sense of isolation, stigmatization and guilt [5, 6]. Block [7] cites that the diagnosis of cancer evokes a sub-existence crisis in every affected individual. So supportive methods are needed to handle the disease successfully, which could lead the patient to regaining a certain control over the situation.

Anti-Tumor Therapy of Gynecological Cancer

Basic methods in treatment of cancer are the biomodular methods, i.e. the surgeon therapy (radical intervention or palliative intervention or combined intervention), chemotherapy (systematic or regional or combined , therapeutic or palliative, neoadjuvantive or adjuvantive), immunotherapy (separate i.e. monotherapy or in combination with chemotherapy, so called immunochemotherapy) and radiotherapy (inter or outer). These basic methods are then complemented with specific methods (hematopoietic stem cell transplantation) [1-3, 8].

Classic medicine has been focused on the biology of the tumor for a long time and has not considered psychological and social factor too much which comes to interaction with cancer [3, 9,10]. There are still more studies in last 50 years which show favorable influence of psychosocial remedy to the course of cancer. According to Tschuschke [4], we need to understand psychological intervention, such as supporting and supplementing methods, not as a substitute of curing methods.

So if we want to interpret the anti-tumor therapy complexly, it should include 3 sections [3, 4, 9]:

1. biological section (surgical treatment, chemotherapy, immunotherapy, radiotherapy, hematopoietic stem cell transplantation).
2. psychological section (psychological intervention, systematically applied by professional psychologists and h psychotherapists).
3. social section (social foothold – the presence of another person who can influence the individual positively, family).

Biological and psychological social sections are in constant interaction (Image 1) and sometimes it is hard to distinguish which one of them is of more importantance (see Figure 1) [4].

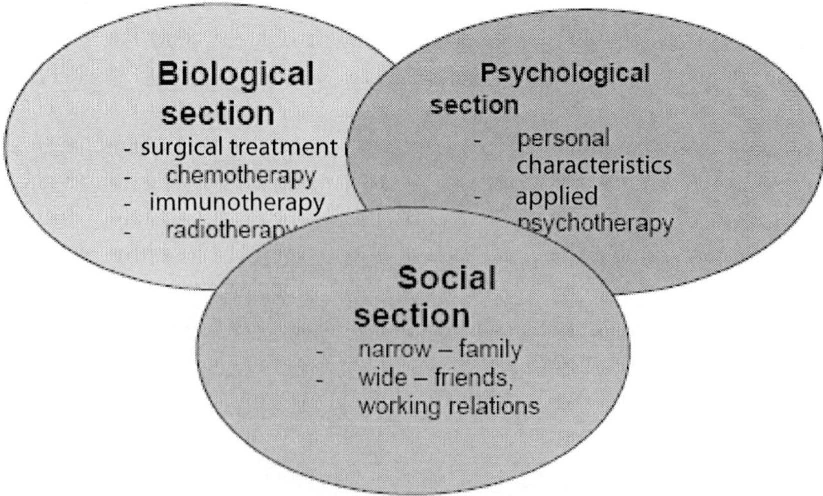

Figure 1. General principle of anti-tumor treatment (modified by Tschuschke [4].

Phases of Experiencing Gynecological Cancer

Cancer is marked in its course by characteristic phases of experience [3, 4, 9, 10]. Tschuschke [4] and Fawzy [11] divide it into phases of diagnosis, treatment, relapse, advanced stage of disease and terminally – palliative stage: 1. diagnosis of cancer, 2. treatment of cancer, 3. remission of cancer, 4. relapse of cancer, 5. advanced stage of cancer, 6. terminally – palliative stage.

- Diagnosis of cancer: This phase represents the shock and fear, patient is confronted with his own mortality and questions of his future existence.
- Treatment of cancer: Crisis regarding painful and burning curing interventions, negative effects of treatment, diminution of psychological and psychic strength.
- Remission of cancer: Feeling of fear of remise can predominate. Hypochondriac anxieties are common mainly before the control examinations
- Relapse of cancer: First relapse of disease is experienced as the most stressing event in the whole course of the disease. It is similar but surely more intensive to the diagnosis of disease. Patient is frustrated that his disease won over the treatment.
- Advanced stage of cancer: Repeated treatment is ineffective, new forms of treatment are sought , use of some very aggressive forms is unrealistic. Crisis repeats, it is manifested with panic and fear. Often patients withdraw to alternative methods, feeling the classic medicine failed.
- Terminally – palliative stage: It is necessary to focus on unpleasant symptoms, provide a psychic relief.

Psychological Disorders and Cancer

Cancer diagnosis and treatment often produce psychological stresses resulting from the actual symptoms of the disease, as well as perceptions of the disease and its stigma [12, 13]. Depression is seen in many cancer patients [14, 15]. Depression occurs in approximately 25% of palliative-care patients [14, 15]. It is widely recognized by clinicians that depression is a difficult symptom to identify amongst patients with advanced illnesses. Depression, the psychiatric syndrome that has received the most attention in individuals with cancer, has been a challenged to study because symptoms occur on a spectrum that ranges from sadness to major affective disorder and because mood change is often difficult to evaluate when a patient is confronted by repeated threats to life, is receiving cancer treatments, is fatigued, or is experiencing pain [16]. However, depression in cancer patients has been essential to study because co-morbid illnesses complicate the treatment of both and may lead to poor adherence to treatment recommendations and less desirable outcomes of both conditions [16]. The severity of medical illness, as manifested by significant pain, declining performance status, or the need for ongoing treatment, is associated with a high risk of co-morbid depression. Whether high rates of depression associated with some cancers are caused by the pathophysiologic effect of the tumor (i.e., paraneoplastic syndromes associated with breast, testis, or lung cancers), treatment effects, or other unidentified factors remains to be described. Cancer, exclusive of site, is associated with a rate of depression that is higher than in the general population [16]. Massie and Derogatis et al. [16] present that although many research groups have assessed depression in cancer patients since the 1960s, the reported prevalence (major depression, 0-38 %, depression spectrum syndromes, 0-58 %) varies significantly because of varying conceptualizations of depression, different criteria used to define depression, differences in methodological approaches to the measurement of depression, and different populations studied [16].

Psychological Disorders and Gynecological Cancer

The incidences of depression in individuals with cancer are different. Cancer types highly associated with depression include breast cancer(1,5-46%) [17, 18]. A lower prevalence of depression is reported among patients with gynecological cancer (12-23%) [19-21]. Pinder et al. [22] found a 13 % prevalence of depression in advanced breast cancer patients (N=139), increased levels of depression were found in those with lowest socioeconomic status, poorest performance status, and closer proximity to death. Evans et al. [23] studied 83 women with gynecological cancer and found a 23 % prevalence of depression and 24 % prevalence of adjustment disorder with depressed mood. Golden et al. [24] found a 23 % rate of major depression in 83 hospitalized women with cervical, endometrial, and vaginal cancer. Montazeri [25] features that QoL as a predictor of survival, similar to known medical factors, QoL data in a metastatic breast cancer patients was found to be prognostic and predictive of survival time. Psychological distress-anxiety and depression were found to be common among breast cancer patients even years after the disease diagnosis and treatment. Psychological factors were also found to predict subsequent QoL or even overall survival in breast cancer patients. Supportive care-clinical treatments to control emesis, or interventions such as counseling, providing social support and exercise could improve QoL. Symptoms - pain, fatigue, arm morbidity and postmenopausal symptoms were among the most common symptoms reported by breast cancer patients. As recommended, recognition and management of these symptoms is an important issue since such symptoms impair HRQoL [25].

Slovacek et al. [26] studied 41 female patients with a metastatic breast cancer in a program of the palliative cancer care. The mean age for all 41 subjects was 58 years old (aged 41 – 80 years old). Dates were obtained during the year 2008. The study evaluated incidence and relevance of depression symptoms and level of health-related quality of life (HRQoL). The statistical evaluation presents that mean ZSDS (Zung self-rating depression score) certifies the presence of signs of moderately depression symptoms among patients with a metastatic breast cancer. The incidence of depression was 61% (25 of all 41 subjects). The relevance of depression is characterized: severely depressed was proved in 5 of all 25 subjects, the moderately depressed in 10 subjects of all 25 subjects and mildly depressed in 10 of all 25 subjects. The HRQoL among patients with a metastatic breast cancer is on very low level. The mean EQ-5D score (dimension of QoL) was 55%. The mean EQ-5D VAS (subjective health condition) was 59.2% [26].

Ovarian cancer has non-specific symptoms, and no screening tool is available for early diagnosis; therefore, only 19% of ovarian cancers are found at an early stage. Given the late diagnosis, women with ovarian cancer often have a prolonged course of treatment and significant morbidity that lasts into survivorship. However, distressing symptoms and their effects on quality of life have been relatively understudied, particularly in survivors of the disease [27]. Ovarian cancer is the fourth-leading cause of cancer mortality among women. Previous research has shown that initial ovarian cancer screening has the potential to cause depressive symptoms among women at increased risk for the disease but no study has evaluated depressive symptoms shortly after screening [28]. Ovarian cancer presents a range of physical and psychological symptoms during stages of diagnosis, treatment, and survival [29]. Women at risk for ovarian cancer who attend screening programs are vulnerable to high levels of depression and anxiety, particularly young women with poor social support. Multiple physiological stressors of surgical menopause, steroid therapy, and pain present during active treatment that place women at a high risk of depression and anxiety during this time. Symptoms of anxiety and depression are also prevalent immediately after chemotherapy and during palliative care. Screening for psychological distress may be useful to identify women who will benefit from psychological counseling [29]. They should be referred to a mental health professional affiliated with the hospital at which they are receiving oncology services. Brief group or individual supportive psychotherapies are effective in relieving psychological distress. Face-to-face psychological intervention should be tailored to the patient's degree of physical mobility. Pain, discomfort, and severe mood symptoms should be addressed pharmacologically, when possible, by a psychiatric consultant knowledgeable in oncology psychiatry. Survivors experience chronic fear of recurrence, sexual dysfunction, and identity disturbance. Reports that ovarian cancer can result in positive life changes, such as closer interpersonal relationships, are encouraging and may provide hope to patients who become despairing about the future [29]. Goncalves et al. [30] performed a study which investigates the presence of psychological disorders longitudinally in women with a new diagnosis of ovarian cancer and the factors that predicted development and maintenance of these disorders. Patients were assessed in a prospective longitudinal study at the beginning of chemotherapy treatment, mid-treatment, end of treatment and 3 months follow-up for depression, anxiety, perceived social support, neuroticism and cognitive strategies to control unwanted thoughts. A total of 121 patients were recruited and 85 patients were assessed at all four time points. Three different longitudinal profiles of anxiety and depression cases were found: non-cases (never cases), occasional cases (cases on at least one but not all four occasions) and stable cases (cases on all four occasions). Most of the women were occasional cases of anxiety (52%, 44), whereas for depression, the majority of women were non-cases (55%, 47). A subset of patients were stable cases of anxiety (22%, 19). Neuroticism and marital status were significant independent predictors of an anxiety case profile. Neuroticism and use of anti-depressants were independent predictors of a depression case profile. Social support was not related to psychological morbidity [30]. Hipkins et al. [31] performed a prospective study in women with ovarian cancer to determine the changes in psychological status in the 3 months following completion of chemotherapy. Sixty-three consecutive patients were assessed at the completion of chemotherapy (Time 1) and 57 at 3 months follow-up (Time 2). Relevant disease and patient characteristics were recorded and patients were assessed at Time 1 for anxiety, depression and their perception of emotional support, an index of their psychosocial environment. Anxiety and depression were re-assessed at Time 2. The results indicate significant initial psychological morbidity, with a clinical case for anxiety (38%) and depression (33%) being common. Follow-up at Time 2 shows that patients undergo a significant reduction in cases (19%) and symptoms of depression but an increase in cases of anxiety (47%). The principal factors associated with symptoms of anxiety at Time 2 were poorly perceived social support, increased intrusive thoughts and, to a lesser extent, younger age. Medical parameters, such as the stage of disease, response of the cancer to treatment, Ca125 (a tumor r glycoprotein) and Karnofsky Performance statuses (a measure of how well the patient is) were not associated with worse psychological outcome [31]. Slovacek et al. [32] studied 30 patients with a metastatic ovarian cancer in a program of palliative cancer care. The mean age for all 30 subjects was 62.1 years old (aged 41 – 88 years old). Dates were obtained during the year 2008. The study is evaluated incidences and relevance of depression symptoms. The statistical evaluation presents that mean Zung´s self-rating depression score (ZSRDS) certifies the presence of signs of mild depression among patients with a metastatic ovarian cancer. The incidence of depression was 83.3% (25 of all 30 subjects). The relevance of depression is characterized: severely depressed was proved in 9 of all 30 subjects, moderately depressed in 5 subjects of all 30 subjects, mildly depressed in 11 of all 30 subjects and normal range in 5 of all 30 subjects [32].

Conclusion

Depression is common in the general population and in adults and children with cancer and frequently coexists with anxiety and pain [10]. It has been challenging to study because symptoms occur on a spectrum that ranges from sadness to major affective disorder and because mood change is often difficult to evaluate when a patient is confronted by repeated threats to life, is receiving cancer treatments, is fatigued, or is experiencing pain. Untreated depression results in significant morbidity and mortality [10].

It is common in the clinical practice to evaluate a patient´s health condition and the success of the treatment based only on one type of marker, the most often by means of somatic, laboratory or detecting markers [26, 32]. But the trend in modern medicine is to evaluate a patient´s health condition in a more complex way, using other aspects. The QoL means more dimensional evaluation of a number of life aspects. Different aspects can be affected in a different way in a different phase of the disease and its treatment [26, 32]. That is why this information enriches our knowledge concerning patient´s needs and it can significantly contribute to the medical treatment improvement. It can also help us to reveal the mechanisms which modify the origin and the course of disease [26, 32].

Psychological and psychosocial intervention have its own firm and indispensable post in a complex care about oncological patients. Its importance is focused mainly on the personal profile of oncological patients, social support and applied psychotherapy in these specific cohort of patients. Both types of interaction help oncologists to perceive changes in a status of health of patients in a wider view [3]. This is the information that enriches our knowledge of patient's urges and can help to improve the medical care. They also enable to reveal the mechanisms that modify the rise and course of disease. Mainly abroad there are very good experiences with so called "Cancer Quality of Life Team" [26, 32]. These teams are personally composed of physicians – the oncologist, nurses with a specialization in oncology and radiotherapy-educated in problematics of QoL among oncological patients, the psycho-oncologist, the psychotherapist , the social staff member and the data manager. The reason to make such a special team is that care of oncological patients and their families prepares the background to which the patient can return after the anti-tumor therapy and which influences their adaptation [26, 32].

Acknowledgments

Supported by the Research Project of the Ministry of Health of the Czech Republic No. 00179906.

References

[1] Slováček L, Slováčková B. Palliative therapy in oncological patients. *Voj zdrav Listy* 2003, 72:1-4.

[2] Slováček L, Slováčková B, Jebavý L, Blažek M, Kačerovský J. Palliative therapy of oncological patients in terminal stage of malignant tumorous disease from overview of the internist. *Prakt Lék* 2003, 83: 711-4.

[3] Slováček L, Slováčková B, Huňka A. Psychological intervention in oncological patients. *Zpravodaj vojenské farmacie* 2006, 16: 6-9.

[4] Tschuschke V. Psycho-oncology. Prague: Portál, 2004.

[5] Block HI. The role of the self in healthy cancer survivorship: a view from the front lines of treating cancer. Advances: *J. Mind-Body Health* 1997, 13: 6-23.

[6] Dunkel-Schetter C, Feinstein LG, Taylor SE, Falke RL. Patterns of coping with cancer. *Health Psychol* 1992, 11: 79-87.

[7] Maguire P. Improving the detection of psychiatric problems in cancer patients. *Soc. Sci. Med.* 1985, 20: 819-23.

[8] Klener P. Clinical oncology. Praque: Grada, 2002.

[9] Chovancová Z, Vašková J. Diagnosis of tumor. Prague: Grada, 1998.

[10] Křivohlavý J. Psychology of disease. Prague: Grada, 2002.

[11] Fawzy IF. Psychosocial interventions for patients with cancer: what works and what doesn´t ? *Eur. J. Cancer* 1999, 35: 1559-64.

[12] Winell J, Roth AJ. Depression in cancer patients. Oncology (Williston Park) 2004, 18: 1554-60, discussion 1561-2.

[13] Lloyd-Williams M, Reeve J, Kisaane D. Distress in palliative care patients: Developing patient-centered approaches to clinical management. *Eur. J. Cancer* 2008, 44: 1133-8.

[14] Lloyd-Williams M, Riddleston H. The stability of depression scores in patients who are receiving palliative care. *J. Pain Symptom. Manage* 2002, 24: 593-7.

[15] Lloyd-Williams M. Is it appropriate to screen palliative care patients for depression? *Am. J. Hosp. Palliat. Care* 2002, 19: 112-4.

[16] Massie MJ. Prevalence of Depression in Patients with Cancer. *Journal of the National Cancer Institute Monographs* 2004, 32: 57-71.

[17] Sneeuw KCA, Aaronson NK, van Wouwe MCC, Sergeant JA, van Dongen JA, Bartelink H. Prevalence and screening of psychiatric disorder in patients with early stage breast cancer. *Qual Life Res* 1993, 2: 50-1.

[18] Sachs G, Rasoul-Rockenschaub S, Aschauer H, Spiess K, Gober I, Staffejn A. et al. Lytic effector cell activity and major depressive disorder in patients with breast cancer: a prospective study. *J. Neuroimmunol.* 1996, 784: 482-5.

[19] Evans DL, McCartney CF, Nemeroff CB et al. Depression in women treated for gynecological cancer: clinical and neuroendocrine assessment. *Am. J. Psychiatry* 1986, 143: 447-51.

[20] Golden RN, McCartney CF, Haggerty JJ et al. The detection of depression by patient self-report in women with gynecological cancer. *Int. J. Psychiatry Med.* 1991, 21: 17-27.

[21] Aass N, Fossa SD, Dahl AA et al. Prevalence of anxiety and depression in cancer patients seen at the Norwegian Radium Hospital. *Eur. J. Cancer* 1997, 33: 1597-1604.

[22] Pinder KL, Ramirez AJ, Black ME. Psychiatric disorder in patients with advanced breast cancer: prevalence and associated factors. *Eur. J. Cancer* 1993, 29A: 524-7.

[23] Evans DL, McCartney CF, Nemeroff CB et al. Depression in women treated for gynecological cancer: clinical and neuroendocrine assessment. *Am. J. Psychiatry* 1986, 143: 447-51.

[24] Golden RN, McCartney CF, Haggerty JJ et al. The detection of depression by patient self-report in women with gynecological cancer. *Int. J. Psychiatry Med.* 1991, 21: 17-27.

[25] Montazeri A. Health-related quality of life in breast cancer patients: a bibliographic review of the literature from 1974 to 2007. *J. Exp. Clin. Cancer Res.* 2008, 27: 32.

[26] Slovacek L, Slovackova B, Slanska I, Petera J. Health-related quality of life and depression symptoms among patients with metastatic breast cancer in a program of palliative cancer care. *Neoplasma* 2009, 56: 467-72.

[27] Fox SW, Lyon D. Symptom clusters and quality of life in survivors of ovarian cancer. *Cancer Nurs.* 2007, 30: 354-61.

[28] Tiffen J, Sharp L, O´Toole C. Depressive symptoms prescreening and post-screening among returning participants in an ovarian cancer early detection program. *Cancer Nurs.* 2005, 28: 325-30.

[29] Hamilton AB. Psychological aspects of ovarian cancer. *Cancer Invest.* 1999, 17: 335-41.

[30] Goncalves V, Jayson G, Tarrier N. A longitudinal investigation of psychological morbidity in patients with ovarian cancer. *Br. J. Cancer* 2008, 99: 1794-1801.

[31] Hipkins J, Whitworth M, Tarrier N et al. Social support, anxiety and depression after chemotherapy for ovarian cancer: a prospective study. *Br. J. Health Psychol.* 2004, 9: 569-81.

[32] Slováček L, Slánská I, Slováčková B, Petera J, Filip S, Priester P, Kopecký J, Jebavý L. Screening for depression in survivors of metastatic ovarian cancer in a program of palliative cancer care: a prospective study. *Bratisl Lek Listy* 2009, 110: 655-9.

Index

2

20th century, 176
21st century, 59, 113

A

abuse, 31, 32, 34, 35, 36, 37, 38, 42, 46, 50, 52, 53, 55, 56, 57, 58, 59, 60, 61, 62, 84, 137
academic performance, 37
access, 8, 15, 16, 24, 25, 32, 34, 38, 65, 70, 96, 123, 127, 132, 135, 154, 155
accommodation, xi, 175, 176, 187
accommodations, 77
ACF, 36, 57
acquired immunodeficiency syndrome, 159
active treatment, xii, 140, 191, 205
adaptation, 102, 206
adipose, 121, 125
adipose tissue, 121, 125
adjustment, 4, 47, 48, 61, 79, 186, 204
administrators, x, xi, 75, 123, 125, 161, 162, 163, 165, 170, 171, 172
adolescent development, 58
adolescents, 57, 58, 59, 61
adults, vii, viii, 24, 32, 40, 45, 46, 47, 57, 58, 63, 65, 68, 74, 75, 78, 81, 83, 85, 98, 118, 119, 127, 128, 142, 178, 187, 188, 189, 192, 206
advancement, 65, 113
advantages, 43, 44, 45
adverse effects, 69, 140
affective disorder, 203, 206
affirmative action, 38
Africa, viii, 31, 32, 39, 43, 44, 48, 49, 58, 59, 60, 61, 62
age, ix, xi, 2, 9, 10, 16, 33, 37, 38, 41, 44, 51, 68, 70, 76, 80, 88, 114, 117, 119, 121, 131, 132, 133, 139, 140, 175, 176, 177, 178, 179, 182, 189, 198, 204, 206
ageing population, xi, 175, 176, 187, 188
aggression, 7, 37, 42, 57, 136, 194
aging population, 81, 187
aging process, 176
AIDS, v, viii, 31, 32, 43, 44, 47, 48, 49, 51, 52, 53, 54, 56, 57, 58, 59, 60, 62, 67, 83, 149, 150, 158
American Psychiatric Association, 34
American Psychological Association, 82
amygdala, 62
amyotrophic lateral sclerosis, 147
analgesic, 177, 186, 196
anger, 37, 42
ANOVA, 51, 52, 53, 55
anoxia, 193
antidepressants, 81
antisocial behavior, 37, 43
anxiety, 7, 32, 35, 37, 41, 43, 47, 49, 50, 51, 52, 56, 57, 60, 62, 146, 188, 204, 205, 206, 208
anxiety disorder, 47, 62, 188
arrest, 34, 134
arthritis, 36, 119, 188
aspiration, 8, 140, 141
aspiration pneumonia, 8, 141
assessment, 6, 7, 15, 33, 70, 75, 79, 85, 89, 90, 121, 123, 124, 126, 136, 138, 155, 186, 208
asthma, 36, 119, 148, 157
attachment, 37, 40, 43, 57, 58, 61
attachment theory, 58, 61
autonomy, 64, 74, 94, 176
autopsy, 4, 49, 56, 146
avoidance, 34, 35, 43
avoidance behavior, 35, 43
awareness, vii, viii, 8, 40, 49, 63, 71, 87, 88, 95, 150

B

Baby Boom Generation, 118
back pain, 179
barriers, 28, 67, 68, 69, 82, 84, 135, 149, 151
basal ganglia, 193
base, 57, 90, 92, 95, 96, 118
behavioral manifestations, 3, 34
behavioral problems, 37
behaviors, viii, 7, 10, 11, 25, 27, 38, 39, 43, 56, 57, 63, 64, 66, 68, 69, 71, 74, 75, 79, 82, 85
belief systems, 46
benchmarking, 165, 169, 170
benchmarks, 171
bending, 21
beneficial effect, 56
benefits, 43, 44, 45, 47, 48, 97, 141
bias, 80
Big Brother, 46
birth weight, 199
Blacks, 39
blame, 70
bleeding, 36, 95, 98, 100
blood, 4, 35, 36, 40, 94, 95, 99, 119, 124, 147, 154, 155, 156
blood flow, 35
blood pressure, 35, 36, 40, 119, 124
blood transfusion, 94, 147, 154
blood transfusions, 94, 147
BMI, ix, 117, 118, 119, 120, 122, 147
body image, 68, 72, 83
body mass index, ix, 117, 147
body weight, 121
bonding, 60
bonds, 78
bone, 36, 90, 95, 98, 99
bone marrow, 90, 95, 98, 99
bone marrow transplant, 90, 98, 99
bones, 36
boredom, 35
bounds, 136
bowel, xi, 5, 35, 122, 175, 177, 179
brain, 3, 4, 34, 35, 36, 61
brain damage, 3
breast cancer, 204, 207, 208
breathing, 134, 138, 155, 186, 187
brothers, 16, 17, 32, 62, 138
Bureau of Labor Statistics, 129
businesses, 162

C

cachexia, 133, 147
caesarean section, 195
cancer, vii, ix, x, xii, 1, 5, 6, 24, 27, 75, 90, 95, 98, 99, 100, 131, 132, 135, 137, 138, 140, 142, 146, 148, 149, 150, 151, 158, 159, 201, 202, 203, 204, 206, 207, 208
cancer care, vii, 1, 27, 151, 204, 206, 208
cancer screening, 205
cardiovascular disease, 119, 149
caregivers, vii, x, 1, 2, 5, 7, 8, 9, 10, 11, 12, 13, 14, 15, 16, 17, 18, 19, 20, 21, 22, 24, 25, 26, 27, 28, 31, 44, 69, 70, 71, 72, 73, 74, 76, 78, 79, 80, 103, 104, 105, 106, 112, 114, 146, 148, 150, 151, 159, 193, 194, 195, 197, 198
caregiving, 7, 127
case studies, ix, 75, 76, 117, 121, 123
case study, 22, 91, 100, 115, 137
casting, 97
cataract, 179, 186
catecholamines, 40
catheter, 122, 125, 166, 170, 192, 195, 197
CDC, 129
cell differentiation, 201
cerebrovascular disease, 3
challenges, iv, vii, ix, 6, 7, 9, 18, 27, 32, 40, 42, 46, 47, 90, 91, 97, 115, 117, 118, 120, 121, 123, 125, 126, 127, 128, 137, 139, 141, 186
chemical, 33, 141
chemicals, 35
chemotherapy, 88, 89, 100, 202, 205, 208
child abuse, 32, 35, 36, 37, 38, 50, 52, 56, 58, 59, 60
child development, 59
child maltreatment, 37, 58
childhood, 36, 47, 59, 61, 62
childhood sexual abuse, 59
children, viii, 11, 15, 31, 32, 36, 37, 38, 39, 41, 43, 44, 45, 46, 47, 48, 49, 51, 52, 56, 57, 58, 60, 61, 62, 71, 119, 135, 176, 193, 194, 196, 197, 198, 199, 206
China, 2, 58
cholesterol, 119
chronic diseases, 75, 146
chronic illness, 146, 176, 186
chronic obstructive pulmonary disease, x, 145, 146, 147, 157, 158, 159
cleaning, 103, 104, 106
clients, 24, 74
clinical depression, 40
Clinical validation, 188
close relationships, 73

closure, 91, 122
clothing, 106, 124
clusters, 68, 208
coefficient of variation, 167
cognitive capacity, 37
cognitive impairment, 66, 81, 133, 177
cognitive process, 70
cognitive processing, 70
cognitive testing, 4
college students, 40, 57
commercial, 45, 167
common symptoms, 204
communication, 3, 5, 7, 26, 33, 70, 75, 78, 82, 93, 125, 137, 146, 148, 149, 151, 154, 158, 159
communication abilities, 7
communication skills, 26, 151
communities, 44, 48, 64
community, vii, 2, 9, 27, 29, 38, 39, 40, 44, 46, 48, 49, 69, 95, 96, 98, 118, 119, 121, 137, 146, 149, 154, 157, 176, 189
community service, 46
community support, 137
compilation, vii
complaints, 49, 178
complement, 102
complexity, 7, 64, 68, 76, 92, 94, 146
complications, 89, 90, 133, 147
composition, 105
confidentiality, 48, 74
confinement, 28, 142
conflict, 34, 48, 79
congestive heart failure, 158
consciousness, 95, 138
consensus, 44, 73, 96, 98, 148, 195, 197
consent, viii, 69, 74, 87, 88, 99, 177
constipation, 34, 122, 179
construct validity, 49
construction, 68, 69, 77, 86, 132
consulting, 15, 192
consumers, 81, 89, 91, 126
content analysis, 127
control group, 36, 51, 52, 56
convention, 60
conversations, 70, 71, 106
coordination, 8, 113, 151
correlation, xi, 168, 175, 179, 182
correlations, xi, 176, 182
cortisol, 58
cost, vii, x, 1, 2, 22, 36, 37, 45, 60, 114, 126, 127, 129, 136, 150, 161, 165, 170, 171, 172, 199
cost saving, 150
counseling, 19, 33, 51, 66, 204, 205
creativity, 38
criminal activity, 37
criminal behavior, 37
cross-sectional study, xi, 175
cultural values, 69
culture, 38, 61, 64, 65, 67, 68, 69, 79, 80, 92, 93, 95, 96, 97, 197, 198
cure, 14, 33, 90, 92, 93, 94, 96, 152
curriculum, 46, 75, 86
Czech Republic, 201, 207

D

daily living, vii, 1, 5, 6, 26, 27, 118, 119, 176
data analysis, 27, 62, 179
data collection, 199
database, 165, 166, 171
deaths, 5, 6, 43, 136, 137, 146, 149, 157
decision makers, 149
decision-making process, 148
deficiencies, 165
deficiency, 165
deficit, 37, 186
dementia, vii, ix, 1, 2, 3, 4, 5, 6, 7, 8, 9, 10, 11, 12, 14, 15, 16, 18, 19, 21, 22, 24, 25, 26, 27, 28, 29, 74, 75, 81, 82, 85, 86, 113, 119, 128, 131, 132, 133, 134, 135, 136, 137, 138, 139, 140, 141, 142, 143, 146, 147
demographic data, xi, 175, 177, 179, 182
denial, 11
dentures, 106
Department of Health and Human Services, 62, 173
Department of Labor, 130
Department of Veterans Affairs, 125
dependent variable, 164
depressants, 205
depression, xi, 3, 7, 14, 16, 37, 40, 47, 49, 50, 52, 56, 58, 59, 73, 83, 146, 175, 177, 178, 181, 182, 186, 188, 189, 190, 203, 204, 205, 206, 207, 208
depressive symptoms, 205
detachment, 64
detection, 207, 208
developed countries, 2
developing countries, 2
developmental psychopathology, 61
deviation, 167
diabetes, 119, 128, 179
diagnosis, vii, x, xii, 1, 4, 5, 7, 14, 15, 16, 25, 27, 28, 67, 92, 94, 96, 97, 135, 136, 145, 147, 148, 149, 150, 159, 199, 201, 203, 204
dialysis, 192
diarrhea, 34

dignity, 91, 129, 132, 136, 154, 193
direct cost, 37, 38
direct costs, 37, 38
directives, 132, 133, 141, 148, 151
disability, 118, 127, 146, 147, 154, 186, 198
disadvantages, 45, 71
discomfort, 26, 33, 64, 70, 194, 205
discrimination, 31, 32, 34, 38, 39, 44, 48, 50, 52, 53, 55, 56, 78, 83, 129, 132
diseases, x, xi, 3, 5, 6, 75, 99, 119, 135, 136, 145, 146, 148, 149, 151, 158, 175, 176
disorder, 36, 37, 47, 58, 203, 204, 206, 207, 208
dissociative disorders, 37
distractions, 151
distress, x, 13, 31, 32, 33, 34, 35, 47, 48, 51, 52, 53, 55, 56, 57, 95, 96, 145, 149, 195, 196, 197, 204, 205
disturbances, 68
diversity, 79, 99, 114
doctors, x, 91, 93, 124, 134, 140, 142, 145, 147, 152
domestic chores, 48
domestic labor, 43
domestic violence, 37, 42
drug abuse, 36
drug addict, 36
drug addiction, 36
drug therapy, 177
drug toxicity, 121
drug treatment, 37
drugs, x, 37, 146, 147, 150, 152, 154, 155, 195
ductus arteriosus, 196
dyspareunia, 69
dysphagia, 140
dyspnea, 155, 193

E

ecological systems, 68
economic consequences, 37
economic independence, 44
economic values, 43
education, x, 37, 42, 43, 44, 46, 49, 68, 70, 76, 81, 82, 83, 85, 97, 102, 103, 119, 126, 136, 145, 149, 151, 156, 177, 178, 179, 180
educational system, 38
educators, 43, 46, 149
elderly population, 133
elders, 46, 48, 66, 75, 82, 84, 120, 128
emergency, xii, 12, 191
emotion, 57, 70, 90, 113
emotional distress, 13, 31
emotional health, 65
emotional intelligence, 70
emotional problems, 60, 73
emotional reactions, 78
empathy, 50, 198
employees, 102
employment, 7
empowerment, 65
EMS, 189, 196
encouragement, 45, 51
enforcement, 37
England, 83, 98, 114, 142, 188, 189
enslavement, 39
environment, 10, 34, 38, 43, 56, 57, 58, 64, 65, 67, 68, 76, 77, 79, 80, 89, 103, 104, 121, 156, 170, 205
environmental issues, 34
environmental threats, 33
epidemic, 118, 119, 128
epidemiology, 58
equipment, vii, ix, 1, 22, 26, 27, 117, 121, 124, 125, 126
estrangement, 34
ethical issues, 4, 83
ethics, 74, 105, 198
Europe, 78, 82, 115, 164
eustress, 34
euthanasia, xii, 138, 191, 195
everyday life, 74
evidence, viii, 6, 28, 40, 41, 61, 63, 66, 87, 88, 90, 95, 96, 120, 121, 123, 125, 127, 136, 141, 142, 143
evolution, 79, 80, 97, 152, 196
examinations, 196, 203
exclusion, 32, 38, 39
execution, 74
exercise, 64, 147, 187, 188, 204
exercise programs, 187
expenditures, 37, 165
experiences, 9, 15, 18, 28, 31, 32, 34, 39, 84, 91, 97, 112, 121, 129, 136, 140, 150, 188, 198, 206
expertise, 9, 24, 26, 72, 74, 95, 96, 132, 139
exposure, 34, 51, 58, 97, 149
external validation, 42

F

facilitators, 151
factor analysis, 158
faecal incontinence, 132
faith, 33
false alarms, 138

families, viii, 6, 16, 24, 25, 26, 28, 33, 41, 44, 45, 48, 57, 73, 78, 83, 84, 87, 88, 89, 90, 92, 96, 97, 99, 133, 136, 142, 148, 151, 157, 176, 196, 206
family members, vii, viii, 6, 43, 44, 45, 48, 56, 63, 69, 133, 137, 148, 149, 151, 158, 176, 177
family support, 26, 33, 192
family system, 43, 44
famine, viii, 31
fear, 16, 34, 35, 37, 39, 64, 71, 72, 82, 148, 153, 203, 205
fears, 38, 70, 74, 77, 176, 197
federal government, 123
federal regulations, 123, 124
feelings, 35, 38, 41, 70, 73, 176, 187
fetal distress, 195
fetus, 193, 195, 199
fibrosis, 147
financial, 26, 27, 46, 50, 113, 162, 165, 171, 172, 187
financial data, 171, 172
financial support, 46, 187
flexibility, 11, 24, 26, 171
flight, 34
food, 5, 8, 9, 21, 31, 34, 44, 48, 62, 106, 107, 109, 110, 111, 139, 140, 147, 165, 197
food intake, 9, 139
food services, 165
force, 68
Ford, 75, 81, 128
formal education, 179, 180
foul language, 69
foundations, 43
France, xii, 191, 195, 196
freedom, 10, 14, 34, 50, 66, 74, 81, 176, 186
freedom of expression, 66
frequencies, 51, 107
friendship, 45, 51
funding, 23, 25, 76, 126, 137, 138
funds, 45, 120
fungal infection, 121
future orientation, 79

G

gallbladder disease, 119
General Accounting Office, 130
general education, 102
General Health Questionnaire, 49, 59
general practitioner, 4, 9, 28, 91, 137, 142, 150
generalized anxiety disorder, 47
genes, 41
genitals, 67
genocide, 56
gerontology, 64, 65, 75, 82
gestation, 193, 198
gestational age, 198
graph, 35, 163
gravity, 151
growth, xii, 62, 65, 137, 187, 201
guardian, 46, 50
guidance, xi, 45, 47, 50, 74, 123, 124, 125, 126, 159, 161, 162, 170, 171, 194
guidelines, 72, 73, 74, 79, 85, 96, 100, 125, 127, 137, 143, 159
guilt, xii, 17, 96, 201

H

happiness, xi, 40, 41, 65, 175, 178, 181, 182, 186, 188, 189
Health and Human Services, 173
health care, vii, viii, ix, x, 1, 2, 32, 33, 34, 38, 74, 75, 77, 79, 87, 88, 103, 113, 114, 117, 124, 127, 150, 151, 161, 162, 164, 165, 187, 188
health care costs, 150
health care sector, 164
health care system, vii, 1, 2, 38, 114
health condition, 119, 121, 128, 204, 206
health information, 74
health insurance, 34
health practitioners, 70
health problems, 7, 37, 73, 186
health services, viii, 63, 72, 149, 199
health status, 6, 62, 65, 119, 133, 186, 188, 199
heart attack, 135
heart disease, x, 119, 138, 145, 149, 179
heart failure, 150, 158
heart rate, 35, 196
height, 118, 120
heterogeneity, 151
high blood pressure, 36, 119
high school, 46
higher education, 71
hippocampus, 35
history, 4, 15, 39, 62, 78, 80, 82, 84, 86, 122, 177, 179, 180, 195, 196
HIV, viii, 31, 32, 44, 47, 48, 49, 56, 59, 60, 62, 83
HIV/AIDS, viii, 31, 44, 48, 49, 57, 59, 60, 62, 83
holistic care, x, 146, 149
home care services, 149
homelessness, 34
homeostasis, 97
homes, vii, viii, ix, x, xi, 12, 33, 47, 48, 63, 64, 65, 66, 67, 68, 69, 70, 71, 72, 76, 78, 79, 80,

81, 82, 83, 84, 86, 101, 102, 103, 104, 105, 112, 113, 114, 117, 118, 120, 123, 124, 125, 126, 127, 128, 129, 135, 137, 161, 162, 163, 164, 165, 166, 167, 168, 169, 170, 171, 172, 175, 176, 177, 179, 186, 187, 188, 189
honesty, 96
Hong Kong, xi, 175, 176, 187, 188, 189
hopelessness, 31, 47
hormones, 67
hospice, 5, 6, 33, 91, 92, 97, 98, 132, 133, 135, 136, 143, 149, 150, 157, 159
hospital death, 149
hospitalization, 90, 148, 193
human, 32, 38, 39, 41, 43, 45, 59, 62, 65, 66, 67, 68, 81, 194, 198
human capital, 45
human motivation, 41
human right, 198
human rights, 198
husband, 10, 12, 17, 19, 20, 22, 26, 138
hybrid, 103
hygiene, 121, 138, 176, 182
hyperactivity, 37
hyperlipidemia, 119
hypertension, 119, 179, 186

I

identification, 28, 89, 127, 162
identity, viii, 60, 63, 64, 68, 72, 77, 78, 79, 81, 83, 84, 205
illicit drug use, viii, 31
images, 39, 69, 192
immigrants, 189
immune system, 33, 40
immunodeficiency, 159
immunotherapy, 202
impacts, 37, 40, 46, 118, 136
impairments, 66
improvements, 176
in transition, 110, 111, 112
incarceration, 34
incidence, vii, 2, 27, 95, 204, 206
income, 34, 42, 126
independence, 38, 44, 50, 56, 178
indirect costs, 38
individual action, 39
individual character, 38
individual characteristics, 38
individual differences, 39
individuals, 2, 32, 34, 40, 41, 42, 64, 66, 68, 69, 71, 73, 75, 78, 80, 90, 91, 96, 119, 120, 123, 129, 131, 140, 178, 203, 204
induction, 100
industrialized countries, 36
industry, x, xi, 65, 129, 161, 162, 163, 165, 180
inefficiency, 162
inequity, 45
infants, 198, 199
infection, 8, 47, 49, 72, 134, 180, 193
information sharing, 75
informed consent, viii, 87, 88
initiation, 97, 140, 198
injuries, 36, 125, 129
insertion, 140, 141
insomnia, 47
inspectors, 73
Institute of Justice, 37, 59
institutionalisation, 137
institutionalized care, xi, 175, 176
institutions, 64, 66, 78, 81, 103, 164
integration, viii, 40, 44, 87, 88, 91, 92, 93, 94, 95, 96, 97
intelligence, 38, 66, 71, 81
intensive care unit, xii, 147, 155, 157, 158, 191, 193, 198
intercourse, 67, 68
interdependence, 40
interdependence theory, 40
interface, 90
internal consistency, 178
Internet, 18, 166, 171
internist, 140, 207
interpersonal relations, 35, 205
interpersonal relationships, 35, 205
intervention, 45, 60, 72, 73, 75, 76, 137, 187, 189, 202, 205, 206, 207
intervention strategies, 75
intimacy, 43, 61, 73, 74, 78, 81, 85, 86
investment, 165, 193
Ireland, 81, 138
irritability, 34, 35
ischemia, 193
isolation, xii, 11, 26, 37, 121, 201
issues, vii, viii, ix, 4, 6, 14, 15, 16, 18, 19, 22, 25, 28, 29, 34, 61, 63, 67, 70, 75, 79, 81, 82, 83, 87, 88, 90, 92, 94, 95, 96, 97, 98, 99, 105, 118, 121, 127, 131, 136, 137, 141, 142, 151, 179, 195, 196, 197

J

Japan, 31, 59
Jordan, 25, 28, 136, 142
jurisdiction, 157

K

karyotype, 196
kinship, 43, 48

L

labour market, 115
language development, 37
languages, 50, 152
later life, xi, 69, 70, 120, 175, 176, 186, 188
lateral sclerosis, 147
Latin America, 2
lead, xii, 13, 25, 71, 79, 102, 126, 148, 176, 191, 195, 201, 203
leadership, 45, 76, 96, 97, 113, 114
left ventricle, 196
legislation, 65, 148, 197
LIFE, 86, 154, 155, 156
life changes, 205
life course, 84
life expectancy, 6, 132, 133, 176, 195, 196
life experiences, 34, 140
life narratives, 77
life satisfaction, xi, 175, 177, 178, 181, 186, 189
lifetime, xii, 37, 38, 39, 201
light, 10, 12, 34, 64, 75, 198
loneliness, xi, 73, 175, 178, 179, 181, 186
longevity, 177
longitudinal study, 40, 47, 59, 133, 205
love, 12, 14, 18, 23, 40, 41, 50, 81
lung cancer, x, 146, 148, 149, 158, 203
lymphoma, 88, 96, 100

M

machinery, 94, 151
magazines, 69
major depression, 59, 204
major depressive disorder, 207
majority, viii, 21, 22, 23, 51, 63, 65, 95, 136, 137, 141, 148, 150, 179, 186, 205
malignancy, 90, 100
malnutrition, 31, 140
maltreatment, 36, 37, 58, 59, 62
mammals, 35
man, 12, 73, 138
management, ix, 6, 7, 8, 24, 26, 33, 34, 69, 76, 96, 97, 98, 121, 127, 131, 132, 136, 137, 151, 156, 167, 170, 186, 187, 188, 189, 195, 196, 197, 204, 207
mania, 188
manufacturing, 162
marginalization, 69
marital status, 119, 140, 177, 179, 205
markers, 6, 132, 206
market share, 162
marriage, 12, 15, 34, 66, 68
marrow, 90, 95, 98, 99
Maryland, 189
mass, ix, 117, 128, 147
mathematical programming, 163, 167
measurement, ix, 34, 83, 101, 104, 105, 106, 107, 110, 111, 184, 189, 204
meat, 21, 191
mechanical ventilation, x, xii, 145, 146, 147, 148, 149, 150, 154, 155, 156, 157, 191, 192, 197
media, 32, 39, 118
Medicaid, 120, 165, 166, 171, 172, 173
medical, vii, ix, xii, 1, 9, 10, 25, 26, 33, 56, 65, 66, 70, 76, 77, 80, 90, 91, 94, 96, 98, 106, 117, 120, 124, 125, 133, 137, 147, 148, 150, 151, 156, 158, 164, 179, 191, 193, 194, 195, 197, 198, 203, 204, 206
medical care, 66, 91, 98, 120, 158, 206
Medicare, 7, 65, 120, 143, 165, 166, 171, 173
medication, 16, 69, 75, 106, 109, 110, 111, 121, 127, 138, 177, 180, 186
medicine, ix, 33, 90, 131, 132, 152, 159, 192, 198, 202, 203, 206
mellitus, 179
membership, 39, 164
membranes, 193
memory, 3, 5, 15, 16, 135
memory loss, 16
menopause, 205
mental disorder, 177
mental health, 24, 32, 37, 47, 48, 51, 52, 54, 55, 56, 58, 61, 64, 70, 72, 73, 81, 103, 127, 186, 188, 205
mental health professionals, 81
mental illness, 37
mentor, 45, 46, 51, 52, 55, 56, 57, 60, 61
mentoring, 32, 45, 46, 47, 48, 50, 51, 52, 53, 54, 56, 58, 60, 61
mentoring program, 46
mentorship, 48, 51, 56
metabolism, 121
metastasis, xii, 201
methodology, 56, 74, 91, 136, 165
metropolitan areas, 78
Microsoft, 167
mildly depressed, 204, 206
miscarriage, 194

misunderstanding, 66
modeling, 51, 167, 168, 171, 172
models, 38, 43, 46, 65, 76, 91, 92, 93, 97, 113, 132, 163, 164, 165, 171
moderates, 40
modernization, viii, 63, 66
monitoring, 103, 155, 196
mood change, 203, 206
morbidity, 66, 149, 204, 206, 208
morphine, 150, 155, 193, 194
mortality, 43, 57, 59, 133, 146, 147, 157, 158, 176, 193, 203, 205, 206
mortality rate, 133, 147
motivation, 41, 75, 76
motor neuron disease, 159
multiple factors, 68
multiple myeloma, 88

N

naming, 11, 89
narcissism, 41, 42
narratives, 77, 84
nasogastric tube, 197
National Health Service, 159
National Institutes of Health, 127
National Survey, 36, 62, 82
natural disaster, 34
negative attitudes, 39, 68, 71, 93, 96, 121, 124
negative effects, 79, 203
negative experiences, 133
negative externality, 126
neglect, 34, 36, 37, 38, 58, 60, 62
Netherlands, ix, 101, 102, 103, 104, 112, 114, 173
neuroleptics, 155
neurological disease, 60
neurologist, 15
New England, 83, 98, 142
New South Wales, 18
New Zealand, 98, 100
newspaper coverage, 127
non-Hodgkin's lymphoma, 88, 100
normal aging, 84, 176
North America, 98
nostalgia, 79
nurses, 65, 70, 73, 84, 91, 93, 94, 96, 98, 102, 112, 113, 114, 115, 120, 121, 124, 128, 129, 148, 152, 166, 170, 186, 187, 198, 206
nursing care, 22, 84, 102, 172, 187
nutrition, 8, 104, 121, 127, 140, 141, 192, 193, 197, 198
nutritional status, 133, 140

O

obesity, ix, 117, 118, 119, 120, 121, 123, 124, 125, 126, 127, 128, 129, 147
obstacles, 64, 69, 80, 95
occupational health, 22
occupational therapy, 73, 85
old age, ix, 9, 16, 80, 131, 132, 139, 176, 189
openness, 95, 97
operations, xi, 161, 162, 170, 171
opportunities, 40, 46, 73, 100, 152
organizational culture, 68
organize, 4, 70, 75, 152
organs, xii, 201
orgasm, 66
osteoarthritis, 119
outpatients, 60
ovarian cancer, 204, 208
oversight, 130
overweight, 118, 119, 127, 128
oxygen, 134, 146, 147, 151, 154

P

pagers, 151
pain, viii, ix, xi, 7, 8, 24, 33, 34, 35, 36, 87, 88, 89, 91, 96, 99, 102, 131, 132, 135, 136, 137, 138, 147, 148, 150, 151, 154, 155, 175, 177, 179, 180, 181, 182, 186, 187, 188, 189, 190, 192, 195, 197, 203, 204, 205, 206
pain management, 33, 136, 137, 186, 187
paints, 39
palliative, vii, viii, ix, x, xii, 1, 5, 6, 7, 8, 22, 24, 25, 26, 27, 32, 33, 58, 87, 88, 89, 90, 91, 92, 93, 94, 95, 96, 97, 98, 99, 100, 115, 131, 132, 133, 135, 136, 137, 138, 141, 142, 143, 145, 146, 147, 148, 149, 150, 152, 154, 158, 191, 192, 193, 194, 195, 196, 197, 198, 199, 202, 203, 204, 205, 207, 208
palpitations, 35
panic disorder, 37
paraneoplastic syndrome, 203
parental care, 32, 56
parental support, 32, 47, 52
parenting, 43, 50, 51
parents, xii, 16, 26, 31, 32, 37, 39, 43, 44, 45, 46, 47, 48, 49, 50, 51, 55, 56, 58, 71, 191, 192, 193, 194, 195, 196, 198, 199
parole, 45
participants, 9, 10, 18, 46, 50, 71, 90, 93, 151, 177, 178, 179, 186, 187, 208
pathology, 195

patient care, 89, 129, 130
peer group, 163
peer review, 91
peer support, 47, 75
perceived control, 70
performance, x, xi, 34, 51, 161, 162, 163, 164, 165, 166, 168, 169, 170, 171, 172, 203, 204
performance indicator, 162
performers, 169, 171
perinatal, 194, 197
peripheral blood, 99
permeability, 196
perpetrators, 69
personal history, 78
personal hygiene, 121
personal relations, 61, 65
personal relationship, 61, 65
personal values, 78
personality, 3, 11, 41, 47, 48, 57, 59, 60
personality disorder, 47
pessimism, 148, 157
Philadelphia, 62, 117
photographs, 12
physical abuse, 61
physical attractiveness, 69
physical environment, 76
physical health, 7, 36, 59, 62, 65
physical therapy, 40, 193
physical well-being, 187
physicians, 26, 129, 141, 148, 149, 151, 159, 198, 206
pilot study, 105, 165, 189
platform, 33
policy, viii, 63, 71, 72, 73, 74, 76, 79, 81, 83, 85, 125, 126, 154, 186
population, viii, ix, xi, 37, 45, 48, 61, 73, 101, 102, 105, 117, 119, 121, 126, 127, 129, 133, 162, 175, 176, 187, 188, 198, 203, 206
positive attitudes, 68, 71, 93
positive correlation, xi, 176, 182
positive feedback, 34
positive interactions, 124
positive mental health, 47, 51, 56
positive relationship, 42, 46, 166
posttraumatic stress, 37
post-traumatic stress disorder, 58
poverty, 31, 34, 45, 47
practical knowledge, 78
predators, 84
pregnancy, xii, 36, 37, 191, 193, 194, 195, 199
prejudice, 39, 68
prejudices, 39, 66
premature infant, 196
prematurity, 194, 198
preparation, iv, 90, 95, 196
preschoolers, 58
pressure sore, 21, 166, 170
preterm infants, 198
prevention, 46, 60, 80, 89, 156
primary caregivers, 44
principles, ix, 6, 59, 73, 74, 131, 132, 136, 197, 198
prioritizing, xi, 161, 162, 170
probability, viii, 7, 31, 48, 119
procurement, 164
productivity, 37, 165
professionals, vii, viii, xii, 1, 4, 6, 8, 9, 25, 26, 33, 70, 72, 74, 80, 81, 87, 88, 89, 90, 91, 92, 93, 95, 96, 97, 141, 176, 187
profit, 162, 164, 166, 168, 171
profitability, 171
prognosis, x, 3, 4, 88, 90, 100, 137, 145, 149, 150, 151, 192, 193
programming, 163, 167
project, vii, viii, 1, 9, 36, 63, 64, 67, 72, 74, 77, 84, 97, 196
proliferation, xii, 201
proposition, 32
prostheses, 156
protection, 51, 61, 62, 74
protective factors, 38
psychiatric patients, 59
psychiatrist, 15
psychiatry, 9, 139, 188, 205
psychobiology, 62
psychological development, 45
psychological distress, 40, 57, 205
psychological health, xi, 56, 175, 179, 186
psychological problems, 186
psychological stress, 203
psychological variables, 75
psychological well-being, 40, 61, 178, 187
psychologist, 19, 156
psychology, 33, 35, 57, 58, 82
psychopathology, 58, 59, 61
psychosocial support, 58, 96
psychosomatic, 33, 47, 52
psychotherapy, 206
public health, 164
publishing, 27, 28, 159

Q

qualifications, 42
qualitative research, 5, 199
quality improvement, 65

quality indicators, 120, 166
quality of life, iv, vii, x, xi, xii, 33, 65, 69, 70, 75, 83, 84, 88, 89, 90, 94, 95, 98, 137, 145, 146, 147, 154, 158, 159, 175, 176, 177, 186, 187, 188, 192, 199, 204, 208
quality of service, 166, 171
Queensland, 18, 87, 99
questioning, 72
questionnaire, xi, 40, 49, 150, 175

R

race, 38, 39, 119, 121, 193
radiotherapy, 202, 206
reactions, 26, 34, 69, 70, 78, 129
reading, 69, 76, 193
reciprocity, 40, 44, 57
recognition, vii, 1, 2, 6, 11, 25, 26, 27, 28, 41, 65, 67, 97, 133, 135, 204
recommendations, iv, ix, 86, 117, 125, 136, 203
reconstruction, 77, 79
recovery, 33, 146
recreation, 127
recreational, 67, 68, 104, 187
recurrence, 205
regression model, 164
regulations, 123, 124
rehabilitation, 33, 36, 99, 118, 146, 156
reinforcement, 45, 151
rejection, 38, 39
relationship satisfaction, 57
relatives, 10, 17, 19, 25, 26, 138, 148, 150, 151, 152, 154, 155, 193
relaxation, 35, 187
relevance, xi, 48, 60, 176, 204, 206
reliability, 49, 50, 51, 105, 178, 188, 189
relief, 21, 24, 89, 132, 135, 137, 138, 150, 152, 186, 189, 203
religious beliefs, 66, 71
requirements, 48, 102, 121, 124, 128
researchers, 135, 171
resilience, 32, 38, 47, 48, 59
resistance, 33, 58
resolution, 178
resource allocation, 31
resource utilization, ix, 117
resources, vii, xi, 2, 14, 24, 25, 26, 33, 34, 41, 48, 74, 75, 76, 79, 80, 126, 129, 132, 137, 139, 154, 157, 162, 165
respirator, 193
respiratory arrest, 134
respiratory failure, x, 145, 147, 150, 159
respiratory therapist, 152, 156
response, xii, 28, 35, 42, 43, 51, 69, 72, 83, 89, 126, 134, 140, 147, 156, 171, 191, 206
rights, viii, 60, 63, 65, 67, 73, 74, 75, 76, 79, 80, 196, 198
risk, x, 36, 37, 45, 46, 48, 57, 58, 59, 73, 74, 77, 78, 83, 119, 121, 122, 125, 128, 133, 141, 145, 146, 147, 158, 171, 186, 193, 195, 203, 205
risk factors, 128
risks, 125, 140, 141, 158, 194
risk-taking, 37
rituximab, 88, 100
routines, 113, 115
Royal Society, 142
rules, 25, 114, 115
Rwanda, 60

S

sadness, 203, 206
safety, ix, 12, 22, 25, 65, 117, 121, 165
school, 31, 32, 34, 37, 38, 39, 45, 46, 47, 48, 49, 57
school achievement, 34
school enrollment, 31
schooling, 32, 106, 110, 111, 193
screening, 178, 189, 190, 204, 207
scripts, 28, 69, 85
self-actualization, 41
self-assessment, 70
self-concept, 34, 178
self-confidence, 41
self-efficacy, 75, 186
self-esteem, 32, 37, 38, 41, 42, 43, 49, 50, 56, 57, 59, 60, 61, 65, 73, 77
self-expression, 187
self-regard, 41
self-sufficiency, 197
self-understanding, 57
self-worth, 41, 42, 50, 65
senile dementia, 147
sensation, 140
sensitivity, 124, 151
service organizations, 1, 24, 137, 165
service provider, 9, 25
service quality, 170
services, vii, viii, x, 1, 2, 6, 8, 9, 14, 16, 18, 19, 20, 22, 23, 24, 25, 26, 27, 29, 33, 37, 38, 63, 65, 72, 74, 76, 79, 89, 95, 96, 98, 103, 104, 105, 118, 133, 135, 136, 137, 139, 145, 149, 157, 162, 164, 166, 171, 188, 189, 193, 197, 199, 205
sex, 36, 39, 50, 59, 64, 66, 67, 68, 69, 71, 73, 74, 77, 78, 79, 81, 83, 84

sexism, 40
sexology, 63, 64, 67, 78, 82
sexual abuse, 57, 59, 84
sexual activities, 73, 74, 80
sexual activity, 65, 66, 68, 69, 72, 74, 84
sexual behavior, 66, 68, 69, 71, 75, 76, 82, 83, 86
sexual behaviour, 85
sexual desire, 73, 77, 79
sexual development, 68
sexual experiences, 78
sexual health, viii, 59, 63, 72, 74, 75, 79, 81, 82, 84, 86
sexual identity, viii, 63, 64, 68, 72, 77, 78, 81, 83, 84
sexual orientation, 78
sexual problems, 66, 80
sexuality, vii, viii, 63, 64, 65, 66, 67, 68, 69, 70, 71, 72, 73, 74, 75, 76, 77, 78, 79, 80, 81, 82, 83, 84, 85, 86
shame, 12, 26, 47, 49
shock, xii, 58, 201, 203
shortness of breath, 35
showing, 11, 52, 53, 55, 123, 148, 178, 196
siblings, 31, 194, 196
side effects, xii, 75, 147, 201
signals, 34, 96
signs, 5, 11, 35, 187, 194, 196, 198, 204, 206
skin, 12, 38, 121, 122, 125, 126, 128, 130, 194
sleep disturbance, 186
smoking, 119
social activities, 73, 104, 106
social attitudes, 71
social behavior, 37, 38, 43
social care, 2, 8, 28, 159, 187
social context, viii, 63, 64
social development, ix, 101
social environment, 34, 56, 57, 58
social exclusion, 32
social group, 39, 40
social image, 68
social integration, 40
social interactions, 83
social network, 26, 47, 61
social norms, 68
social organization, 83
social perception, 38
social policy, 71
social problems, ix, 101, 104
social relations, 40, 46
social relationships, 40, 46
social security, 43
Social Security, 65
social services, 103
social structure, 39, 68
social support, 32, 34, 40, 41, 43, 50, 51, 52, 57, 59, 61, 62, 73, 176, 186, 204, 205, 206
social support network, 176
social withdrawal, 34
social workers, 73, 115
socialization, 43, 51, 127, 186
society, 37, 38, 44, 66, 68, 119, 120, 176, 186, 198
socioeconomic status, 204
software, 167, 172
solution, viii, 72, 76, 87, 88, 150
South Africa, 32, 39, 44, 48, 59, 60
South Dakota, 120
special education, 37
specialists, vii, 1, 14, 96, 112, 149
specialization, 102, 206
speech, 3, 73, 151
spending, 2, 35, 68
spinal cord, 36
spiritual care, 33
spirituality, 136, 149
stability, 38, 42, 51, 64, 77, 207
stabilization, 43, 46
staff members, 70, 71, 75, 122
staffing, ix, 113, 117, 121, 123, 126, 128, 129, 165, 166
standard deviation, 167
state, x, 14, 33, 35, 40, 41, 43, 46, 56, 72, 89, 120, 123, 161, 165, 166, 170, 171, 196
states, 43, 68, 120, 123, 151, 165, 171, 172, 193
Statistical Package for the Social Sciences, 179
statistics, 36, 167
stereotypes, 39, 66
stereotyping, 32, 47
steroids, 193
stigma, 31, 44, 45, 47, 58, 60, 203
storage, 196
stress, viii, 17, 33, 34, 35, 37, 40, 41, 58, 60, 61, 87, 88, 89, 90, 91, 96, 99
stressful events, 40
stressors, 32, 33, 34, 40, 205
stroke, 21, 119, 179, 186, 189
structure, viii, 63, 67, 72, 176, 189, 194
style, 77
subacute, 189
sub-Saharan Africa, viii, 31, 32, 43, 48, 56, 59
subsidy, 45
substance abuse, 37, 46
suicidal ideation, 188
suicide, 37, 58, 188
suicide attempts, 37
supervision, 75, 103

supervisor, 104
surveillance, x, 145, 149
survey, 5, 47, 48, 76, 78, 96, 119, 121, 124, 136, 141, 142, 148, 157, 165, 171, 189
survival, x, 41, 43, 88, 98, 132, 133, 137, 140, 141, 143, 145, 146, 148, 149, 150, 157, 193, 197, 204, 205
survivors, 98, 199, 204, 208
Sweden, 71, 86
symptoms, ix, x, 4, 5, 6, 7, 8, 32, 35, 37, 47, 52, 61, 89, 131, 132, 135, 136, 146, 147, 149, 150, 151, 152, 156, 187, 203, 204, 206, 208
syndrome, xii, 56, 159, 191, 203

T

tangles, 3
Tanzania, 60
target, 84, 149, 151, 153, 169, 170
taxonomy, 35
teachers, 32, 38, 46
team members, 97
teams, 74, 79, 136, 193, 194, 195, 196, 197, 206
techniques, xi, xii, 4, 8, 9, 42, 139, 161, 163, 191, 193
technology, viii, 87, 88, 94, 96, 176
teeth, 106
telephone, 34, 119
temperament, 58
tension, 35, 44
terminal illness, vii, 1, 6, 27, 89, 133, 192
terminal patients, 151
terminally ill, viii, 6, 87, 88, 98, 100, 140
territorial, 94
test-retest reliability, 49, 178
therapeutic effects, 187
therapeutic intervention, 90, 187
therapeutic interventions, 90, 187
therapist, 45, 72, 155, 156
therapy, xii, 40, 73, 85, 88, 89, 146, 147, 151, 154, 155, 156, 177, 186, 187, 189, 191, 193, 201, 202, 205, 206, 207
thoughts, 10, 35, 41, 66, 68, 93, 187, 205
threats, 33, 35, 42, 203, 206
thrush, 138
tissue, xii, 121, 125, 201
total parenteral nutrition, 192
toxicity, 121
tracheostomy, 150, 156, 158
trainees, 75, 76, 164
training, viii, 24, 45, 63, 72, 73, 74, 75, 76, 79, 81, 82, 84, 85, 86, 102, 106, 124, 125, 129, 136, 140, 151, 156, 189
training programs, 75, 124
traits, 39, 59
trajectory, x, 6, 89, 90, 99, 133, 136, 145, 146, 158
transaction costs, 115
transformation, 176
transformations, 65
transfusion, 94, 154
transgression, 69
transition period, 102
transplant, 98, 147
transplantation, 90, 98, 99, 202
transport, 106, 107, 108, 111, 122, 196
transportation, 34
trauma, 16, 61, 126
treatment, iv, viii, 33, 36, 37, 42, 58, 75, 80, 82, 87, 88, 89, 90, 91, 94, 98, 99, 103, 106, 127, 140, 142, 148, 152, 153, 154, 155, 186, 192, 193, 197, 198, 202, 203, 204, 206
trial, 60, 100, 113, 141, 149, 158, 188, 189
tumor, 202, 203, 206, 207
turnover, 164
two-sided test, 109
type 2 diabetes, 119

U

ulcers, 121, 125, 140
UN, 38, 48, 57, 60, 62
underlying mechanisms, 62
unhappiness, 31
United Kingdom, 2, 112, 148
United States, ix, 2, 29, 36, 39, 45, 46, 58, 60, 71, 83, 86, 112, 117, 127, 129, 133, 162, 165
universality, 99
unwanted thoughts, 205
urban, 44, 58, 62
US Department of Health and Human Services, 62

V

validation, 42, 188, 189, 190
valuation, 46, 173, 199
variables, 70, 71, 75, 163, 164, 166, 168, 171, 172, 179, 183, 184
varieties, ix, 101, 103
vascular dementia, 119, 128
vascularization, 121, 125
ventilation, x, xii, 146, 147, 148, 150, 154, 155, 156, 157, 158, 191, 192, 197
ventricle, 196

Viagra, 80
Vice President, 76
violence, 11, 34, 37, 42, 57, 61
violent behavior, 11, 37
violent behaviour, 11
violent crime, 37
violent criminals, 42
vision, 67, 73, 78, 189
vocational education, 103
vulnerability, 32, 59

W

Wales, 18
walking, xi, 21, 106, 120, 121, 156, 175, 177, 178, 181, 186
war, viii, 31, 43, 44, 45, 104, 105, 106, 136, 147, 197
Washington, 59, 60, 82, 83, 127, 128, 129, 130
water, 122, 138
weight loss, 9, 133, 139, 147, 170
welfare, 37, 45, 59
welfare system, 37
well-being, viii, 28, 38, 40, 56, 60, 61, 63, 64, 65, 66, 72, 73, 74, 80, 142, 147, 178, 187
wellness, 75, 84, 177
West Africa, 59
WHO, 32, 56, 62, 88, 100
wilderness, 35
windows, 134
withdrawal, 3, 34, 148, 157, 158, 193, 198
work ethic, 42
workers, 9, 23, 26, 40, 73, 75, 78, 91, 115, 124, 125, 129, 186, 196
workforce, 13, 26
workload, 44
workplace, 48, 51, 85, 125
worldwide, vii, viii, 2, 27, 29, 31
worry, 24, 34, 35, 49

Y

Y-axis, 35
young adults, 47
young people, 45, 46
young women, 205

Z

Zimbabwe, 58